# Current Concepts in Ophthalmology

Andrzej Grzybowski

Editor

# Current Concepts
# in Ophthalmology

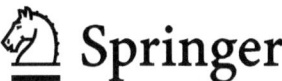 Springer

*Editor*
Andrzej Grzybowski
Department of Ophthalmology
University of Warmia and Mazury
Poznan
Poland

ISBN 978-3-030-25388-2      ISBN 978-3-030-25389-9   (eBook)
https://doi.org/10.1007/978-3-030-25389-9

This Springer imprint is published by the registered company Springer Nature Switzerland AG
The registered company address is: Gewerbestrasse 11, 6330 Cham, Switzerland

# Contents

**1  Updates in Refractive Surgery** . . . . . . . . . . . . . . . . . . . . . . . . . . . . . . . . . 1
M. Joan T. D. Balgos and Jorge L. Alió

**2  Recent Developments in Cornea and Corneal Transplants** . . . . . . . . 35
Caterina Sarnicola, Enrica Sarnicola, Paolo Perri, and
Vincenzo Sarnicola

**3  Recent Developments in Cataract Surgery** . . . . . . . . . . . . . . . . . . . . . 55
Andrzej Grzybowski and Piotr Kanclerz

**4  Recent Developments in Glaucoma** . . . . . . . . . . . . . . . . . . . . . . . . . . . . 99
Nathan M. Kerr and Keith Barton

**5  Recent Advances in Uveitis** . . . . . . . . . . . . . . . . . . . . . . . . . . . . . . . . . . 121
Xia Ni Wu, Lazha Ahmed Talat Sharief, Roy Schwartz, Þóra
Elísabet Jónsdóttir, Anastasia Tasiopoulou, Ahmed Al-Janabi,
Noura Al Qassimi, Amgad Mahmoud, Sue Lightman,
and Oren Tomkins-Netzer

**6  Recent Developments in Maculopathy** . . . . . . . . . . . . . . . . . . . . . . . . . 141
Francesco Bandello, Marco Battista, Maria Brambati,
Vincenzo Starace, Alessandro Arrigo, and Maurizio Battaglia Parodi

**7  Recent Developments in Vitreo-Retinal Surgery** . . . . . . . . . . . . . . . . 165
Sana Idrees, Ajay E. Kuriyan, Stephen G. Schwartz,
Jean-Marie Parel, and Harry W. Flynn Jr

**8  Clinical Updates and Recent Developments
in Neuro-Ophthalmology** . . . . . . . . . . . . . . . . . . . . . . . . . . . . . . . . . . . . 201
Amrita-Amanda D. Vuppala and Neil R. Miller

**9    Recent Advances in Pediatric Ophthalmology**.................... 251
Ken K. Nischal

**10   Recent Developments in Ocular Oncology**...................... 275
Bertil Damato

**Index**......................................................... 295

# Chapter 1
# Updates in Refractive Surgery

M. Joan T. D. Balgos and Jorge L. Alió

## Introduction

The correction of refractive errors—hyperopia, myopia, astigmatism, and presbyopia—is of interest to eye practitioners worldwide. Functionally, good vision allows one to do his activities of daily life without assistance. Cosmesis and convenience, especially for people who live active lifestyles, require a decrease or elimination in dependency on spectacles and contact lenses. Refractive surgery aims to improve the refractive state of the eye caused by ammetropia—whether due to the globe's axial length or through a difference in the refractive power of the cornea and the lens—or by pathologies such as keratoconus. Modern means for achieving this include topical medications, surgical remodeling of the cornea, intraocular lens implantation, and crystalline lens extraction and replacement with an intraocular implant.

## Pharmacologic Treatment of Presbyopia

Several classes of eyedrops that address presbyopia are being developed or are currently under clinical evaluation [1]. One such type of eyedrop involves parasympathomimetics. Whether in combination with a non-steroidal anti-inflammatory drug or with tropicamide, these drops have been reported to stimulate parasympathetic innervation and induce ciliary body stimulation and miosis, resulting in an increased

M. J. T. D. Balgos
Vissum, Alicante, Spain

J. L. Alió (✉)
Vissum, Alicante, Spain

Division of Ophthalmology, Universidad Miguel Hernández, Alicante, Spain
e-mail: jlalio@vissum.com

© Springer Nature Switzerland AG 2020
A. Grzybowski (ed.), *Current Concepts in Ophthalmology*,
https://doi.org/10.1007/978-3-030-25389-9_1

depth of focus [2]. Pilot studies have reported improvement of both uncorrected distance visual acuity (UDVA) and uncorrected near visual acuity (UNVA), and some are currently in phase IIb trials. Most of the effect diminished after several hours; adverse effects include headache, ocular stinging, and nausea [3–5].

Another set of eyedrops targets the crystalline lens to treat presbyopia. Pirenoxine eyedrops have been shown to suppress crystalline lens hardening in rats. The same effect was also reported in a small randomized controlled study on 18 Japanese males with early presbyopia—no improvement was noted in patients with advanced presbyopia [6]. A 1.5% lipoic acid choline ester-based eyedrop is also in development. It is said to reduce crystalline protein disulfide bonds—softening the lens and preserving its shape-changing ability during accommodation. Phase I and II studies have reported good outcomes [7].

# Corneal Inlays

Corneal inlays are implanted in the non-dominant eye, under a stromal flap or within a corneal pocket made by femtosecond laser [8]. Inlays that alter corneal curvature are implanted more superficially and inlays with small aperture or those that have a different index of refraction are implanted deeper to avoid changes in the cornea curvature and to allow a proper diffusion of nutrients in the corneal stroma [9]. The material used in corneal inlays allows for sufficient nutrient flow into the stroma [9–12]. Table 1.1 enumerates the advantages and disadvantages of corneal inlay implantation for presbyopia treatment.

**Corneal reshaping inlays** enhance near and intermediate vision through a multifocal effect, changing the shape of the anterior curvature of the cornea and making it hyper-prolate to increase power. **Refractive inlays** alter the refractive index with a bifocal optic. **Small aperture inlays** improve depth of focus [9, 12].

The *Raindrop™ (ReVision Optics, Lake Forest, California, USA),* is a reshaping inlay that is no longer commercially available. It changes the anterior corneal surface and creates a hyper-prolate region, resulting in a multifocal

**Table 1.1** Advantages and disadvantages of corneal inlays

| Advantages | Disadvantages |
| --- | --- |
| Minimally invasive | Requires monovision |
| Reversible | Decreased distance visual acuity |
| No need to remove corneal tissue | Decreased contrast sensitivity |
| Quick recovery | Perception of halos |
| Does not affect visual field testing | Corneal topography changes |
| Can be combined with other refractive procedures | (long-term) |
| Enables normal visualization of central and peripheral | Induces HOAs |
| fundus | Corneal haze (with long-term |
| | implantation) |
| | Dependent on inlay centration |
| | Dry eye |

cornea [9, 12, 13]. In emmetropic presbyopes, the Raindrop has been shown to improve monocular and binocular UNVA [8, 14]. UIVA was also said to improve [14], however both UDVA and CDVA were found to decrease [8, 14]. It was associated with significant increases in total RMS, coma-like RMS and spherical-like RMS for a 4 mm pupil size. The Raindrop has been associated with monocular contrast sensitivity loss, but with no binocular loss. Common reasons for inlay explantation were vision dissatisfaction, inlay misalignment, decreased visual acuity, epithelial ingrowth, and recurrent central corneal haze.

The *Flexivue Microlens™ (Presbia Cooperatief U.A., Amsterdam, Netherlands)* is a transparent hydrophilic refractive inlay (Fig. 1.1) [13, 15, 16]. Its central zone is plano and its peripheral zone has powers ranging from +1.25 to +3D for reading. A central opening facilitates the transfer of nutrients and oxygen through the cornea [ 9, 12, 13, 16, 17]. Light rays are designed to pass through the central zone during distance vision, and rays pass through the peripheral refractive zone during near vision [15, 16]. In emmetropic presbyopes the Flexivue has been found to improve UNVA [16]. UDVA is said to decrease in the operated eye, although binocular UDVA and CDVA is not significantly affected [15, 16]. Higher order aberrations [16] and mean spherical aberration [15] increased after surgery, and contrast sensitivity decreased in the operated eye [16].

The *Icolens™ (Neoptics AG, Huenenberg, Switzerland)* is a refractive inlay made of a copolymer of hydroxyethyl methacrylate and methyl methacrylate [13, 18] (Fig. 1.2). It has a bifocal design with a peripheral positive refractive zone for near and a central zone for distance vision. This implant improves UNVA, albeit with a decrease in UDVA and CDVA [18].

The *Kamra Inlay™ (Acufocus Inc., Irvine, CA, USA)* is a small aperture inlay made of carbon nanoparticles, whose microperforations allow nutritional flow through the cornea (Fig. 1.3). It is implanted in the non-dominant eye, in a lamellar pocket. [9, 12, 13, 19] The Kamra improves near vision by increasing the depth of field through the principle of small aperture optics [9, 12, 13].

The Kamra can be implanted simultaneously with LASIK for hyperopes, myopes and emmetropes [20, 21]. Improvement in near and intermediate visual

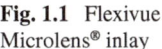

**Fig. 1.1** Flexivue Microlens® inlay

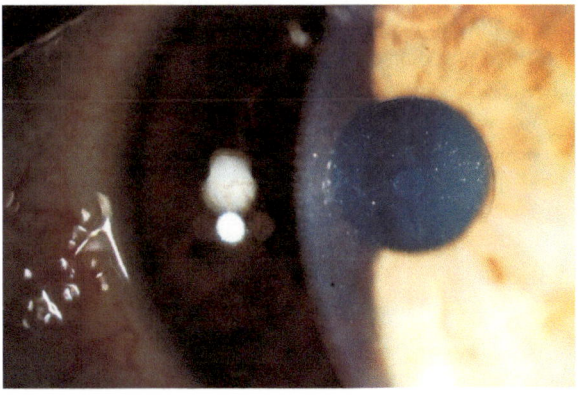

**Fig. 1.2** Icolens® inlay [18]

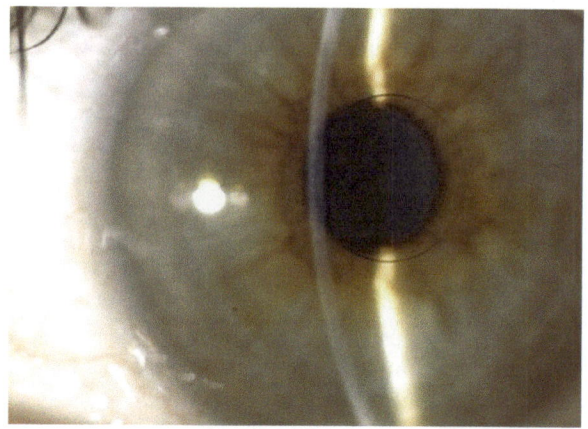

**Fig. 1.3** Kamra® inlay [26]

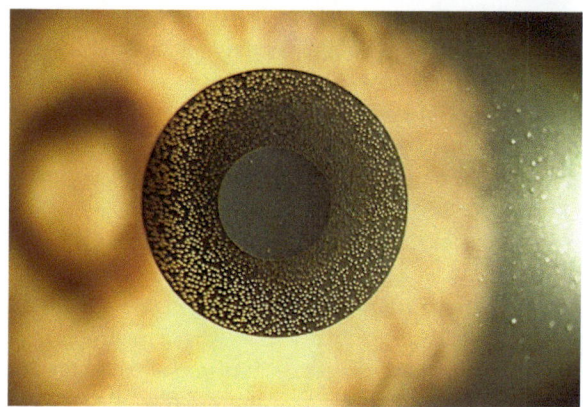

acuity have been reported [20, 21], with some compromise in uncorrected monocular distance visual acuity [22] and corrected distance visual acuity. When implanted in pseudophakic patients with monofocal IOLs—there is also improvement in NVA, and decrease in DVA [23]. Monocular contrast sensitivity is mildly reduced after implantation of the KAMRA inlay [24]. Halos, glare, and night-vision disturbance are also associated with the KAMRA [20, 21]. An advantage of Kamra inlays is their removability—with no permanent changes in corneal topography and aberrometry, and recovery of preoparative corrected and uncorrected NVA and DVA up to 6 months after removal [25].

## *Conclusion*

The idea of using intracorneal inlays to obtain multifocality is interesting, it is an active subject in ophthalmologic research. However these inlays have never gained full popularity due to issues of corneal immune reaction and centration during implantation. Other concerns that need to be addressed include late complications of corneal stromal opacity, hyperopic shift, and corneal irregularity—all of which have led to high explantation rates. As other technology for establishing multifocality is being developed, we believe that the use of these inlays will decline.

## Pseudophakic Presbyopic IOL's: Conceptual Issues and Optical Profiles

Presbyopia is the loss or insufficiency of the accommodative ability of the eye, and it causes difficulties with reading and performing tasks that require near vision. It affects individuals at the peak of their professional and creative activity, and as such, there is an increasing demand for correcting presbyopia and eliminating the need to use spectacles or contact lenses. This has been further bolstered by advances in cataract and refractive surgery and implant design.

*Multifocal IOL's* provide pseudoaccomodation—they are designed to focus light onto multiple foci and do not change power with ciliary body contraction as with accommodation [27, 28]. *Bifocal IOL's* focus light onto two discrete focal points, and *trifocal IOL's* focus light onto three focal points [27, 29, 30]. Multifocal IOL's may also be classified according to their design. *Rotationally symmetrical IOL's* can be further divided into diffractive, refractive, or combined IOL designs [27, 31]. *Rotationally asymmetric or varifocal IOLs* are characterized by an inferior segmental near add [32, 33]. There is a larger section for distance vision, and a smaller reading segment with only one transition zone [34]. *Extended depth of focus lenses* (EDOF) focus incoming light waves in a continuous and extended longitudinal plane in order to give good vision at all distances [35, 36]. *Accommodative lenses* have monofocal optics which, through several mechanisms, change power with accommodative effort [37].

Several obstacles that need to be overcome by presbyopic IOL implants include visual symptoms. Glares, haloes, starbursts, dysphotopsia and shadows occur due to the effect of the lens design on light [38–40]. A large angle kappa, leading to temporal IOL decentration, has been implicated as a contributor to photic phenomena in refractive multifocal lenses [41]. Decreased contrast sensitivity is due to the splitting of available light—especially by multifocal IOLs [41]. Neuroadaptation is a phenomenon in which patients implanted with multifocal IOL implants learn to adapt to image perception changes and visual symptoms induced by the lens design. This may take several months [42]. A case series on the causes of multifocal IOL explantation and exchange reported that while uncorrected distance visual acuity may have been 20/20 or better, the visual side effects were significant enough to warrant lens exchange. The most common reasons for explantation were decreased contrast sensitivity, photic phenomena, neuroadaptation failure, incorrect IOL power, excessive preoperative expectation, IOL decentration, and anisometropia [43]. Careful preoperative evaluation and planning is also necessary for implantation of pseudophakic presbyopic implants, as lens selection should be based on a multifactorial approach. The inherent anatomy and physiology of the

eye, and the pertinent ophthalmic history –especially a previous refractive surgery, irregular astigmatism, or ocular surface disease- should be considered, along
with the patient's lifestyle, visual needs, and expectations [41]. Hence a thorough
knowledge and understanding of the optical qualities and profiles of each presbyopic pseudophakic lens is necessary in order to aid the surgeon in pre-operative
planning and implant selection, and in advising the patient about subsequent postoperative expectations.

## Optical Profiles of Presbyopic Pseudophakic Lenses

### Diffractive Multifocal IOL's

*Diffractive IOLs* have rings on the surface, forming a discontinued optical density, such that light particles that hit these rings are directed equally towards discrete focal points [27, 31]. Apodized diffractive IOL's have a gradual and uniform
decrease in diffractive step heights from the center to the periphery [30]. These
ensure that light is equally distributed in both focal points independently of pupil
size, and theoretically creates a smooth transition of light between the focal points
[41]. **Apodized diffractive lenses** have a gradual decrease in refractive step heights
from center to periphery, resulting in distance-dominant good vision for people with
large pupils [41].

The *AT LISA® tri 839 MP (Carl Zeiss Meditec, Jena, Germany)* is a one-
piece trifocal diffractive aspheric IOL [31] (Fig. 1.4). Patients who were bilaterally
implanted with the AT LISA Tri showed significant reduction in sphere, cylinder,
and spherical equivalent. There was continuous and acceptable visual acuity for all
distances. The defocus curves for the AT LISA tri show that it provides excellent
near VA between 33 and 40 cm, with the ideal distance for near vision at 36 cm.
Intermediate VA is excellent between 67 and 100 cm, and the ideal distance is at
80 cm [31]. Contrast sensitivity improved within the first month post-surgery, especially for medium spatial frequencies [31]. Ocular aberrometric analysis showed

**Fig. 1.4** AT LISA® tri
839 mp IOL [31]

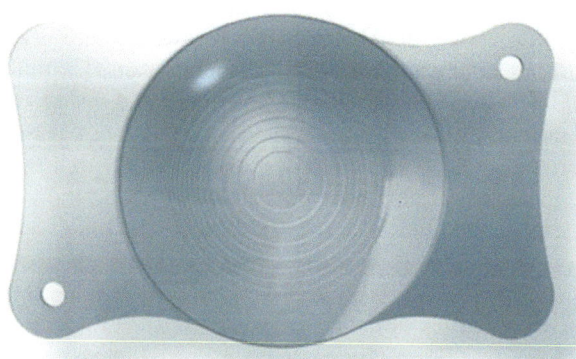

significant decrease in RMS total aberrations, RMS tilt, primary coma and RMS spherical aberration. There was a significant mean decrease in total internal aberrations. Most importantly, no significant changes were found in internal aberrations between 1, 3, and 6 months post-surgery—signifying the rapid restoration of visual function as early as the first month after surgery. The AT LISA tri induced negative values of internal spherical aberration—more negative than that previously induced by the crystalline lens—cancelling out the corneal spherical aberrations and resulting in lower ocular spherical aberration values [31].

The *FineVision® Micro F (PhysIOL, Liège, Belgium)* is a one-piece, pupil-dependent, trifocal IOL. It has an aspheric posterior surface, with a convoluted diffractive anterior surface (Fig. 1.5). By varying the height of the diffractive step the amount of light distributed to the near, intermediate and distant foci are adjusted according to the pupil aperture. The IOL distributes 43% of light energy to far vision, 28% to near vision, and 15% to intermediate vision [31]. Binocular defocus curve at 6 months for this lens showed a wide range of useful vision, with excellent contrast sensitivity under scotopic conditions. There was statistically insignificant reduction of HOA, yet statistically significant increase in Strehl ratio after 6 months [31].

The **SeeLens (Hanita Lenses, R.C.A. Ltd., Kibbutz Hanita, Israel)** is an apodized diffractive IOL with an asymmetrical light distribution. It has concentric rings located 4 mm from the the middle, and is independent of pupil size. Its design theoretically allows for an optimum distribution of energy in different light conditions and minimizes spherical aberrations [31]. Our experience with bilateral implantation of this lens in 20 patients resulted in statistically significant improvements in UDVA, CDVA, UNVA and CNVA within the first post-operative month. Mean defocus curves for the SeeLens showed that there are two peaks of maximum vision, one at distance and one at near. Defocus of −1.5D was needed to provide aceptable intermediate vision. Contrast sensitivity function was within physiologic levels, albeit reduced in scotopic conditions. Only the RMS of the internal high-order aberrations, coma aberration, third-order and fourth-order aberrations were significantly decreased. Visual quality measured with the Hartmann-Shack aberrometer showed an increase in Strehl ratio [31].

**Fig. 1.5** FineVision®
Micro F IOL [31]

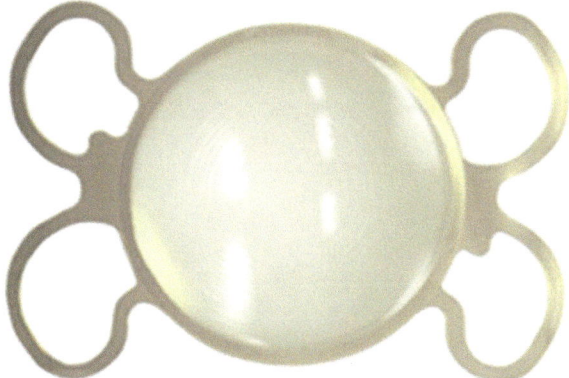

## Refractive Multifocal IOL's

*Refractive IOLs* use concentric zones of different dioptric powers to achieve multifocality. They are pupil dependent and may be affected by decentration, thus the number of zones that redistribute the light for distance and near vision vary [41].

The **Rezoom *(AMO, Santa Ana, CA)*** uses a refractive design which has different zones within the concentric rings for focusing at varying distances (Fig. 1.6). Studies using an eye model with a 3 mm pupil showed that its near MTF did not change in spite of decentration up to 1 mm. Clinical experience with the Rezoom has shown that it provides good distance and intermediate vision, however near

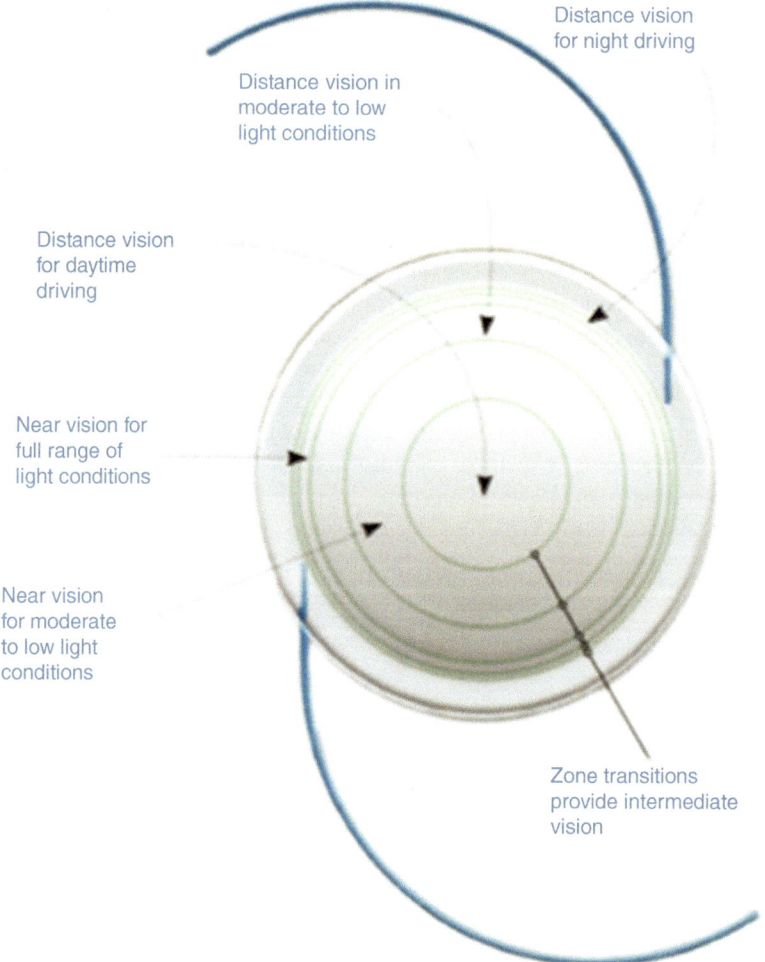

Distance vision for night driving

Distance vision in moderate to low light conditions

Distance vision for daytime driving

Near vision for full range of light conditions

Near vision for moderate to low light conditions

Zone transitions provide intermediate vision

**Fig. 1.6** A diagram of the Rezoom and a display of the focal points for each zone [31]

vision tasks require spectacle use especially with small pupil size, and it is still associated with photic phenomena [31].

The *M-Flex 630F (Rayner, East Sussex, UK)* is a center distance dominant lens with five refractive zones that alternate between two powers (Fig. 1.7) [44]. Reports from clinical studies showed good monocular and binocular UIVA and UDVA, with fair UNVA. Contrast sensitivity was at par with that of monofocal IOL's, and the incidence of visual disturbances was low. These did not change even after 12 months of follow up, and neither was there the occurrence of posterior capsular opacification requiring Nd:YAG laser capsulotomy [45].

## Extended Depth-of-Focus Lenses

Extended depth-of-focus or EDOF lenses comprise a relatively more recent class of presbyopia correcting IOL implants. These focus incoming light waves in an extended longitudinal plane and not onto discrete points as with traditional multifocal lenses. The elongated focus eliminates the overlapping of near and far images caused by traditional multifocal IOLs—improving intermediate vision while leaving far vision unaffected [35, 36, 46]. Strategies used to achieve extended depth-of-focus include the induction of spherical aberration in specific portions, the echelette design, or the use of small apertures [35]. Several of these lenses are in clinical use, and some of the new generation of multifocal IOL's induce extended depth-of-focus to a certain extent. In 2017, the American College of Ophthalmology Task Force published a consensus statement which outlines criteria for defining an EDOF IOL and serve as a guide for appraising studies that evaluate EDOF lenses [47].

The *MiniWell (SIFI, Italy)* is a progressive multifocal aspheric EDOF IOL (Fig. 1.8). It has a monofocal outer zone, and the inner and middle zones have spherical aberrations with opposite signs in order to induce depth of focus and generate multifocality [48]. In vitro testing for this lens showed a comparable performance with the Symfony in terms of far and intermediate-near vision at a 3.0 mm pupil diameter [49]. HOA levels were also found to be maintained regardless of pupil size [50]. Published clinical results on the Miniwell presented good performance at intermediate. There were no relevant differences in near visual acuity between this lens and multifocal IOL's, with few visual disturbances at night and similar contrast sensitivity as diffractive multifocal lenses [48, 51]. The personal experience of the authors, however, conflict with these results. Our own results in

**Fig. 1.7** The M-Flex 630-F [31]

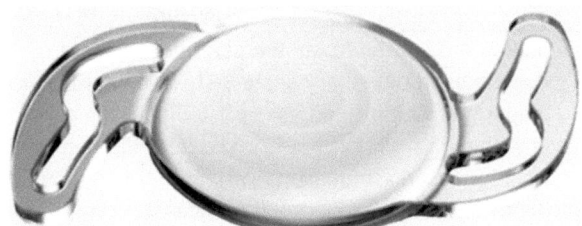

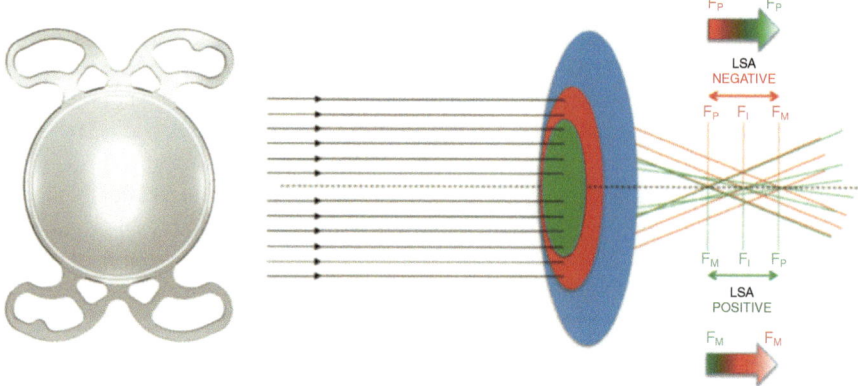

**Fig. 1.8** A diagram of the MiniWell IOL design and mode of action [48]

10 bilaterally implanted patients have been poor near and distance vision, even requiring lens exchange. We think that this is because a huge number of patients in the reported studies so far had undergone Miniwell implantation blended with a monofocal IOL, and so it would be interesting to find large-scale studies reporting outcomes with bilateral implantation.

The *Wichterle Intraocular Lens-Continuous Focus (WIOL-CF; Medicem, Kemenné Zehrovice, Czech Republic)* is a single haptic-less, full-optic hydrogel lens with a meniscoid anterior surface and a polyfocal hyperbolic posterior surface that creates a refractive gradient towards the optic center. This was said to be enhanced with pupil constriction during accommodative effort—making this lens both an accommodative and an EDOF lens hybrid [52]. While this lens had aceptable outcomes for UNVA and UDVA, MTF and HOA [53], it was recently withdrawn from the market [54].

**Small-aperture IOL's** achieve an extended and continuous range of vision due to an embedded opaque annular mask. This mask blocks unfocused paracentral light rays and allows the entry of paraxial light rays, similar to a pinole [36, 55]. The *IC-8 small-aperture IOL (Acufocus, Inc)*, has a 3.2 mm central mask with a 1.36 mm central aperture (Fig. 1.9). It is commercially available in Europe, Australia and New Zealand. When implanted bilaterally, an extended range of focus is attained with excellent intermediate and near vision albeit with higher scores for halos [56]. Unilateral implantation in the non-dominant eye, with micromonovision or monovision as the target, has good near and intermediate visual outcomes, with lower halo scores and higher patient satisfaction [56, 57]. Another such device on the market is the *Xtrafocus Pinhole Implant (Morcher, GmbH)*, which is a black hydrophobic acrylic implant (Fig. 1.10) that is placed as a piggyback lens in the ciliary sulcus. This implant has no dioptric power—it is purely a diaphragm-pinhole and its occluder has a concave-convex design to prevent contact with the primary IOL [55]. The IC-8 has demonstrated good tolerance to defocus and induced astigmatism [58]; both the IC-8 and Xtrafocus have been used for patients with highly-aberrated corneas with irregular astigmatism [59, 60]. Long-term follow-up data is pending, and would be interesting to see, for these implants.

**Fig. 1.9**  The IC-8 Small
Aperture IOL [55]

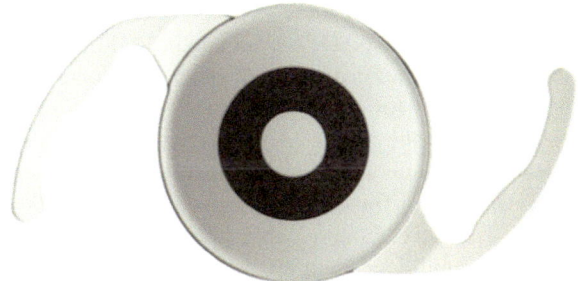

**Fig. 1.10**  The Xtrafocus
Pinhole Implant [60]

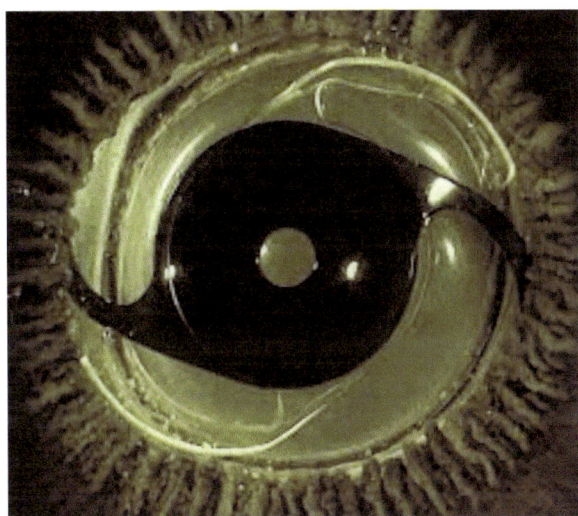

## Hybrid Lenses

It is important to note that there are overlaps between focality classes, and a refractive bifocal IOL may also be an EDOF IOL as well as a diffractive IOL. Some IOL's are considered hybrids as they are designed with either diffractive or refractive surfaces with an additional design in order to induce chromatic aberrations. Other IOL's use both diffractive and refractive technology.

The *AcrySof® Restor® SN6AD3 (Alcon Laboratories, Inc., Fort Worth, Texas)* is a one-piece multifocal IOL that uses both apodized diffractive and refractive technology. The central 3.5 mm of the optic zone has 12 concentric steps with gradually decreasing step height. This diffractive apodized region is surrounded by the refractive area (Fig. 1.11). The Restor is an aspheric lens, and provides negative spherical aberration in order to improve contrast sensitivity. The SN6AD3 model comes with a near add of 4D, and the SN6AD1 comes with a near add of 3D for improved intermediate vision, as has been found by De Vries et al. [31, 61] Defocus curve outcomes for the SN6AD3 also show two peaks of maximal vision at far and near, with a trough for intermediate vision. Mean intraocular aberrations after implantation of the SN6AD3 resulted in higher values of total and tilt RMS compared to a monofocal IOL, while there were lower values of total, spherical and spherical-like RMS [62]. The SN6AD1 has an apodized diffractive center to focus light for near distance while the peripheral refractive zone focuses light for distance vision. Mean defocus curves for this leans shows two peaks of maximum vision for distance and near, like the SN6AD3, although an acceptable intermediate vision is maintained. Normal photopic and low mesopic contrast sensitivity was reported for both ReSTOR lenses. The SN6AD1 induced lower values of spherical aberration [31].

The *Panoptix® (Alcon Laboratories, Fort Worth, Texas, USA)* is a single-piece, aspheric, pupil-dependent apodized IOL. This IOL has a 4.5 mm unapodized diffractive area in the center with 15 diffractive zones and an outer refractive rim. Light is then distributed to four focal points—half to the distance focus and half to the near focus. An additional feature is a negative spherical aberration on the anterior face, in order to compensate for the positive spherical aberration of the human cornea [63]. Optical bench studies of this lens showed pupil-independent good intermediate distance performance, with distance and near resolution comparable to that of a traditional multifocal IOL [64, 65]. This was in agreement with clinical studies. Furthermore, with the Panoptix there was no significant decrease in contrast sensitivity, HOA values and halo perception. Significant changes with these results were encountered in mesopic or photopic conditions [66–68].

The *Lentis® Mplus LS-313(Oculentis GmbH, Berlin, Germany)* is a single-piece, refractive rotationally asymmetric, varifocal, IOL. This is a pupil-dependent IOL with an inferior surface-embedded segment (Fig. 1.12). It has two definite corrective zones for far and near vision, with a seamless transition between each zone [69]. The Lentis

**Fig. 1.11** AcrySof® Restor
SN6AD3 [31]

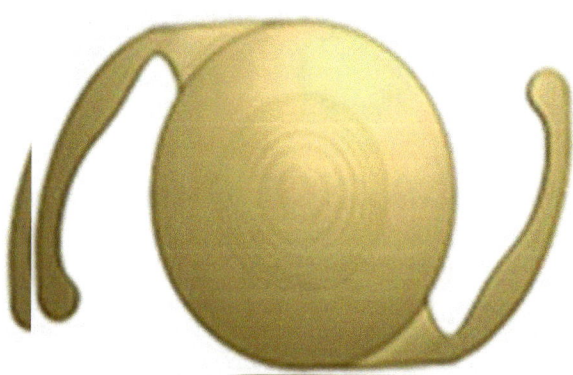

**Fig. 1.12** Lentis® Mplus
LS-313 IOL [31]

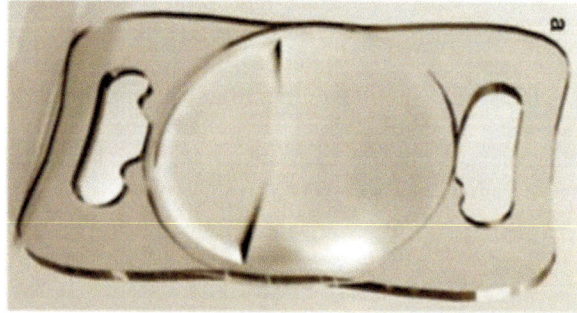

MPlus had significantly better CDVA than other multifocal IOL's, and comparable UDVA and CDVA to that of a monofocal lens. Its defocus curve also showed good visual acuity from −4D to −1D. *Ex vivo* studies with an optical bench analysis corroborates these findings [70] There are also less reports of photic phenomena with this lens [71]. A large magnitude intraocular primary vertical coma has been reported with this lens [69], probably due to its vertically asymmetric optical geometry. This, however, confers an extended depth-of-focus which gives good vision at all distances, as evidenced by its defocus curves [69, 72]. Caution is advised, however, when measuring for higher order berrations as some machines and measuring tools used might not accurately predict through-focus optical quality [69].

The ***Tecnis® Symfony (Abbot Medical Optics, Inc., Santa Ana California, USA)*** is a diffractive non-apodized achromatic IOL. This IOL has a biconvex wavefront-designed anterior aspheric surface and a posterior achromatic diffractive surface featuring an echelette design (Fig. 1.13) [63], thus it elongates the focus and corrects the corneal chromatic and spherical aberration [63, 73]. *Ex vivo* evaluation of this lens with a USAF target showed a pupil-dependent good range of vision from far to 50 cm albeit with a drop at near [74], and pupil-dependent MTF degradation [75]. Furthermore, the lens itself showed a higher absolute value of spherical aberration compared to trifocal IOL's [74, 76]. Clinical studies found that, while bilateral implantation of Symfony resulted in good UDVA, UIVA and UNVA, better UIVA and UNVA was found when targeted for monovision [73]. When compared with other lenses- such as the Panoptix or FineVision- the other lenses had better near vision, equivalent distance vision. The Panoptix and Symfony had similar results for intermediate vision. This lens showed no statistically significant improvement in terms of light distortion, visual symptoms, contrast sensitivity and aberrometry [63, 77].

**Accommodating IOLs**

Accommodating IOLs supposedly undergo a progressive dioptric power change in response to active ciliary body contraction during an accommodative effort [78]. Several designs have been used in order to achieve the required power change but presently there is still no conclusive evidence of the targeted dioptric power change in any of the IOLs that are available or in development.

*Position-changing IOL's* have a single optic which provides near and intermediate vision by anterior axial movement [37]. One such example is the ***CrystaLens®***

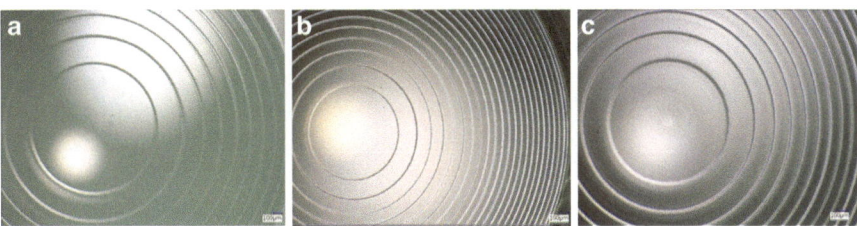

**Fig. 1.13** The appearance of the concentric rings for the Symfony (**a**), compared with a trifocal IOL (**b**) and bifocal IOL (**c**) [74]

*(Bausch & Lomb, Rochester, NY, USA)*, the first FDA-approved accommodating IOL, and has gone through several different designs [79]. Its optic is biaspheric to increase depth of focus, and hinges transmit ciliary body contraction to enable axial movement (Fig. 1.14). The anterior surface also changes its radius of curvature to improve near vision [80]. Significantly better UNVA was reported with the Crystalens® HD over a monofocal IOL, although there was no significant difference in CNVA. No difference was noted in intraocular aberrometric coefficient between the two lens types [80]. When compared with a low-addition-power (+1.5D) rotationally asymmetric trifocal IOL, the Lentis® M-Plus, both had comparable postoperative UNVA and CNVA. In the defocus curve, there was significantly better visual acuity with the multifocal IOL at several defocus levels. There were, however, less reports of lens tilting with the Crystalens® HD, with statistically insignificant differences in mean ocular higher order aberrations [17]. The Crystalens is, however, associated with a higher risk of posterior capsular opacity [81, 82]. Capsular contraction syndrome, or Z-syndrome, is a post-operative complication that is uniquely associated with the Crystalens®. Asymmetric capsular contraction causes the plate haptics to vault in opposite directions, inducing astigmatism [83, 84].

The *1CU® (Human Optics, Erlangen, Germany)* is a single piece biconvex IOL with four flexible haptics (Fig. 1.15) that bend to allow anterior movement of the optic during accommodative effort [86]. It was discontinued due to poor near vision outcomes [87] and significant reports of glare [82]. Another single-optic lens is the *TetraFlex® (Lenstec Inc, St. Petersburg, Fla, USA)*, which has flexible angulated closed-loop haptics (Fig. 1.16) that also allow forward movement within the capsular bag [86]. This lens has also been found to increase HOA's within the capsular bag [88]. The *BiocomFold 89A (Morcher GmbH, Sttgart, Germany)* is a

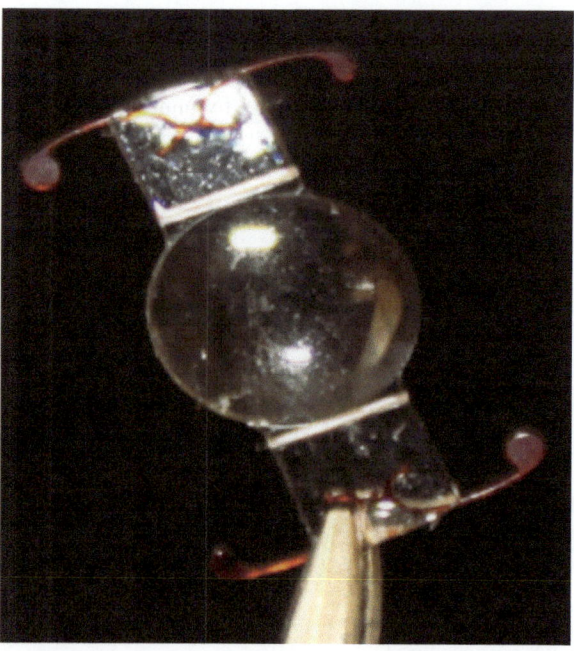

**Fig. 1.14** A schematic diagram of the Crystalens® IOL [97]

bag-in-the-lens implant. However, it has been found to produce limited and clinically insignificant axial movement compared to standard bag-implanted accommodating implants [89]. Other accommodating single-optic position-changing IOL's that have been developed include the *C-Well (Acuity Ltd, OrYehuda, Israel), OPAL (Bausch&Lomb, Rochester, NY, USA) and Tek-Clear (Tekia, Irvine, CA, USA)*. There is, however, little published clinical data on these lenses [82]. The main limitation with single-optic accommodating IOL's is that there is limited amplitude of accommodation, which is further impeded by capsular fibrosis. There are also reports of higher association with posterior capsular opacity, especially with the 1CU®—necessitating Nd:YAG capsulotomy. The YAG procedure had no effect on accommodative amplitude [82, 90].

**Dual optic IOL's** have a mobile front optic connected to a stationary rear optic by a spring-type haptic [86]. The now-discontinued *Synchrony® (Visiogen Inc, Abbott Medical Optics, Santa Ana, California, USA)* had an anterior biconvex optic with a high plus power and a posterior concave optic with a low minus power

**Fig. 1.15** Schematic diagram of the 1CU IOL [82]

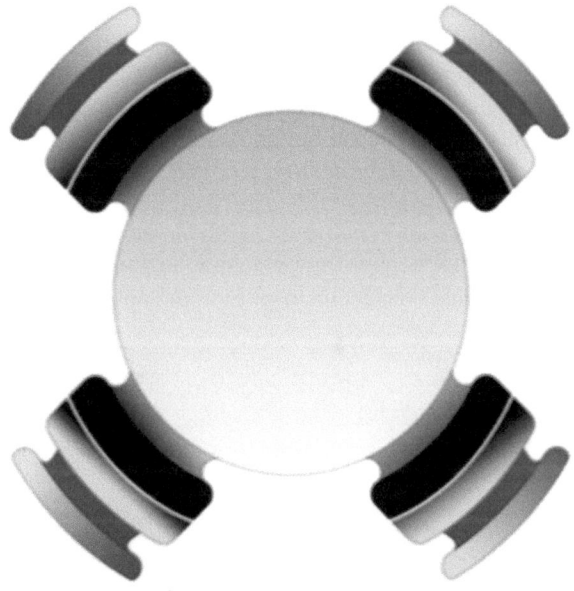

**Fig. 1.16** Schematic diagram of the Tetraflex® IOL [82]

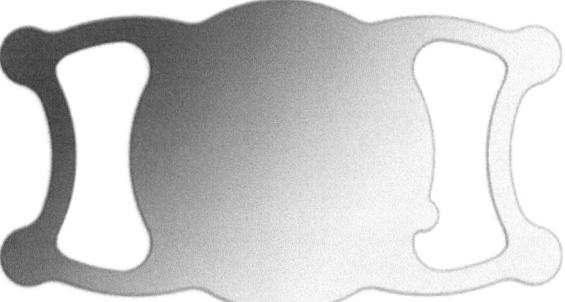

(Fig. 1.17). Tension caused by the capsular bag compresses the optics and an attempt to accommodate releases this strain energy [81, 91]. The *Synchrony*® has similar outcomes as the Crystalens® HD—with no statistically significant differences in UDVA, CDVA, near or intermediate visual outcomes between the 2 IOLs [81]. The *Sarfarazi (Bausch & Lomb, Rochester, NY, USA)* has 2 optic lenses connected by three haptics (Fig. 1.18). The change in dioptric power is also brought about by the displacement of the anterior optic. *Ex vivo* testing has shown that this is capable of attaining an amplitude of accommodation of up to 4.0D [82]. This lens has never been released commercially and there is no published paper on its clinical results.

Dual-optic lenses, specifically the Synchrony Lens, completely occupy the capsular bag, leading to a lower incidence of PCO. This also theoretically facilitates lens movement during accommodative effort and has been clinically shown with a wider range of defocus curves compared to single-optic lenses [81]. Studies have shown that there is no reduction in accommodative ability over a year-long follow-up period [92], and so it would be interesting to see long-term results with these lenses. While dual-optic accommodating IOL's have significantly better ocular quality than single-optic lenses, with comparable distance-vision outcomes, their near-vision outcomes are still limited [81] and patients may require training in order to attain good visual performance [92]. Yet another significant finding with dual-optic lenses is magnification of the viewed image, because of the increased distance between the retina and the image space nodal point during accommodative effort and movement of the anterior lens [93].

**Shape-changing IOL's** can change lens curvature to change dioptric power. The *FluidVision*® *(Powervision, Belmont, California, USA)* has optics filled with silicone oil. During accommodation, this oil is pushed into the optic through fluid channels that connect the haptics to the optic, inflating the lens and increasing the

**Fig. 1.17** Schematic diagram of the Synchrony® IOL [97]

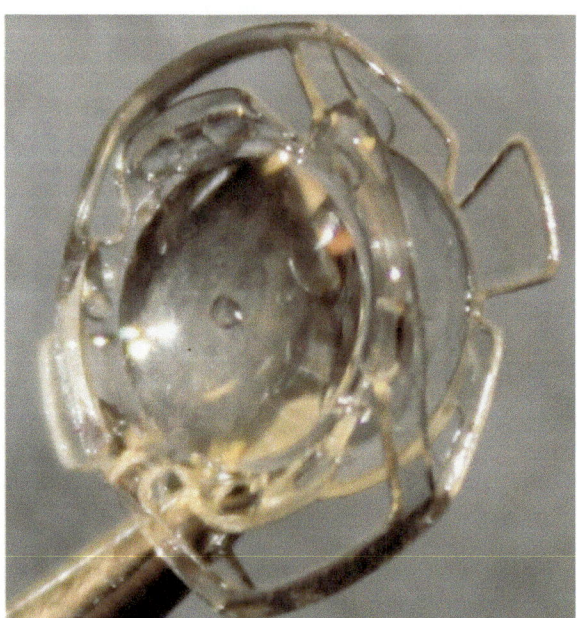

**Fig. 1.18** Schematic diagram of the Sarfarazi® IOL [97]

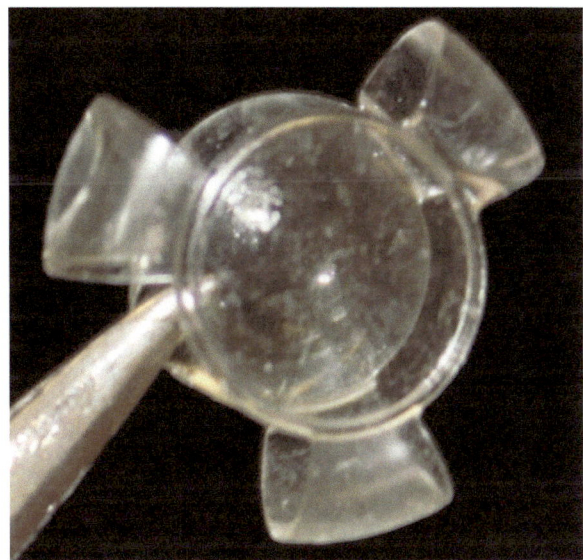

**Fig. 1.19** Nulens IOL [149]

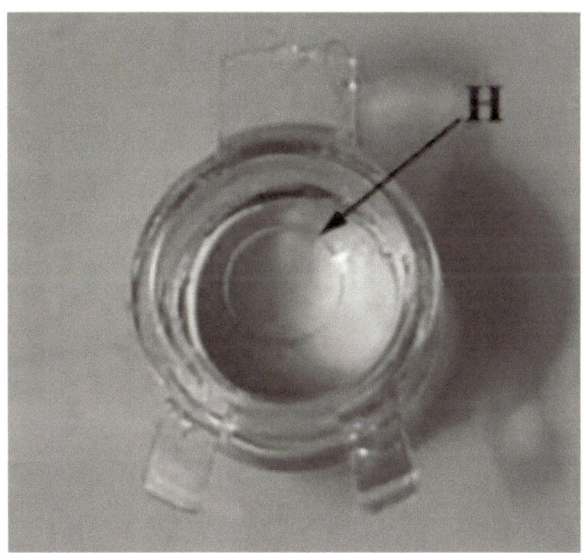

dioptric power for near vision [94]. The *NuLens® (DynaCurve, Herzliya Pituah, Israel)* is a conceptual sulcus-implanted lens that consists of PMMA haptics, a PMMA anterior reference plane that provides distance vision correction, a small chamber that contains a solid silicone gel, and a posterior piston with an aperture in the center (Fig. 1.19). When pressure is applied on the posterior piston, the gel-filled chamber bulges to increase or decrease optical power [95]. The *Juvene accommodating IOL (LensGen, Irvine, CA)* is a 2-component IOL with a fixed foldable lens—consisting of a base optic similar to that of an aspheric monofocal lens and a 360-degree haptic (Fig. 1.20). The foldable lens is injected through a

3.2 mm incision after which another fluid-based shape-changing lens is inserted and secured to the first with 3 tabs. The fluid lens has a flexible anterior suface which can change curvature in response to capsular forces with accommodation [52]. Clinical trials involving this lens are anticipated to start soon, and these would be interesting to see.

**Power-changing IOL's** dynamically change in refractive power. The ***Lumina®*** ***(Akkolens International, Breda, Netherlands)*** is a conceptual sulcus-implanted, continuous variable, lens design that has 2 partially overlapping aspherical optics. Each optic has an elastic U-shaped loop with a spring function, and non-elastic connections to the main body of the lens (Fig. 1.21). The anterior optic has a fixed power of 5.0D, and the power of the posterior optic depends on the required correction of the eye. The IOL's focal length changes as the optics shift in opposite directions in a plane that is perpendicular to the optical axis [52]. When the IOL is compressed by ciliary muscle contraction, as with accommodation, the optics

a                                                b

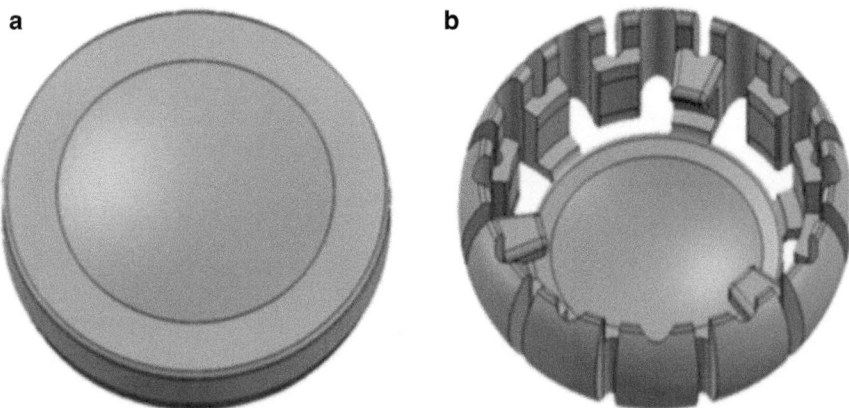

**Fig. 1.20** The Juvene IOL. One part is the base optic (**a**). The modular second implant (**b**) contains a silicone optic which changes curvature when the ciliary muscles contract and the zonules relax [52]

**Fig. 1.21** Lumina IOL. (Image courtesy of Mr. Aleksey Simonov, Akkolens International b.v. Breda, The Netherlands)

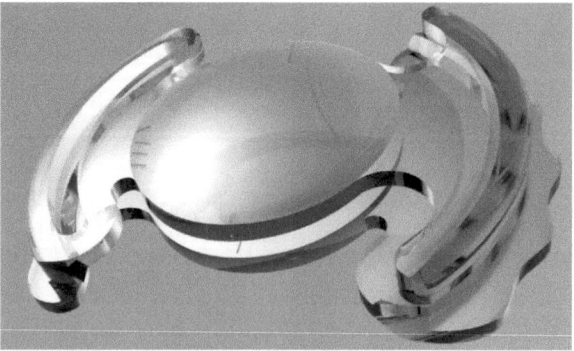

move centripetally in opposite directions to increase optical lens power. Ciliary muscle relaxation forces the elements back to their original state to decrease optical power [96]. Preliminary clinical tests with a monofocal IOL control have shown that the Lumina IOL significantly improves near, intermediate and far vision without affecting contrast sensitivity, with an accommodative power between 1.5 and 6.0D. Defocus curves showed improved near vision between −4.5 and −0.5D [96]. Nd:YAG capsulotomy did not adversely affect visual acuity and accommodation. Furthermore, the location of the IOL in the sulcus would also in theory avoid the effect of capsular fibrosis and contraction.

Other experimental IOL concepts are still in development. *Magnet-driven active shift IOL's* involve the implantation of magnets under the superior and inferior rectus muscles and in the capsular bags with the lens. The repellent action of these magnets are expected to drive the lens and capsular bag forward during accommodation—decreasing the effect of PCO and capsular fibrosis [97]. While implantation of this design has been reported in human eyes, no published data have been found. The *LiquiLens (Vision Solutions Technologies, Inc, Rockville, MD)* contains two solutions with different refractive indices. These solutions are inmiscible, and the current prototype has a bifocal effect which is driven by gravity [52]. An *electroadaptive accommodating IOL* is also in the works. It contains nematic liquid crystals sandwiched between transparent electrodes. Physiologic changes in light are triggered by accommodative effort and this activates microsensors [52].

## Conclusion

Presbyopic lenses are approached with optical multifocality based on refractive and diffractive optical principles, or monofocality which enables progressive dioptric power change in response to an active accommodative effort—as with the accommodating. Multifocality always requires neuroadaptation, which is the main reason for inadequate patient satisfaction and should significantly improve with the most recent models. Accommodating lenses are mostly in the experimental and pre-clinical development. Some of them, especially the sulcus-based lenses, have published consistent results that seem to be promising for future use in cataract and lens surgery. Experimental lenses are still in development but with no clinical trial to date.

## Refractive Laser Procedures

The advent of refractive corneal surgery was ushered by the emergence of the excimer and later the femtosecond laser. Ablative refractive surgery aims to change refraction through the removal of small amounts of tissue from the anterior surface of the cornea [98]. The development and evolution of the excimer laser, and the emergence of diagnostic wavefront technology, has made possible the execution of corneal surface ablation with increasingly accurate and predictable results [99]. The excimer laser emits photons at 193 nm, resulting in ablative photodecomposition which breaks the peptide backbone and vaporizes corneal collagen molecules. It can ablate corneal tissue without causing significant damage to adjacent tissue due to low tissue penetration and short pulse duration. The femtosecond laser, on the other hand, has a solid-state Nd:Glass laser source and uses ultra-fast focused pulses at near-infrared wavelenghts to create photo disruption at their focal point. A high-intensity electric field is generated, which forms a mixture of free electrons and ions called the plasma state. This plasma state expands and displaces the surrounding tissue, forming a cavitation bubble in the focal volume of the laser beam. Cutting is completed when these bubbles fuse [100].

*Photorefractive keratectomy (PRK)*, the oldest excimer laser procedure, involves the removal of the central corneal epithelium—achieved mechanically after a brief application of alcohol in order to loosen the epithelium. The exposed anterior stroma is then reshaped using the excimer laser. Myopia is treated with central corneal flattening, hyperopia with steepening, and astigmatism with an astigmatic pattern [100]. Epithelium removal leads to significant post-operative pain. There is relatively slow visual recovery and risk of haze development with PRK. However, PRK is still performed in corneas with superficial scarring, epithelial dystrophies, recurrent erosions, thin corneas, in post-keratoplasty patients, and for keratorefractive treatment of low to moderate myopia [100, 101] or hyperopia [102]. The use of mitomycin C coupled with the introduction of more improved surface ablation techniques and machines have both increased the range of treatment, and lowered the risk of corneal haze and regression after PRK [100]. Long-term studies on PRK outcomes report good safety and satisfaction with this procedure [78, 101]. Targeted refraction within ±1.00D is reached in 55–81% of eyes, and refractive stability is attained within one year. The treatment of low to moderate myopia was associated with night-time visual disturbances and haze [100]. Refractive predictability is lower, and the occurrence of haze higher, for treatment of eyes with high myopia [101]. PRK for low to moderate hyperopia is marked by an initial temporary myopic overshoot, with a subsequent hyperopic regression over a 24-month follow-up [102].

*Laser-assisted in situ keratomileusis (LASIK)* was first reported in 1990 by Pallikaris, who initially used a microkeratome to cut a hinged corneal flap, followed by excimer ablation of the stromal bed and subsequent flap repositioning [100, 103]. It is arguably the most-used refractive surgical procedure. LASIK is associated with high safety and refractive predictability, even on long-term follow-up, and excellent patient satisfaction rates [78, 100, 104]. The advantages of LASIK over PRK include faster visual recovery, less post-operative discomfort, better and more predictable wound healing, and less risk for corneal haze. Although there is faster improvement in UDVA with LASIK than with PRK, long-term efficacy outcomes are comparable for both procedures [105]. The advantages of flap creation with the femtosecond laser, as opposed to the conventional microkeratome assisted LASIK, has increased the safety, precision and predictability of performing LASIK—with better planning of flap diameter and depth. There is reduced risk of flap button hole or free cap formation, better flap stability, reduced post-operative dry eye symptoms [106, 107]. Studies on LASIK for myopia and myopic astigmatism show good post-operative unaided visual acuity, with goodsafety outcomes and refractive stability [78, 104, 107]. Myopic regression, however, has been reported in a study with a 12-year observation period [108]. LASIK for treating for treating low to moderate hyperopia was also found to have good safety and refractive outcomes. However, regression has been reported even up to follow-up periods of 5 years [109, 110]. Ectasia after corneal refractive surgery is characterized by a progressive increase in myopia and loss of UDVA or CDVA, with or without increasing astigmatism, with keratometric steepening of the cornea, topographic asymmetric inferior corneal thinning, and central or paracentral thinning. While corneal ectasia after refractive surgery is rare, with reported estimates ranging from 0.4 to 0.6%, it is potentially devastating and occurs more commonly after LASIK [111]. LASIK results in a weakening of the cornea's biomechanical strength, mainly because the creation of the flap affects the integrity of the corea. Patients should be carefully screened for pre-operative risk factors for ectasia, which include abnormal topographic patterns (such as in forme fruste keratoconus), corneal thickness and calculated residual stromal bed thickness [111]. Management of symptomatic corneal ectasia involves visual rehabilitation, conservative management with glasses or rigid gas permeable contact lenses and scleral lenses, corneal cross-linkting to halt progression, and surgical management with penetrating keratoplasty (PKP) or deep anterior lamellar keratoplasty (DALK) [111].

The development of more advanced diagnostic machines and wavefront technology have enabled an increased knowledge of optical aberrations. This, in turn, has allowed for the customization of the laser refractive procedure with the end goal being minimized degradation of visual quality compared to conventional laser corneal refractive surgery. In wavefront-guided refractive procedures, the excimer laser ablates a customized spatially variant pattern based on measurements taken with an aberrometer. Wavefront-guided LASIK and PRK have been performed clinically and have shown effectivity in treating myopia with and without astigmatism. There was significant improvement in UCVA at 1 year, with good safety profiles—although faster recovery was noted with LASIK as opposed to PRK [99]. Customized refractive procedures utilize information on the ocular aberrations and the topography of the patient as well as the refractive error in order to plan the ablation pattern to be executed. Clinical reports on outcomes with customized PRK and Femtosecond assisted LASIK have found that higher order and spherical aberrations increased with both procedures moreso with PRK than with LASIK, while total aberrations decreased. Sphere and cylinder were decreased from pre-operative values, and UDVA showed similar improvement for both procedures [112]. As more information is being gathered on the impact of optical aberrations on vision and visual quality, more understanding will be gained on the utility and effectivity of these procedures for treating ammetropia. In the meantime, careful patient selection is advised with pre-operative counselling as to the details of both wavefront-guided and customized refractive procedures.

*Small Incision Lenticule Extraction (SMILE)* is an all-femtosecond laser flapless procedure—it involves the creation of a lenticule after which a dissector is passed through a small incision to mobilize the lenticule and allow its removal (Fig. 1.22). It is approved to treat myopic sphere up to −10.00D, cylinder up to −5.00D and spherical equivalent up to −12.50D. This procedure came about as a result of the improvement in precision and technical design of the femtosecond laser such that the creation of lenticules of adequate dimension have been made possible [113, 114]. SMILE is a keyhole or flapless procedure, thus it has a reduced risk of traumatic cap or flap dislocation—albeit it may be more surgically demanding and require a higher learning curve. There is less disruption of the anterior stromal nerve plexus leading to faster dry eye recovery [100]. Preservation of the anterior stromal lamellar, and avoidance of vertical cuts contribute to better corneal biomechanics—and less propensity to develop corneal ectasia [100, 101, 113]. Reports of outcomes for SMILE showed good results—with a high percentage of eyes with good UDVA and CDVA and within ±1.00D or ± 0.50D of intended correction, regular corneal topography, no induced spherical aberration, and good patient satisfaction [100, 114–117]. Several studies have reported no significant differences in post-operative UDVA and CDVA, nor in post-operative refraction between SMILE and LASIK [118, 119]. Higher refractive correction in the corneal periphery was achieved with SMILE rather than with LASIK [118], which has been postulated to explain lower values of spherical, coma, and total HOA's with SMILE [118]. One disadvantage of SMILE, compared to LASIK, is its slightly slower visual recovery. Lenticule dissection and extraction is the most challenging step and intra-operative complications associated with SMILE include epithelial abrasions, incision tears, difficult lenticule extraction, cap perforation, and suction

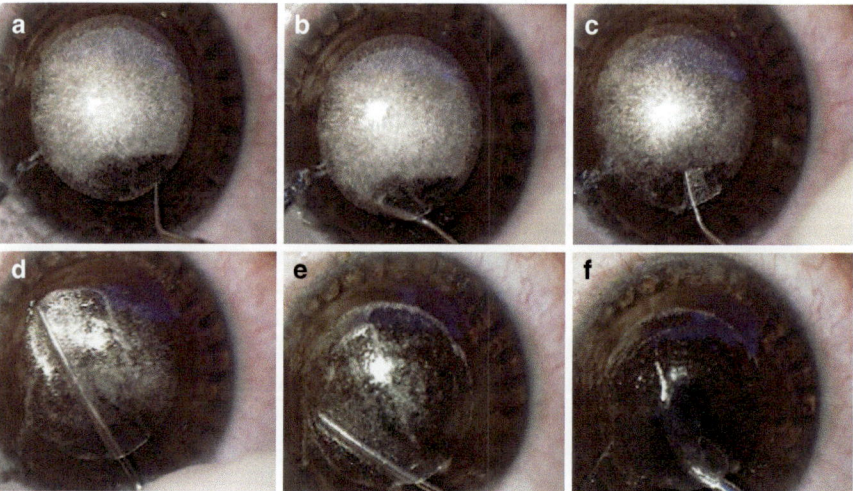

**Fig. 1.22** Small incision lenticule extraction (SMILE). A femtosecond laser is used to create a lenticule with a superior incision. The dissector is used to define the inferior and then the superior edges of the lenticule, and to release any adhesions from the cap and the underlying cornea. (**a–e**) Once the lenticule has been released, it is extracted with a pair of forceps (**f**) [124]

loss. These complications were not significantly associated with visual or refractive sequelae [100, 117, 120]. Post-operative complications include trace haze, some epithelial dryness, interface inflammation, retained lenticular fragments, and epithelial ingrowth [114, 121]. In spite of the current limitations for SMILE in terms of its treatment range, it has plenty of potential uses in the future all of which are being currently investigated– including the treatment of a higher range of myopia and hyperopia, as well as the transplantation of the preserved SMILE lenticule [122, 123].

## Phakic Intraocular Lenses

Laser keratorefractive procedures have limited use in the correction of high refractive errors—wound healing and biochemical responses can lead to poor refractive predictability, visual recovery may be prolonged and refraction unstable, and corneas are prone to scarring or haze and irregularity. High refractive errors also require the ablation of more corneal tissue, which may induce progressive ectasia. Intraocular refractive procedures have several advantages over laser refractive procedures—they can treat a broader range of ametropía with more stable post-operative refraction and faster visual recovery, and lead to better visual quality. *Phakic Intraocular Lenses (pIOL)* may be removed surgically hence any refractive result is potentially reversible, and the procedure does not require expensive or special devices [125]. Implantation of pIOL's is reserved for eyes with thin corneas or abnormal topographic findings, and may be classified according to the site of implantation. Refractive multifocal pIOL's have also been devised and pilot studies showed promising results for near, intermediate and distance visual acuity—with good patient satisfaction [126, 127]. Implantation of these lenses, however, is not routinely performed due to the higher rate of cataract formation and endothelial cell loss.

Anterior-chamber pIOL's may be angle fixated or iris fixated. Posterior chamber pIOL's are implanted posterior to the iris. A pIOL's design and location generally predicts its safety profile. A lens closer to the corneal endothelium, angle structures, or crystalline lens is more likely to lead to endothelial cell loss, iris complications or cataract. Anterior chamber pIOL's are more associated with elevated intraocular pressure and endothelial cell loss, whereas posterior chamber pIOLs are associated with cataract formation and lens subluxation [128, 129]. Comprehensive preoperative evaluation is required and measurement of the anterior chamber depth is critical as a shallow anterior chamber can complicate the insertion of the pIOL as well as lead to increased endothelial cell loss. The minimum required anterior chamber depth is between 3.0 and 3.2 mm as measured between the central anterior lens capsule and the endothelium. A patient's age and preoperative refraction should be taken into account as a predictive model as the safety zone between the endothelium and lens becomes much less than the recommended 1.5 mm over time—more than 20 years— due to age-related changes in the anatomy of the anterior segment structures [130, 131]. This has significant effects in the decision to use pIOL's for young patients with very high myopia [131]. A normal anterior chamber angle is necessary for the placement of anterior-chamber angle lenses. The corneal endothelium should also be evaluated, as there is a need to preserve the endothelial cell density to accommodate aging. Correct pIOL sizing avoids postoperative complications such as spinning, decentration, and cataract formation due to an inadequate vault over the crystalline lens. Peripheral iridotomies are required in order to prevent a pupillary block [125].

*Angle fixated pIOL's* were the first to be designed. The ***ZB5M lens*** had a z-flex haptic with four support points, a thin optic and small vaulting angle. It is placed at the angle of the anterior chamber. A study on this lens showed good refractive stability compared to LASIK, with superior improvement in CDVA—possibly due to a magnification of the retinal image. However, a high rate of endothelial cell loss per year was also reported, along with pupil ovalization, uveitis and glaucoma [132]. This lens has already been taken of the market. The ***ZSAL4 (Morcher GmbH, Stuttgart, Germany)*** was designed with longer haptics to decrease pressure on the angle structures and a larger optical zone—with less night halos and glare. Pupil ovalization was reported with the ZSAL4 and the ZB5M [133]. The ***Kelman Duet Implant Phakic IOL (Tekia Inc., Irvine, CA)*** featured a separate optic and haptic to enable optic exchange in case of poor fit or changes in refraction. The **AcrySof Cachet pIOL (Alcon Laboratories, Inc., Fort Worth, TX)** had reported long-term outcomes of good UDVA 20/40 or better in more than 90% of eyes, mean IOL rotation of 10.6°, spherical equivalent of −0.17D, and residual refractive error within ±1.00D for more than 90% [129, 134].

The ***iris-fixated or "iris claw" lens*** was developed due to an increasing number of reported complications with angle-supported pIOL's—although it was initially intended for the correction of aphakia. Several advantages include one size that fits all eyes, optimal distance from the crystalline lens and corneal endothelium, maintenance of the iris vascular supply and good iris function, and excellent stability with good lens centration. The ***Artisan (Ophtec BV, Groningen, the Netherlands)*** has a convex-concave optic with an 0.87 mm vault anterior to the iris (Fig. 1.23), and is available in powers ranging from −3.00 to −23.5D. The ***Artiflex*** was later developed

**Fig. 1.23** The Artisan phakic IOL [141]

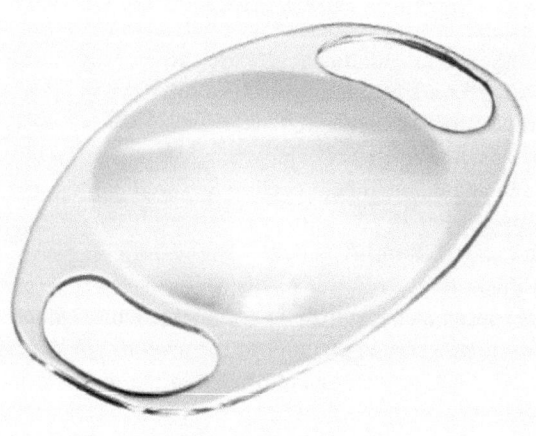

based on the Artisan, but with a flexible, convex-concave silicone optic (Fig. 1.24). It requires a smaller (3.2 mm) self-sealing incision, allowing for rapid visual recovery [125]. Studies on outcomes with the Artisan for both myopia and hyperopia report good UCVA, increased contrast sensitivity, good patient satisfaction rates, and stable long-term refraction [135, 136]. The Artisan has also been used for patients with stable keratoconus [137]. It was found to have a superior safety index when compared prospectively with LASIK for myopia −8 to −10D. For patients with myopia greater than -15D, LASIK was found to be an effective enhancement treatment. As the Artiflex is a foldable lens, clinical trials have reported a faster visual recovery with better UCVA compared to the Artisan [136, 138, 139]. Post-operative anterior chamber measurements for the Artiflex show that the minimum distance between the endothelium and the lens center should be maintained at 1.7 mm to minimize endothelial cell loss [130]. The *Artisan/Verisyse toric pIOL* is less likely to rotate due to its fixation to the iris stroma. It has excellent refractive outcomes—3-year results show UCVA better than 20/40 in 84% of 662 eyes [140].

**Posterior-chamber pIOL's** are placed behind the iris, and as such are cosmetically appealing and only noticeable upon careful examination. They are far from the anterior-chamber angle and the corneal endothelium, hence they are associated with less changes in intraocular pressure and endothelial cell density. The *Visian ICL (STAAR Surgical CO., Monrovia, CA)* is one such lens (Fig. 1.25). It is approved for myopia from −3 to −15D and for myopia −15 to −20D with astigmatism less than or equal to 2.5D [125]. Studies on outcomes for the Visian ICL showed good UDVA and good contrast sensitivity for hyperopia [142], and low-to-moderate to high myopia [143, 144]. Patients with lower levels of preoperative myopia were found to have better uncorrected visual acuity and better satisfaction rates with less overall reports of complications. Pupillary block was more likely to occur for hyperopic eyes [145]. The Visian ICL offered better safety, efficacy and predictability when compared with LASIK [143, 146] and PRK [147] for high myopes.

**Fig. 1.24** The Artiflex phakic IOL [141]

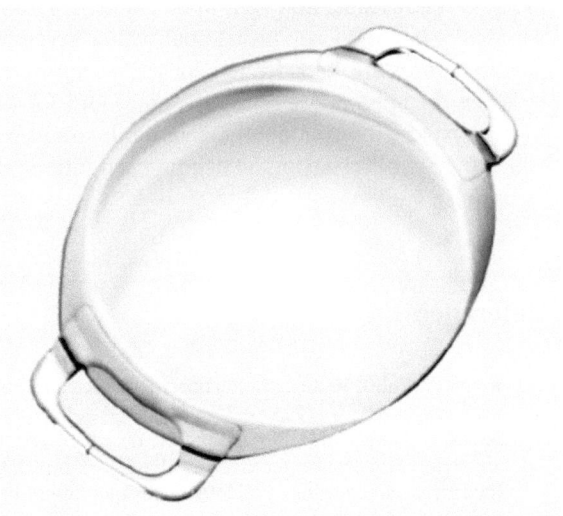

**Fig. 1.25** The Visian ICL [148]

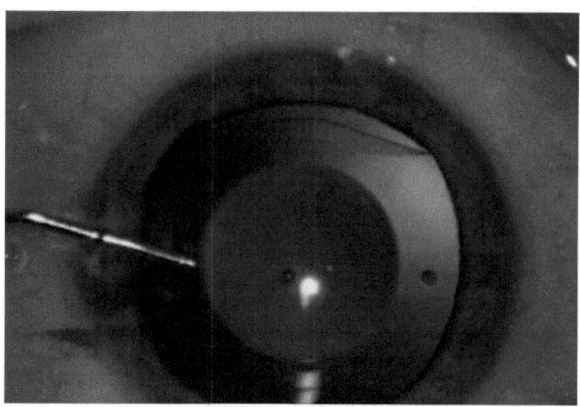

## Conclusion

In the last century we have seen leaps and bounds in the development and evolution of modern refractive surgery. The increasing availability of new technology for diagnosis and assessment of the ocular structures—the wavefront aberrometers and topographers, the optical coherence tomographers—have allowed for an increased understanding in what constitutes good visual quality. The capacity to develop new biocompatible materials have enabled the conception and production of increasingly varied intraocular implants that can be safely delivered into the eye and provide good unassisted vision at all distances. The latest machines used in refractive surgery—the phacoemulsification platforms, the femtosecond laser and excimer laser—have allowed for an unprecedented increase in the safety, precision, reproducibility and efficacy of modern-day refractive procedures. The currently available literature supports this with information on the outcomes of refractive procedures for a large number of patients over a long follow-up time. There is still plenty of knowledge, however, to be gained regarding the intricacies of the different factors that influence visual quality. Furthermore, there is a need to determine how to harness this knowledge in order to improve the available options as well as to select the appropriate refractive procedure for the correct indications in order to give improved vision at all distances. It would be interesting to see how this is addressed by the results of the ongoing and future studies—and the future seems to be promising.

## References

1. Renna A, Alió J, Vejarano L. Pharmacological treatments of presbyopia: a review of modern perspectives. Eye Vis. 2017;4:3.
2. Krader C, Feinbaum C. Simple solution for presbyopia: topical agent acts by reducing pupil size to increase depth of focus. Ophthalmology Times. http://www.ophthalmologytimes.com/modern-medicine-feature-articles/simple-solution-presbyopia. Published 2015. Accessed 10 Mar 2018.

3. Patel S, Salamun F, Matovic K. Pharmacological correction of presbyopia. In: Poster Presentation European Society of Cataract and Refractive Surgery Congress XXXI. http://www.escrs.org/amsterdam2013/programme/posters-details.asp?id=19804. Published 2013. Accessed 28 Mar 2018.
4. Renna A, Vejarano L, De la Cruz E, Alió J. Pharmacological treatment of presbyopia by novel binocularly instilled eye drops: a pilot study. Ophthalmol Therapy. 2016;5:63–73.
5. Cole J. Can an eye drop eliminate presbyopia? Rev Optom. https://www.reviewofoptometry.com/article/ro0617-can-an-eye-drop-eliminate-presbyopia. Published 2017. Accessed 10 Mar 2018.
6. Tsuneyoshi Y, Higuchi A, Negishi K, Tsubota K. Suppression of presbyopia progression with pirenoxine eyedrops: experiments on rats and non-blinded, randomized clinical trial of efficacy. Sci Rep. 2017;7:6819.
7. Krader C. Topical drops show promise as treatment for presbyopia. Ophthalmol Times Eur. 2016;12(6):18–20.
8. Garza E, Gomez S, Chayet A, Dishler J. One-year safety and efficacy results of a hydrogel inlay to improve near vision in patients with emmetropic presbyopia. J Refract Surg. 2013;29:166–72.
9. Konstantopoulos A, Mehta J. Surgical compensation of presbyopia with corneal inlays. Expert Rev. 2015;12(3):341–52.
10. Mulet M, Alió J, Knorz M. Hydrogel intracorneal inlays for the correction of hyperopia. Ophthalmology. 2009;116:1455–60.
11. Alió J, Shabayek M, Montes-Mico R, Mulet M, Ahmed A, Merayo J. Intracorneal hydrogel lenses and corneal aberrations. J Refract Surg. 2005;21:247–52.
12. Lindstrom R, Macrae S, Pepose J, Hoopes P. Corneal inlays for presbyopia correction. Curr Opin Ophthalmol. 2013;24:281–7.
13. Arlt E, Krall E, Moussa S, Grabner G, Dexl A. Implantable inlay devices for presbyopia : the evidence to date. Clin Ophthalmol. 2015;9:129–37.
14. Whitman J, Dougherty P, Parkhurst G, et al. Treatment of presbyopia in emmetropes using a shape-changing corneal inlay: one-year clinical outcomes. Ophthalmology. 2016;123:466–75.
15. Malandrini A, Martone G, Menabuoni L, et al. Bifocal refractive corneal inlay implantation to improve near vision in emmetropic presbyopic patients. J Cataract Refract Surg. 2015;41:1962–72.
16. Limnopoulou A, Bouzoukis D, Kymionis G, et al. Visual outcomes and safety of a refractive corneal inlay for presbyopia using femtosecond laser. J Refract Surg. 2013;29(1):12–8.
17. Alió J, Plaza-Puche A, Montalban R, Javaloy J. Visual outcomes with a single-optic accommodating intraocular lens and a low-addition-power rotational asymmetric multifocal intraocular lens. J Cataract Refract Surg. 2012;38:978–85.
18. Baily C, Kohnen T, Keefe M. Preloaded refractive-addition corneal inlay to compensate for presbyopia implanted using a femtosecond laser: one-year visual outcomes and safety. J Cataract Refract Surg. 2014;40:1341–8.
19. Naroo S, Bilkhu S. Clinical utility of the KAMRA corneal inlay. Clin Ophthalmol. 2016;10:913–9.
20. Tomita M, Kanamori T, Waring G, et al. Simultaneous corneal inlay implantation and laser in situ keratomileusis for presbyopia in patients with hyperopia, myopia, or emmetropia: six-month results. J Cataract Refract Surg. 2012;38:495–506.
21. Tomita M, Kanamori T, Waring G, Nakamura T, Yukawa S. Small-aperture corneal inlay implantation to treat presbyopia after laser in situ keratomileusis. J Cataract Refract Surg. 2013;39:898–905.
22. Igras E, Caoimh R, Paul O, William P. Long-term results of combined LASIK and monocular small-aperture corneal inlay implantation. J Refract Surg. 2016;32(6):379–84.
23. Huseynova T, Kanamori T, Waring G, Tomita M. Outcomes of small aperture corneal inlay implantation in patients with pseudophakia. J Refract Surg. 2014;30(2):110–5.
24. Lin L, Vilupuru S, Pepose J. Contrast sensitivity in patients with emmetropic presbyopia before and after small-aperture inlay implantation. J Refract Surg. 2016;32:386–93.

25. Alió J, Abbouda A, Huseynli S, Knorz M, Homs M, Durrie D. Removability of a small aperture intracorneal inlay for presbyopia correction. J Refract Surg. 2013;29(8):550–6.
26. Dexl A, Seyeddain O, Riha W, Hohensinn M, Hitzl W, Grabner G. Reading performance after implantation of a small-aperture corneal inlay for the surgical correction of presbyopia:two-year follow-up. J Cataract Refract Surg. 2011;37:525–31.
27. Gooi P, Ahmed I. Review of presbyopic IOLs: multifocal and accommodating IOLs. Int Ophthalmol Clin. 2012;52(2):41–50.
28. Kohnen T. Multifocal IOL technology: a successful step on the journey toward presbyopia treatment. J Cataract Refract Surg. 2008;34(12):2005.
29. Rosen E, Alió J, Dick H, Dell S, Slade S. Efficacy and safety of multifocal intraocular lenses following cataract and refractive lens exchange: meta-analysis of peer-reviewed publications. J Cataract Refract Surg. 2016;42:310–28.
30. Davison J, Simpson M. History and development of the apodized diffractive intraocular lens. J Cataract Refract Surg. 2006;32(5):849–58.
31. Duran-Garcia M, Multifocal Intraocular Lenses AJ. Types and models. In: Alió J, Pikkel J, editors. Multifocal intraocular lenses. The art and the practice. 1st ed. London: Springer Healthcare; 2014.
32. Alió J, Plaza-Puche A, Javaloy J, et al. Comparison of a new refractive multifocal intraocular lens with an inferior segmental near add and a diffractive multifocal intraocular lens. Ophthalmology. 2012;119:555–63.
33. Alió J, Plaza-Puche A, Javaloy J, Ayala M. Comparison of the visual and intraocular optical performance of a refractive multifocal IOL with rotational asymmetry and an apodized diffractive multifocal IOL. J Refract Surg. 2012;28:100–5.
34. McNeely R, Pazo E, Spence A, et al. Comparison of the visual performance and quality of vision with combined symmetrical inferonasal near addition versus inferonasal and superotemporal placement of rotationally asymmetric refractive multifocal intraocular lenses. J Cataract Refract Surg. 2016;42:1721–9.
35. Rocha K. Extended depth of focus IOLs: the next chapter in refractive technology? J Refract Surg. 2017;33(3):46.
36. Breyer D, Kaymak H, Ax T, Kretz F, Auffarth G, Hagen P. Multifocal intraocular lenses and extended depth of focus intraocular lenses. Asia-Pac J Ophthalmol. 2017;6:339–49.
37. Beiko G. Status of accommodative intraocular lenses. Curr Opin Ophthalmol. 2007;18(1):74–9.
38. Liu J-P, Zhang F, Zhao J-Y, Ma L-W, Zhang J-S. Visual function and higher order aberration after implantation of aspheric and spherical multifocal intraocular lenses: a meta-analysis. Int J Ophthalmol. 2013;6(5):690–5.
39. Rosen E, Alió J, Dick H, Dell S, Slade S. Efficacy and safety of multifocal intraocular lenses following cataract and refractive lens exchange: metaanalysis of peer-reviewed publications. J Cataract Refract Surg. 2016;42:310–28.
40. Alio JL, Grzybowski A, El Aswad A, Romaniuk D. Refractive lens exchange. Surv Ophthalmol. 2014;59:579–98. https://doi.org/10.1016/j.survophthal.2014.04.004.
41. Sachdev G, Sachdev M. Optimizing outcomes with multifocal intraocular lenses. Indian J Ophthalmol. 2017;65:1294–300.
42. Alió J, Plaza-Puche A, Férnandez-Buenaga R, Pikkel J, Maldonado M. Multifocal intraocular lenses: an overview. Surv Ophthalmol. 2017;62:611–34.
43. Kamiya K, Hayashi K, Shimizu K, Negishi K, Sato M, Bissen-Miyajima H. Multifocal intraocular lens explantation: a case series of 50 eyes. Am J Ophthalmol. 2014;158:215.220.e1.
44. Lichtinger A, Rootman D. Intraocular lenses for presbyopia correction: past, present and future. Curr Opin Ophthalmol. 2012;23(1):40–6.
45. Prieto J, Bautista M. Visual outcomes after implantation of a refractive multifocal intraocular lens with a +3.00 D addition. J Cataract Refract Surg. 2010;36:1508–16.
46. Akella S, Juthani V. Extended depth of focus intraocular lenses for presbyopia. Curr Opin Ophthalmol. 2018;29:318–22. https://doi.org/10.1097/ICU.0000000000000490.

47. MacRae S, Holladay J, Glasser A, et al. Special report: American Academy of Ophthalmology Task Force consensus statement for extended depth of field intraocular lenses. Ophthalmology. 2017;124:139–41.
48. Savini G, Schiano-Lomoriello D, Balducci N, Barboni P. Visual performance of a new extended depth-of-focus intraocular lens compared to a distance-dominant diffractive multifocal intraocular lens. J Refract Surg. 2018;34(4):228–35.
49. Domínguez-Vicent A, Esteve-Taboada J, Del Águila-Carrasco A, Monsálvez-Romin D, Montés-Micó R. In vitro optical quality comparison of 2 trifocal intraocular lenses and 1 progressive multifocal intraocular lens. J Cataract Refract Surg. 2016;42(1):138–47.
50. Bellucci R, Curatolo M. A new extended depth of focus intraocular lens based on spherical aberration. J Refract Surg. 2017;33(6):389–94.
51. Savini G, Balducci N, Carbonara C, et al. Functional assessment of a new extended depth-of-focus intraocular lens. Eye. 2019;33:404–10. https://doi.org/10.1038/s41433-018-0221-1.
52. Pepose J, Burke J, Qazi M. Accommodating intraocular lenses. Asia-Pac J Ophthalmol. 2017;6:350–7.
53. Siatiri H, Mohammadpour M, Gholami A, Ashrafi E, Siatiri N, Mirshahi R. Optical aberrations, accommodation, and visual quality with a bioanalogic continuous focus intraocular lens after cataract surgery. J Curr Ophthalmol. 2017;29(4):274–81.
54. Kim Y, Kang K, Yeo Y, Kim K, Siringo F. Consistent pattern in positional instability of polyfocal full-optic accommodative IOL. Int Ophthalmol. 2017;37(6):1299–304.
55. Srinivasan S. Small aperture intraocular lenses: the new kids on the block. J Cataract Refract Surg. 2018;44(8):927–8.
56. Dick H, Elling M, Schultz T. Binocular and monocular implantation of small-aperture intraocular lenses in cataract surgery. J Refract Surg. 2018;34(9):629–31.
57. Dick H, Pioevella M, Vukich J. Prospective multicenter trial of a small-aperture intraocular lens in cataract surgery. J Cataract Refract Surg. 2017;43:956–68.
58. Ang R. Small-aperture intraocular lens tolerance to induced astigmatism. Clin Ophthalmol. 2018;12:1659–64.
59. Schultz T, Dick H. Small-aperture intraocular lens implantation in a patient with an irregular cornea. J Refract Surg. 2016;32(10):706–8.
60. Trindade C, Trindade B, Trindade F, Werner L, Osher R, Santhiago M. New pinhole sulcus implant for the correction of irregular corneal astigmatism. J Cataract Refract Surg. 2017;43(10):1297–306.
61. De Vries N, Webers C, Montés-Micó R, Ferrer-Blasco T, Nujits R. Visual outcomes after cataract surgery with implantation of a +3.00D or +4.00D aspheric diffractive multifocal intraocular lens: comparative study. J Cataract Refract Surg. 2010;36:1316–22.
62. Alió J, Piñero D, Plaza-Puche A, et al. Visual and optical performance with two different diffractive multifocal intraocular lenses compared to a monofocal lens. J Refract Surg. 2011;27:570–81.
63. Cochener B, Boutillier G, Lamard M, Auberger-Zagnoli C. A comparative evaluation of a new generation of diffractive trifocal and extended depth of focus intraocular lens. J Refract Surg. 2018;34(8):507–14.
64. Carson D, Xu Z, Alexander E, Choi M, Zhao Z, Hong X. Optical bench performance of 3 trifocal intraocular lenses. J Cataract Refract Surg. 2016;42:1361–7.
65. Lee S, Choi M, Xu Z, Zhao Z, Alexander E, Liu Y. Optical bench performance of a novel trifocal intraocular lens compared with a multifocal intraocular lens. Clin Ophthalmol. 2016;10:1031–8.
66. Ruiz-Mesa R, Abengózar-Vela A, Ruiz-Santos M. A comparative study of the visual outcomes between a new trifocal and an extended depth of focus intraocular lens. Eur J Ophthalmol. 2018;28(2):182–7.
67. García-Pérez J, Gros-Otero J, Sánchez-Ramos C, Blázquez V, Contreras I. Short term visual outcomes of a new trifocal intraocular lens. BMC Ophthalmol. 2017;17:72. https://doi.org/10.1186/s12886-017-0462-y.

68. Lawless M, Hodge C, Reich J, et al. Visual and refractive outcomes following implantation of a new trifocal intraocular lens. Eye Vis. 2017;4(4):10. https://doi.org/10.1186/s40662-017-0076-8.
69. Akondi V, Pérez-Merino P, Martinez-Enriquez E, et al. Evaluation of the true wavefront aberrations in eyes implanted with a rotationally asymmetric multifocal intraocular lens. J Cataract Refract Surg. 2017;33(4):257–65.
70. Plaza-Puche A, Alió J, MacRae S, Zheleznyak L, Sala E, Yoon G. Correlating optical bench performance with clinical defocus curves in varifocal and trifocal intraocular lenses. J Refract Surg. 2015;31(5):300–7.
71. Veliká V, Hejsek L, Raiskup F. Clinical results of implantation of two types of multifocal rotationally-asymmetric intraocular lenses. Čes a slov Oftal. 2017;73(1):3–12.
72. Alió J, Piñero D, Plaza-Puche A, Chan M. Visual outcomes and optical performance of a monofocal intraocular lens and a new-generation multifocal intraocular lens. J Cataract Refract Surg. 2011;37:241–50.
73. Cochener B, Group CS. Clinical outcomes of a new extended range of vision intraocular lens: International Multicenter Concerto Study. J Cataract Refract Surg. 2016;42:1268–75.
74. Gatinel D, Loicq J. Clinically relevant optical properties of bifocal, trifocal, and extended depth of focus intraocular lenses. J Refract Surg. 2016;32(4):273–80.
75. Yoo Y-S, Whang W, Byun Y, et al. Through-focus optical bench performance of extended depth-of-focus and bifocal intraocular lenses compared to a monofocal lens. J Refract Surg. 2018;34(4):236–43.
76. Camps V, Tolosa A, Piñero D, de Fez D, Caballero M, Miret J. In vitro aberrometric assessment of a multifocal intraocular lens and two extended depth of focus IOLs. J Ophthalmol. 2017;2017:7095734.
77. Escandón-García S, Ribeiro F, McAlinden C, Queirós A, González-Méijome MJ. Through-focus vision performance and light disturbances of 3 new intraocular lenses for presbyopia correction. J Ophthalmol. 2018;2018:6165493. https://doi.org/10.1155/2018/6165493.
78. Kamiya K, Igarashi A, Hayashi K, et al. A multicenter prospective cohort study on refractive surgery in 15,011 eyes. Am J Ophthalmol. 2017;175:159–68.
79. Werner L, Olson R, Mamalis N. New technology IOL optics. Ophthalmol Clin North Am. 2006;19:469–83.
80. Alió J, Piñero D, Plaza-Puche A. Visual outcomes and optical performance with a monofocal intraocular lens and a new-generation single-optic accommodating intraocular lens. J Cataract Refract Surg. 2010;36:1656–64.
81. Alió J, Plaza-Puche A, Montalban R, Ortega P. Near visual outcomes with single optic and dual-optic accommodating intraocular lenses. J Cataract Refract Surg. 2012;38:1568–75.
82. Liang Y-L, Jia S-B. Clinical application of accommodating intraocular lens. Int J Ophthalmol. 2018;11(6):1028–37.
83. Kramer G, Werner L, Neuhann T, Tetz M, Mamalis N. Anterior haptic flexing and in-the-bag subluxation of an accommodating intraocular lens due to excessive capsular bag contraction. J Cataract Refract Surg. 2015;41:2010–3.
84. Page T, Whitman J. A stepwise approach for the management of capsular contraction syndrome in hinge-based accommodative intraocular lenses. Clin Ophthalmol. 2016;10:1039–46.
85. Jardim D, Soloway B, Starr C. Asymmetric vault of an accommodating intraocular lens. J Cataract Refract Surg. 2006;32(2):347–50.
86. Menapace R, Findl O, Kriechbaum K. Accommodating intraocular lenses: a critical review of present and future concepts. Graefes Arch Clin Exp Ophthalmol. 2007;245:473–89.
87. Saiki M, Negishi K, Dogru M, Yamaguchi T, Tsubota K. Biconvex posterior chamber accommodating intraocular lens implantation after cataract surgery: long-term outcomes. J Cataract Refract Surg. 2010;36:603–8.
88. Wolffsohn J, Davies L, Gupta N, et al. Mechanism of action of the tetraflex accommodative intraocular lens. J Refract Surg. 2010;26:858–62.

89. Cleary G, Spalton D, Gala K. A randomized intraindividual comparison of the accommodative performance of the bag-in-the-lens intraocular lens in presbyopic eyes. Am J Ophthalmol. 2010;150(5):619–27.
90. Nguyen N, Sietz B, Reese S, Langenbucher A, Küchle M. Accommodation after Nd:YAG capsulotomy in patients with accommodative posterior chamber lens 1CU. Graefes Arch Clin Exp Ophthalmol. 2005;243(2):120–6.
91. Bohórquez V, Alarcon R. Long-term reading performance in patients with bilateral dual-optic accommodating intraocular lenses. J Cataract Refract Surg. 2010;36:1880–6.
92. Peris-Martínez C, Díez-Ajenjo A, García-Domene C. Short-term results with the Synchrony lens implant for correction of presbyopia following cataract surgery. J Emmetropia. 2013;4:137–43.
93. Ale J, Manns F, Ho A. Magnifications of single and dual element accommodative intraocular lenses: paraxial optics analysis. Ophthalmic Physiol Opt. 2011;31(1):7–16.
94. Kohl J, Werner L, Ford J, et al. Long-term uveal and capsular biocompatibility of a new accommodating intraocular lens. J Cataract Refract Surg. 2014;40:2113–9.
95. Alió J, Ben-nun J, Rodríguez-Prats J, Plaza-Puche A. Visual and accommodative outcomes 1 year after implantation of an accommodating intraocular lens based on a new concept. J Cataract Refract Surg. 2009;35:1671–8.
96. Alió J, Simonov A, Plaza-Puche A, et al. Visual outcomes and accommodative response of the lumina accommodative intraocular lens. Am J Ophthalmol. 2016;164:37–48.
97. Sheppard A, Bashir A, Wolffsohn J, Davies L. Accommodating intraocular lenses: a review of design concepts, usage and assessment methods. Clin Exp Optom. 2010;93(6):441–52.
98. Boyd B, Agarwal S, Agarwal A, Agarwal A. Lasik and beyond Lasik: wavefront analysis and customized ablation. Highlights of Ophthalmology Int'l: Panama; 2002.
99. Manche E, Haw W. Wavefront-guided laser in situ keratomileusis (LASIK) versus wavefront-guided photorefractive keratectomy (PRK): a prospective randomized eye-to-eye comparison (an American Ophthalmological Society thesis). Trans Am Ophthalmol Soc. 2011;109:201–20.
100. Vestergaard A. Past and present of corneal refractive surgery: a retrospective study of long-term results after photorefractive keratectomy and a prospective study of refractive lenticule extraction. Acta Ophthalmol. 2014;92 Thesis(2):1–21.
101. Vestergaard A, Hjortdal J, Ivarsen A, Work K, Grauslund J, Sjølie A. Long-term outcomes of photorefractive keratectomy for low to high myopia: 13 to 19 years of follow-up. J Refract Surg. 2013;29(5):312–9.
102. Spadea L, Sabetti L, D'Alessandri L, Balestrazzi E. Photorefractive keratectomy and LASIK for the correction of hyperopia: 2-year follow-up. J Refract Surg. 2006;22:131–6.
103. Reinstein D, Archer T, Gobbe M. The history of LASIK. J Refract Surg. 2012;28(4):291–8.
104. Kamiya K, Igarashi A, Hayashi K, et al. A multicenter retrospective survey of refractive surgery in 78,248 eyes. J Refract Surg. 2017;33(9):598–602.
105. Hersh P, Brint S, Maloney R, et al. Photorefractive keratectomy versus laser in situ keratomileusis for moderate to high myopia: a randomized protective study. Ophthalmology. 1998;105:1512–23.
106. Torky M, Al Zafiri Y, Khattab A, Farag R, Awad E. Visumax femtolasik versus Moria M2 microkeratome in mild to moderate myopia: efficacy, safety, predictability, aberrometri changes and flap thickness predictability. BMC Ophthalmol. 2017;17:125. https://doi.org/10.1186/s12886-017-0520-5.
107. Aristeidou A, Taniguchi E, Tsatsos M, et al. The evolution of corneal and refractive surgery with the femtosecond laser. Eye Vis. 2015;2:12.
108. Ikeda T, Shimizu K, Igarashi A, Kasahara S, Kamiya K. Twelve-year follow-up of laser in situ keratomileusis for moderate to high myopia. Biomed Res Int. 2017;2017:9391436. https://doi.org/10.1155/2017/9391436
109. Frings A, Richard G, Steinberg J, Druchkiv V, Linke S, Katz T. LASIK and PRK in hyperopic astigmatic eyes: is early retreatment advisable? Clin Ophthalmol. 2016;10:565–70.

110. Jaycock P, O'Brart D, Rajan M, Marshall J. 5-year follow-up of LASIK for hyperopia. Ophthalmology. 2005;112(2):191–9.
111. Wolle M, Randleman J, Woodward M. Complications of refractive surgery: ectasia after refractive surgery. Int Ophthalmol Clin. 2016;56(2):129–41.
112. Sajjadi V, Ghoreishi M, Jafarzadehpour E. Refractive and aberration outcomes after customized photorefractive keratectomy in comparison with customized femtosecond laser. Med Hypothesis Discov Innov Ophthalmol. 2015;4(4):136–42.
113. Reinstein D, Carp G, Archer T, et al. In: Reinstein D, Carp G, Archer T, editors. The Surgeon's Guide to SMILE: small incision lenticule extraction. Thorofare, NJ: SLACK; 2018.
114. Reinstein D, Archer T, Gobbe M. Small incision lenticule extraction (SMILE) history, fundamentals of a new refractive surgery technique and clinical outcomes. Eye Vis. 2014;1:3.
115. Sekundo W, Kunert K, Russmann C, et al. First efficacy and safety study of femtosecond lenticule extraction for the correction of myopia: six-month results. J Cataract Refract Surg. 2008;34(9):1513–20.
116. Sekundo W, Gertnere J, Bertelmann T, Solomatin I. One-year refractive results, contrast sensitivity, high-order aberrations and complications after myopic small-incision lenticule extraction (ReLEx SMILE). Graefes Arch Clin Exp Ophthalmol. 2014;252(5):837–43.
117. Vestergard A, Ivarsen A, Asp S, Hjortdal J. Small-incision lenticule extraction for moderate to high myopia: predictability, safety, and patient satisfaction. J Cataract Refract Surg. 2012;38:2003–10.
118. Kataoka T, Nishida T, Murata A, et al. Control-matched comparison of refractive and visual outcomes between small incision lenticule extraction and femtosecond laser-assisted LASIK. Clin Ophthalmol. 2018;12:865–73.
119. Han T, Xu Y, Han X, et al. Three-year outcomes of small incision lenticule extraction (SMILE) and femtosecond laser-assisted laser in situ keratomileusis (FS-LASIK) for myopia and myopic astigmatism. Br J Ophthalmol. 2019;103:565–8. https://doi.org/10.1136/bjophthalmol-2018-312140.
120. Titiyal J, Kaur M, Rathi A, Falera R, Chaniyara M, Sharma N. Learning curve of small incision lenticule extraction: challenges and complications. Cornea. 2017;36(11):1377–82.
121. Krueger R, Meister C. A review of small incision lenticule extraction complications. Curr Opin Ophthalmol. 2018;29(4):292–8.
122. Liu Y, Teo E, Ang H, et al. Biological corneal inlay for presbyopia derived from small incision lenticule extraction (SMILE). Sci Rep. 2018;8:1831. https://doi.org/10.1038/s41598-018-20267-7.
123. Jacob S, Kumar D, Agarwal A, Agarwal A, Aravind R, Saijimol A. Preliminary evidence of successful near vision enhancement with a new technique: PrEsbyopic Allogenic Refractive Lenticule (PEARL) corneal inlay using a SMILE lenticule. J Refract Surg. 2017;33(4):224–9.
124. Titiyal J, Shaikh F, Kaur M, Rathi A. Small incision lenticule extraction (SMILE) techniques: patient selection and perspectives. Clin Ophthalmol. 2018;12:1685–99.
125. Huang D, Schallhorn S, Sugar A, et al. Phakic intraocular lens implantation for the correction of myopia: a report by the American Academy of Ophthalmology. Ophthalmology. 2009;116:2244–58.
126. Alió J, Mulet M. Presbyopia correction with an anterior chamber phakic multifocal intraocular lens. Ophthalmology. 2005;112(8):1368–74.
127. Baïkoff G, Matach G, Fontaine A, Ferraz C, Spera C. Correction of presbyopia with refractive multifocal phakic intraocular lenses. J Cataract Refract Surg. 2004;30(7):1454–60.
128. Alió J, Toffaha B, Peña-Garcia P, Sádaba L, Barraquer R. Phakic intraocular lens explantation: causes in 240 cases. J Refract Surg. 2015;31(1):30–5.
129. Aerts A, Jonker S, Wielders L, et al. Phakic intraocular lens: two-year results and comparison of endothelial cell loss with iris-fixated intraocular lenses. J Cataract Refract Surg. 2015;41:2258–65.
130. Ferreira T, Portelinha J. Endothelial distance after phakic iris-fixated intraocular lens implantation: a new safety reference. Clin Ophthalmol. 2014;8:225–61.

131. Alió J, Abbouda A, Peña-Garcia P. Anterior segment optical coherence tomography of long-term phakic angle-supported intraocular lenses. Am J Ophthalmol. 2013;156(5):894–901.
132. Rosman M, Alió J, Ortiz D, Pérez-Santonja J. Refractive stability of LASIK with the VISX 20/20 excimer laser vs ZB5M phakic IOL implantation in patients with high myopia (>−10.00D): a 10-year retrospective study. J Refract Surg. 2011;27(4):279–86.
133. Alió J, De la Hoz F, Pérez-Santonja J, Ruiz-Moreno J, Quesada J. Phakic anterior chamber lenses for the correction of myopia: a 7-year cumulative analysis of complications in 263 cases. Ophthalmology. 1999;106:458–66.
134. Gimbel H, Norton N, Amritanand A. Angle-supported phakic intraocular lenses for the correction of myopia: three-year follow-up. J Cataract Refract Surg. 2015;41:2179–89.
135. Qasem Q, Kirwan C, O'Keefe M. 5-year prospective follow-up of Artisan phakic intraocular lenses for the correction of myopia, hyperopia and astigmatism. Ophthalmologica. 2010;224(5):283–90.
136. Karimian F, Baradaran-Rafii A, Hashemian S, et al. Comparison of three phakic intraocular lenses for correction of myopia. J Ophthalmic Vis Res. 2014;9(4):427–33.
137. Sedaghat M, Ansari-Astaneh M, Zarei-Ghanavati M, Davis S, Sikder S. Artisan iris-supported phakic IOL implantation in patients with keratoconus: a review of 16 eyes. J Refract Surg. 2011;27(7):489–93.
138. Dick H, Budo C, Malecaze F, et al. Foldable Artiflex phakic intraocular lens for the correction of myopia: two-year follow-up results of a prospective European multicenter study. Ophthalmology. 2009;116(4):671–7.
139. Ozertürk Y, Kuboaglu A, Sari E, et al. Foldable iris-fixated phakic intraocular lens implantation for the correction of myopia: two years of follow-up. Indian J Ophthalmol. 2012;60(1):23–8.
140. Stulting R, Group UVS. Three-year results of Artisan/Verisyse phakic intraocular lens implantation: results of the United States Food and Drug Administration clinical trial. Ophthalmology. 2008;115(3):464–72.
141. Simões P, Ferreira T. Iris-fixated intraocular lenses for ametropia and aphakia. Med Hypothesis Discov Innov Ophthalmol. 2014;3(4):116–22.
142. Davidorf J, Zaldivar R, Oscherow S. Posterior chamber phakic intraocular lens for hyperopia of +4 to +11 diopters. J Refract Surg. 1998;14(3):306–11.
143. Dougherty P, Taylor T. Refractive outcomes and safety of the implantable collamer lens in young low-to-moderate myopes. Clin Ophthalmol. 2017;11:273–7.
144. Kamiya K, Shimizu K, Igarashi A, et al. Posterior chamber phakic intraocular lens implantation: comparative, multicentre study in 351 eyes with low-to-moderate or high myopia. Br J Ophthalmol. 2017;0:1–5. https://doi.org/10.1135/bjophthalmol-2017-310164.
145. Pesando P, Ghiringhello M, Tagliavacche P. Posterior chamber collamer phakic intraocular lens for myopia and hyperopia. J Refract Surg. 1999;15(4):415–23.
146. Kobashi H, Kamiya K, Igarashi A, Matsumura K, Komatsu M, Shimizu K. Long-term quality of life after posterior chamber phakic intraocular lens implantation and after wavefront-guided laser in situ keratomileusis for myopia. J Cataract Refract Surg. 2014;40:2019–24.
147. Hashemi H, Miraftab M, Asgari S. Comparison of the visual outcomes between PRK-MMC and phakic IOL implantation in high myopic patients. Eye. 2014;28:1113–8.
148. Hassaballa M, Macky T. Phakic intraocular lenses outcomes and complications: Artisan vs Visian ICL. Eye. 2011;25(10):1365–70.
149. Ben-nun J. The NuLens Accommodating Intraocular Lens. Ophthalmol Clinic North Am. 2006;19:129–134.

# Chapter 2
# Recent Developments in Cornea and Corneal Transplants

Caterina Sarnicola, Enrica Sarnicola, Paolo Perri, and Vincenzo Sarnicola

## Cornea

### NGF Treatment for Neurotrophic Keratopathy

Neurotrophic Keratopathy (NK) results from impaired corneal innervation which may lead to persistent epithelial defect, corneal melting and perforation. The risk factor for NK are numerous and can coexist. To date, the available treatments has been working in maintaining a proper lubrication and protecting the integrity of the ocular surface. Medical management includes preservative free artificial tears, serum/plasma drops, and anti-inflammatory agents. Contact lenses, punctal plugs, and lid closure with botulinum toxin has been proven to be helpful. Severe cases can require surgical intervention as amniotic membrane transplantation, conjunctival flaps and tarsorrhaphy.

Recently a human recombinant nerve growth factor (Cenegermin) has been approved as topical treatment for NK. This medication promotes epithelial heal-

C. Sarnicola (✉) · E. Sarnicola
Clinica degli Occhi Sarnicola, Grosseto, Italy

Ophthalmology Department II, Ospedale San Giovanni Bosco and Ospedale Oftalmico, Turin, Italy

P. Perri
Department of Biomedical and Specialty Surgical Sciences, University of Ferrara, Ferrara, Italy
e-mail: Paolo.perri@unife.it

V. Sarnicola
Clinica degli Occhi Sarnicola, Grosseto, Italy

© Springer Nature Switzerland AG 2020                                     35
A. Grzybowski (ed.), *Current Concepts in Ophthalmology*,
https://doi.org/10.1007/978-3-030-25389-9_2

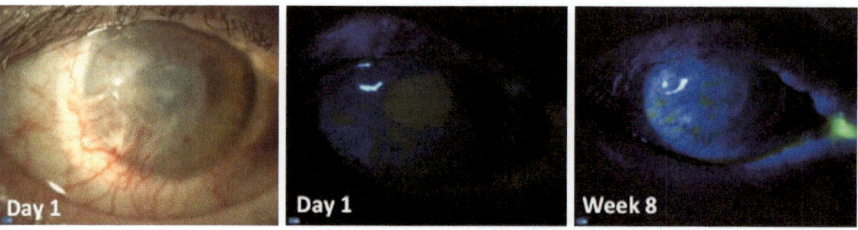

**Fig. 2.1** NGF treatment (Cenegermin) in corneal ulcer due to radiation exposure

ing and nerve health addressing for the first time the underlying pathology of NK (Fig. 2.1).

Two independent, multicentre, randomised, double-masked, vehicle-controlled clinical studies demonstrated the efficacy and safety of Cenegermin in patients affected by moderate or severe NK that were refractory to other non-surgical treatments. In both studies patients received Cenegermin 6 times daily in the affected eye for 8 weeks [1, 2].

## *Highlights on Corneal Infections*

Infectious keratitis are a major cause of blindness and visual impairment globally. The prompt identification of the pathogen organism and an early targeted therapy are crucial to control the infection, but often difficult to obtain. New tools in diagnosis and treatment are the following.

### Diagnostic Investigation

Cultural exam remains the prevalent diagnostic procedure. However other approaches can be effective to identify the causative organism or to have a faster response.

*In vivo* confocal microscopy is helpful to identify fungal hyphae or Acanthamoeba cysts [3].

PCR (Polymerase Chain Reaction) is useful especially to identify Acanthamoeba and Herpesviridae DNA [4]. Ultimately, the use of Next Generation Sequencing (NGS) has been suggested. NGS includes a number of different modern sequencing technologies that allow to sequence DNA and RNA very quickly. These techniques can be advantageous particularly for organisms that are difficult to culture such as atypical or anaerobic bacteria [5].

**Collagen Cross-Linking (CXL) for Corneal Infections**

CXL is a procedure which uses UV light and a photosensitizer (riboflavin) to strengthen chemical bonds in the cornea. The main indication for CXL is to prevent the progression of keratoconus or other ectatic disorders, however, it has been recently proposed to treat corneal infections. In fact, several study has shown that CXL has some antimicrobial effects and has the potential to inhibit enzymatic degradation and corneal melting [6].

There is no agreement yet about when and how to employ CXL to treat keratitis, however, several papers showed the efficacy in bacterial cases whereas there is less evidence in fungal and Acanthamoeba cases [7, 8]. Furthermore, CXL should be avoided in patient with history of herpes because the virus can be activated by ultraviolet light [9].

Further studies are needed to determine the optimized CXL protocol and define the indications in corneal infections treatment.

**Povidone-Iodine (PVI) and Corneal Infections**

PVI is a well known disinfectant and antiseptic agent. Thanks to its broad spectrum of microbicidal activity with no reports of resistance or anaphylaxis, and its reasonable cost, it is widely used in ophthalmic surgery [10]. In addiction, PVI has been shown to be active against Acanthamoeba in vitro and it does not induce resistance or cross-resistance to antibiotics [11].

A recent study conducted in India and Philippines on 172 patients affected by bacterial keratitis, showed no significant difference between the effect of topical PVI 1.25% and topical antibiotics available in developing countries (0.3% ciprofloxacin or neomycin-polymyxin b-gramicidin) [12].

Suggesting that PVI (widely available and inexpensive) should be considered for treatment of bacterial keratitis in countries with limited access to antibiotic therapy.

Additionally, povidone iodine contact lens disinfection systems has been proven effective against a variety of pathogenic microorganisms and may aid in the prevention of potentially sight threatening microbial keratitis [13, 14].

## *Dry Eye Disease*

Dry eye disease (DED) is a common ocular condition that can be the result of insufficient production and/or evaporation of the aqueous tears (Table 2.1).

The definition of dry eye is still under continual revision. According to the 2017 Report of International Dry Eye Workshop, DED is a multifactorial disease of the ocular surface characterized by a loss of homeostasis of the tear film, and accompanied by ocular symptoms, in which tear film instability and hyperosmo-

**Table 2.1** Dry eye etiology

| Aqueous deficient | | Evaporative | |
|---|---|---|---|
| **Sjogren Syndrome DED:**<br>Primary<br>Secondary | **Non-Sjogren Syndrome DED:**<br>Lacrimal deficiency<br>Lacrimal gland duct obstruction<br>Reflex block<br>Systemic drugs | **Intrinsic:**<br>Meibomian oil deficiency<br>Disorders of lid aperture<br>Low blink rate<br>Drug action<br>Accutane | **Extrinsic:**<br>Vitamin A deficiency<br>Topical drugs preservatives<br>Contact lens<br>Ocular surface disease |

*DED* dry eye disease

larity, ocular surface inflammation and damage, and neurosensory abnormalities play etiological roles.

Classic clinical tests are tear break-up time, Schirmer test, corneal esthesiometry, and dye staining.

Newer diagnostic tests measure tear film osmolarity, matrix metalloproteinases levels, and lipid composition. Advanced imaging has also allowed us to measure tear film meniscus height (by OCT), ocular surface health (epithelium and nerve quality by in vivo confocal microscopy), and tear film evaporation (by noninvasive tear break-up time).

There are numerous treatments for DED, depending on the causes. The more common include artificial tears, gel or oinments, tear conserving interventions such as punctal plugs, topical ophthalmic steroids and tetracycline.

Topical cyclosporine-A inhibits T cell activation and decrease IL-6 and HLA-DR. It has been the only pharmacologic treatment specifically approved for DED by the Food and Drug Administration (FDA), but it is discontinued by most patients as it causes burning sensation in the eye.

In 2016 lifitegrast has been approved by the FDA as therapeutic option for dry eye too, as it affects the T-cell-mediated inflammatory pathways, inhibiting the release of cytokines, interferon d, tumor necrosis factor alpha (TNF-$\alpha$), and other interleukins [15, 16].

Neurostimulation is another important addition to our armamentarium in DED treatment to stimulate natural tear production using electrical stimulation. The intra-nasal neurostimolator was shown to be safe and effective for temporarily increasing tear production in adult patients [17].

## Corneal Transplants

Corneal transplantation has developed dramatically in the last 25 years. The surgery moved from full-thickness grafts (penetrating keratoplasty—PK) toward lamellar keratoplasties, anatomically targeted procedures that avoid the removal of healthy corneal tissue and replace only the diseased layer (Fig. 2.2).

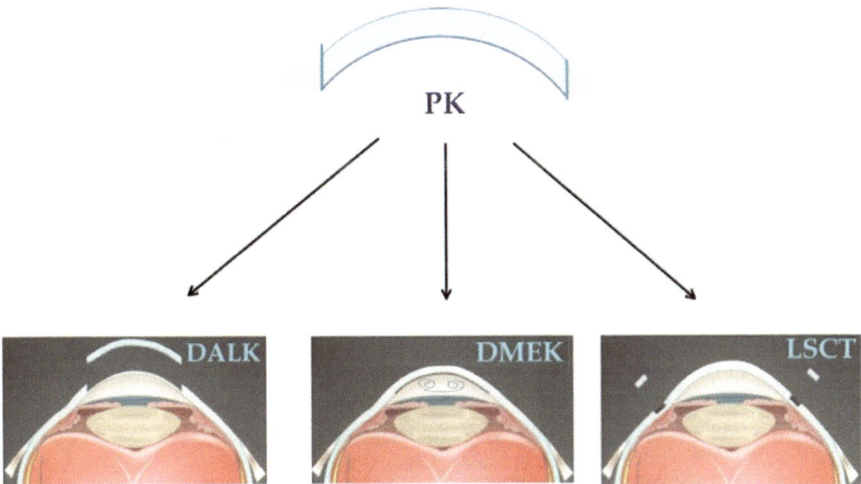

**Fig. 2.2** Evolution from penetrating keratoplasty to lamellar corneal transplant

Deep anterior lamellar keratoplasty (DALK) is replacing penetrating keratoplasty for disorders affecting the corneal stromal layers, while eliminating the risk of endothelial rejection, providing longer graft survival, avoiding an open sky procedure and offering stronger postoperative wound resistance.

Endothelial keratoplasty selectively replaces the corneal endothelium in patients with endothelial disease and results in more rapid and predictable visual outcomes.

Other emerging therapies are ocular surface reconstruction and artificial cornea (keratoprosthesis) surgery, which have become more widely performed because of the advances in these techniques. Together, these advances have resulted in improved outcomes, and have expanded the number of cases of corneal blindness that can now be treated successfully.

A comparison between different corneal transplant techniques is shown in Table 2.2.

## DALK: Deep Anterior Lamellar Keratoplasty

DALK is now the procedure of choice for corneal stromal diseases with a healthy endothelium.

The most common indication to perform a DALK is Keratoconus, other indications are other corneal ectasia [18–21], corneal stromal dystrophies when the endothelium is not affected, corneal scarring [22, 23], corneal melting [24], Descemetoceles [24], penetrating corneal wound without loss of substance [25]. In very experienced hands of surgeons with a low conversion rate to PK, DALK should also be considered in case of dangerous infectious stromal keratitis unresponsive to medical treatment (fungi or Acanthamoeba infections) [26, 27].

**Table 2.2** Comparison between corneal transplant techniques

|  | Indications | Advantages | Disadvantages |
|---|---|---|---|
| PK | Suitable for all indications | − Fast learning curve | − Open-sky surgery related risks |
|  |  | − Relatively fast procedure | − Progressive endothelial cell loss |
|  |  | − Less expensive procedure | − High glaucoma risk |
|  |  |  | − Considerable rejection rate |
|  |  |  | − High postoperative astigmatism |
| DALK | − **Corneal ectasia** (Keratoconus, pellucid marginal degeneration, keratoglobus, post-laser-assisted in situ keratomileusis ectasia, recurrence of ectasia in previous PK) | − Spares the host endothelium | − Steep learning curve |
|  | − **Corneal stromal dystrophies when the endothelium is not affected** (macular corneal dystrophy, granular corneal dystrophy, lattice corneal dystrophy and Avellino dystrophy) | − Less rejection risk | − Stroma interface can affect the visual outcome (manual dissection techniques) |
|  | − **Corneal scarring** (secondary to trauma, infection, chemical injury) | − No endothelial rejection | − Time consuming procedure |
|  | − **Corneal melting** (autoimmune, neurotrophic or infectious) | − Long term graft survival | − Postoperative astigmatism similar to PK |
|  | − **Descemetoceles** | − Less intraoperative complications |  |
|  | − **Penetrating corneal wound without loss of substance** | − Early suture removal |  |
|  | − **Fungi or Acanthamoeba stromal keratitis unresponsive to medical treatment** | − Stronger postoperative wound resistance |  |
| EK | − **Endothelial dystrophy** (Fuchs endothelial dystrophy, posterior polymorphous dystrophy and congenital hereditary endothelial dystrophy) | − Spares the healthy stroma | − More difficult learning curve |
|  | − **Iridocorneal endothelial syndrome** | − Less rejection risk | − Donor selection and manipulation |

**Table 2.2** (continued)

| Indications | Advantages | Disadvantages |
|---|---|---|
| – **Bullous keratopathy** (iatrogenic, post-traumatic or post-infective) | – Early and better visual recovery | – Stroma interface can affect the visual outcome in DSAEK |
| – **Endothelial failure of a prior corneal transplant** | – No induced astigmatism | |
| | – Fewer suture and wound complications | |

*PK* penetrating keratoplasty, *DALK* deep anterior lamellar keratoplasty, *EK* endothelial keratoplasty

- ❏ **Peeling off (Malbran, 1966)**                      ⎤ Manual dissection
- ❏ **Divide and conquer-dissection (Tsubota, 1998)**     ⎦ techniques
- ❏ **Hydrodissection (Sugita, 1997)**
- ❏ **Viscoelastic dissection (Melles, 2000)**
- ❏ **(needle) Big-Bubble dissection (Anwar, 2002)**
- ❏ **Cannula Big Bubble (Sarnicola, Tan, Fogla, 2009)**
- ❏ **Air/visco-Bubble dissection (Sarnicola, 2010)**

**Fig. 2.3** DALK surgical techniques

Over the years different techniques to perform a DALK have been described. DALK techniques still adopted are listed in Fig. 2.3. The most critical step in this surgery is to achieve separation between Descemet membrane and the remaining stroma. To facilitate this step Anwar and Teichmann in 2002 described the Big Bubble technique, this represented an epochal change that has allowed the spread of this surgery [28].

**Needle Big Bubble Technique**

This is the most used DALK procedure. A suction trephine is used to perform a partial thickness corneal trephination at a depth of about 60–80%. A 27- or 30-gauge needle attached to an air-filled syringe is inserted deep into the paracentral stroma through the bottom of the trephination groove and is advanced so that the bevel remains parallel to Descemet membrane (DM) and faces down. At this point, air is injected, forming a large air bubble between DM and the corneal stroma in most cases (60–70%). The stromectomy must be completed then the donor can be sutured [28, 29].

## Cannula Big Bubble

The use of a special blunt cannula has been proposed to let surgeons go as deep as possible into the corneal stroma, without being afraid of DM perforation (Fig. 2.4).

It is common opinion that the deeper the air is injected, the higher the chances of generating a BB. Sarnicola and Toro described the surgical steps for achieving a Big Bubble (BB) using a blunt cannula [30]. After a partial corneal trephination, a smooth spatula is inserted as deep as possible into the peripheral trephination groove. The spatula is moved forward in the attempt to reach the predescemetic plane, deeper and deeper toward the center of the cornea. Once the predescemetic plane is reached, two important signs are frequently observed: reduced resistance of the advancement of the spatula and the appearance of DM folds. The spatula can then be removed, leaving a corneal tunnel into which a 27-gauge cannula attached to a 5 cc air-filled syringe is inserted. The cannula has a port that faces down so that air can push DM posteriorly. After advancing the cannula to the center of the cornea, air can be injected. The literature shows that using a cannula to inject air provides the highest rate of successful BB accomplishment [29, 31].

## Air-Viscobubble Dissection

AVB is a technique designed to manage those cases in which BB formation has failed.

**Fig. 2.4** Cannula Big Bubble. Tunnel formation in the deep stroma using a 27 G spatula (**a**), air insufflation using a 27 G cannula achieving the Big Bubble formation (**b**)

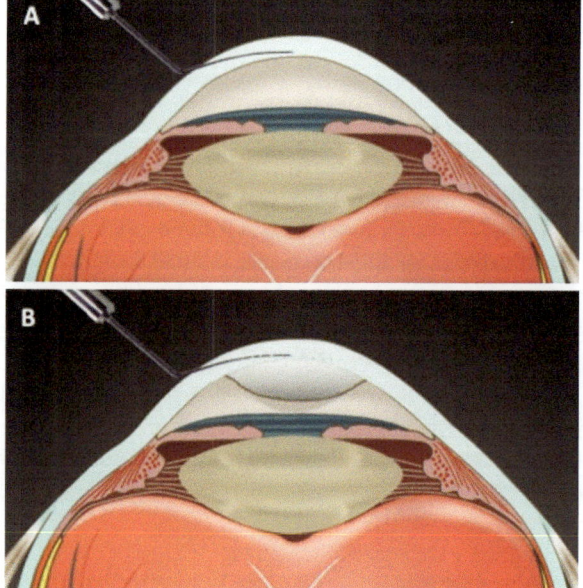

When air dissection does not result in big-bubble formation, superficial kera-tectomy is performed with a Golf knife. A new deeper tunnel is created into the stroma using the same spatula. The same cannula used for the air injection is then attached to a viscoelastic material-filled syringe, and viscodissection is tried as a second approach to separate DM from the corneal stroma. Sarnicola et al. reported the percentage of DALK obtained with this combined technique: AVB helped to attain DM separation from the stroma in 7% of cases that together with the 86% of cases in which DM separation from the stroma had been achieved with the Big Bubble technique using a cannula, resulted in a total achievement of DALK in 93% of cases [29, 32].

**Results and Complications**

The visual outcome after a DALK is similar to PK if the residual stromal bed thick-ness is less then 100 microns. Compare to PK, DALK provides tremendous advan-tages in terms of rejection rate, graft survival, and intraoperative and postoperative complications.

After a DALK procedure, rejection is extremely rare and is easily treatable because it does not involve the endothelium. Epithelial rejection is usually very mild, always reversible with steroid drops, and occurring within the initial postoper-ative weeks. Subepithelial rejection is a belated complication that generally happens within the first postoperative year; this complication is successfully reversible with topical steroids most of the time. Stromal rejection is a more dangerous complica-tion because it can lead to the necrosis of the stroma. It is usually very rare [33, 34].

The endothelium cells count becomes stable after 2 years post-op, this allow a long term graft survival, probably lifetime [34]. Moreover DALK is not an open sky surgery and there are less intraoperative complications.

The most frequent complications of DALK are DM ruptures and double anterior chamber formation. The ability to solve these complications generally improves when surgeons gradually become more expert.

## *Endothelial Keratoplasty (EK)*

Endothelial keratoplasty is the procedure of choice for endothelium disfunction treatment, including endothelial dystrophy (such as Fuchs endothelial dystrophy, posterior polymorphous dystrophy and congenital hereditary endothelial dystro-phy), iridocorneal endothelial (ICE) syndrome, iatrogenic or post-traumatic bullous keratopathy and endothelial failure of a prior corneal transplant [35].

Compare to PK, EK provides tremendous advantages in terms of rejection rate, graft survival, visual outcome and intraoperative and postoperative compli-cations [36].

Several EK procedures have been described, nowadays the most adopted are DSAEK and DMEK (Table 2.3).

**Table 2.3** Advantages and disadvantages of DMEK over DSAEK

| Advantages | – Restores the corneal anatomy |
|---|---|
| | – Less rejection risk |
| | – Better and faster visual recovery |
| | – Higher quality of vision |
| Disadvantages | – Steeper learning curve |
| | – More difficult donor preparation |
| | – Not indicated in case of aphakia and aniridia |
| | – Challenging in case of vitrectomized eyes, eyes with ACIOL or tube shunt |

*DMEK* descemet membrane endothelial keratoplasty, *DSAEK* descemet stripping automated endothelial keratoplasty, *ACIOL* anterior chamber intraocular lens

## Descemet Stripping Automated Endothelial Keratoplasty (DSAEK)

DSAEK was first described by Gorovoy in 2006, he modified the original technique described by Melles using a microkeratome to prepare a more thin and uniform donor tissue [37, 38].

The DSAEK graft includes corneal endothelium, Descemet's membrane and a thin amount of posterior stroma. In the ultrathin-DSAEK the graft thickness is less then 150 μm, the nanothin-DSAEK graft is less then 50 μm. Thinner graft allows a better visual outcome and less rejection risk [39, 40].

The DSAEK procedure involves creation of a 3–5 mm corneal/scleral incision in the recipient eye. A descemetorhexis under cohesive viscoelastic or air removes the endothelium and Descemet's membrane of the recipient eye. Viscoelastic use advantages are a more stable anterior chamber and a better visibility; it is important to use a cohesive viscoelastic that can be easily fully removed from the anterior chamber before graft insertion. Several techniques have been described to insert the graft in the AC. A noncompression forceps was originally used to insert a 60/40 folded graft. Then donor inserters and several glides were suggested to pull the donor tissue in the anterior chamber.

A suture pull-through insertion was even described using a double-armed 10-0 polypropylene, nonabsorbable suture, particularly useful in case of shallow anterior chamber or floppy iris syndrome. An asymmetric 60/40 taco graft, with the endothelial side inward protected by a small amount of viscoelastic (endo-on), is pulled-through the AC [41].

Once the donor is centered, air is injected into the anterior chamber to facilitate the adhesion between the donor stroma and host stroma. Pupillary block risk can be prevented performing an inferior peripheral iridectomy and/or with postoperatively mydriatic drops. Close patient monitoring is needed in the 4–5 h post-op. Air drainage from the paracentesis has to be performed if pupillary block occurs.

Intraoperative complications may be due to the incorrect graft orientation, air management, bleeding and IOL dislocation. Postoperative complications of DSAEK surgery are graft dislocation, pupillary block, primary failure, secondary failure for endothelial cell loss and rejection (which occurs in about 4% of cases) [42].

## Descemet Membrane Endothelial Keratoplasty (DMEK)

The DMEK graft includes corneal endothelium and Descemet's membrane only, allowing the perfect corneal anatomical restoration (Fig. 2.5) [43].

Literature finally showed several advantages of DMEK compared to DSAEK, including better and faster visual outcome, lower rejection rate and higher quality of vision, despite a more difficult surgical technique and a steep learning curve [36].

Aniridia and aphakia still are not indicated cases because of graft con be lost in the vitreous chamber. Vitrectomized eyes, eyes with ACIOLs or tube shunt should be evaluated with caution.

The DMEK graft can be stripped by the surgeon or the eye bank [35].

The initial surgery phases, until the descemetorhexis, are similar to DSAEK. Then the surgery become completely different because DMEK graft has a particular shape: a scroll with endothelium always facing outward (endo-off). This graft feature is very important and has to be always in the mind of the surgeon. It consents to avoid the most frequent complication: the upside down positioning of the graft, the principal graft failure cause.

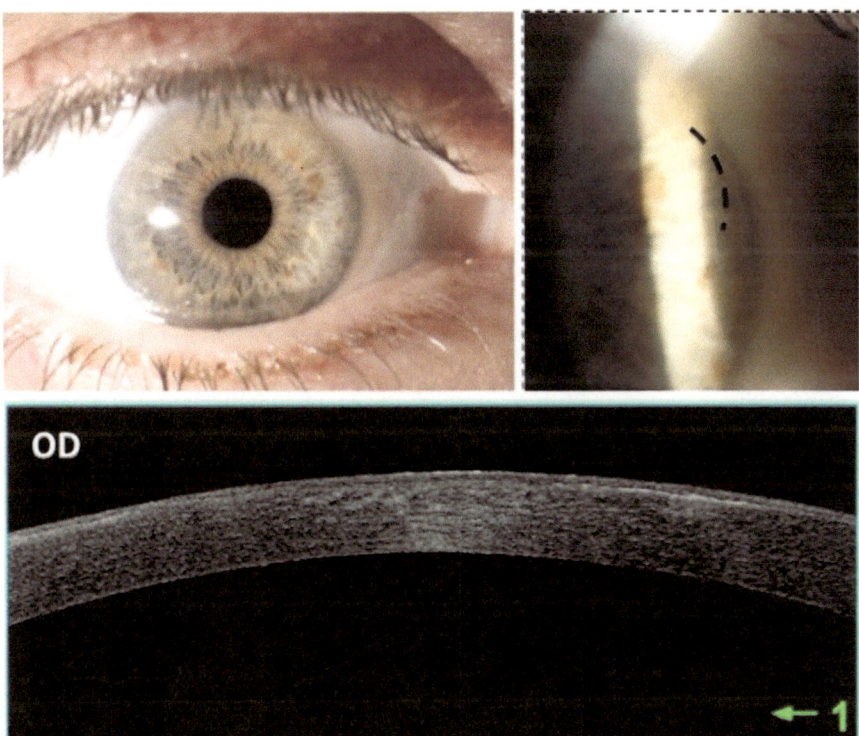

**Fig. 2.5** DMEK post-op. The transplant edge can be detected at the slit lamp examination. AS-OCT shows a restoration of the normal corneal anatomy

Before injecting the graft into the AC it has to be stained with trypan blue to improve tissue visualization and managing. Several injectors have been suggested such as IOL cartridges or glass injectors. Once the graft is inside the AC the main corneal incision must be promptly sutured. Asses the correct orientation of the graft it's a critical step of this procedure. Techniques to determine orientation include pre-stamp the graft with an "S" or "F", the assessment of the Moutsouri's sign, and intraoperative OCT [44, 45]. Unfold the tissue is the challenging step of this surgery. Many techniques have been described, the most adopted are: tapping techniques, air, hydro or mechanical ab interno unfolding techniques, etc. [46–48]. At the end of the surgery air is injected in the AC.

Complications of DMEK can be the upside-down positioning of the graft, graft detachment (which is treated with rebubbling), graft dislocation, primary failure, pupillary block, and rejection (in about 1% of the cases) [49].

## Future Directions: Rho Kinase (ROCK) Inhibitor for Corneal Endothelial Dysfunction

ROCK inhibitor Y-27632 is approved in Japan for the treatment of glaucoma. Kinoshita et al. have largely investigated the role of Y-27632 for corneal endothelium therapy, since it has been shown to promote endothelial cell adhesion and proliferation and to suppress apoptosis [50, 51].

Interesting, ROCK inhibitor has been proved to enhance corneal endothelium wound healing and to decrease the incidence of bullous keratopathy following severe endothelial damage (as in cataract surgery, one of the leading causes of corneal transplantation) [52, 53].

Research has also focused on ROCK inhibitor as adjunct drugs for cell-based therapy. In fact, the injection in anterior chamber of cultured human endothelial cells supplemented with a ROCK inhibitor was followed by an increase in endothelial density and corneal clearance in 11 persons with bullous keratopathy [54].

Recently a novel approach to treat Fuchs endothelial corneal dystrophy (FECD) without endothelial transplantation has been investigated. A 4 to 5 mm area of central endothelium and Descemet membrane is removed without endothelial transplantation. Clinic evidence supports the idea that the corneal endothelium in FECD may be capable of self-regeneration [55]. In about 75% of selected patient with central guttae but a healthy peripheral endothelium, primary descemetorhexis without transplant was successful in restoring corneal transparence [56].

The use of Y-27632 postoperatively seems to facilitate corneal clearance after descemetorhexis without transplantation in FECD [57, 58]. Further investigation is needed to identify appropriate patient selection for this procedure and the optimal descemetorhexis size.

## *Limbal Stem Cell Deficiency and Ocular Surface Transplantation*

The corneal epithelium is entirely regenerated about every seven days. In case of limbal stem cell deficiency (LSCD) the limbal stem cell population located in the limbus is compromised and the cornea loses its ability to regenerate itself, which may result in persistent epithelial defects, chronic inflammation, conjunctivalization, scarring, and loss of transparency.

The causes of LSCD are numerous and various (Table 2.4).

Currently, the diagnosis is based on the history and the clinical features. Corneal impression cytology may reveal the presence of conjunctival goblet cells in the corneal epithelium and confocal microscopy can detect loss of the palisades of Vogt [59].

In case of mild LSCD, mechanical debridement of the conjunctival epithelium and, if needed, an amniotic membrane transplantation, could be sufficient to restore an healthy corneal epithelium. Management of patients with severe or total LSCD has always been challenging because corneal transparency cannot be restored with a keratoplasty; these patients need limbal stem cell transplantation or prosthesis.

In the past few decades tremendous advances in the understanding of stem cells pathophysiology and in the use of immunosuppressive regimens have encouraged the development of several ocular surface transplant procedures. However, before proceeding with a stem cells transplant, causative factors and comorbid conditions must be managed (i.e. autoimmune diseases, ocular inflammation, infections, removal of any ocular surface tumor and iatrogenic insults, eyelid disfunction, inadequate tear film) [60].

Selection of the ocular surface transplant procedure depends on the cause and the extent of LSCD, unilaterality or bilaterality of the deficiency, patient age, living related donor availability, and comorbidity.

Furthermore, in order to asses the best treatment and the prognosis, the staging of the severe ocular surface diseases must consider the condition of both the limbal stem cells and the conjunctiva. According to the classification in Table 2.5, patient with stage I can usually restore a normal epithelium and have localized vascularization that usually do not affect the visual acuity. Patient with more than 50% of limbal stem cells loss and inflamed conjunctiva (stage IIC), as in case of severe

**Table 2.4**  LSCD causes

| Congenital | Aniridia, ectodermal dysplasia |
|---|---|
| Traumatic | Alcali or acid burns, thermal injuries, physical or iatrogenic trauma |
| Autoimmune disorders | Stevens-Johnson syndrome, mucous membrane pemphigoid |

**Table 2.5** Ocular surface diseases classification

| Limbal stem cells lost (%) | Normal conjunctiva (stage A) | Previously inflamed conjunctiva (stage B) | Inflamed conjunctiva (stage C) |
|---|---|---|---|
| <50% (Stage I) | Iatrogenic, OSSN, contact lens (Stage IA) | History of chemical or thermal injury (Stage IB) | Mild SJS, MMP, recent chemical injury (Stage IC) |
| >50% (Stage II) | Aniridia, severe contact lens and iatrogenic (Stage IIA) | History of severe chemical or thermal injury (Stage IIB) | Severe SJS, MMP, recent chemical or thermal injury (Stage IIC) |

Reproduced from Holland EJ, Mannis MJ, Lee WB, editors. Ocular surface disease: cornea, conjunctiva and tear film. Elsevier; 2013. Ch. 38, Table 38.1, p. 318
*OSSN* ocular surface squamous neoplasia, *SJS* Stevens-Johnson syndrome, *MMP* mucous membrane pemphigoid

Stvens-Jhonson Syndrome (SJS), severe Mucous Membrane Pemphigoid (MMP) and recent chemical or thermal injury, have the poorest prognosis for surgical treatment.

## Surgical Options for the Ocular Surface Reconstruction

Conjunctival Limbal Autograft (CLAU)

The conjunctival limbal autograft is the procedure of choice for unilateral limbal stem cell deficiency. Two limbal grafts about 6 mm of limbal arc length, extending about 1 mm into the cornea and 5–8 mm in the conjunctiva, are harvested from the healthy eye and transplanted to the diseased eye. No rejection can occur and no immunosuppression is required. It provides both healthy stem cells and conjunctiva. The procedure only has one chance for the fellow eye to be the donor [61, 62].

Simple Limbal Epithelial Transplant (SLET)

SLET is indicated in unilateral stem cell deficiency. Compared with CLAU, a limited number of stem cells and minimal conjunctiva are transplanted. This technique seems to be less effective in case of severe LSCD or conjunctival disease, but it may potentially be repeated.

In this technique a $2 \times 2$ mm graft is excised from the superior limbus of the healthy eye, cut in small pieces, glued to the recipient cornea and covered with amniotic membrane [63, 64].

Keratolimbal Allograft (KLAL)

The keratolimbal allograft procedure uses one or two cadaveric donor corneoscleral rims as stem cell source. This technique is indicated for bilateral LSCD and provides an excellent number of stem cells. The disadvantages include no tissue typing, increased risk of rejection, need for immunosuppression, and no supply of healthy conjunctiva. This procedure is most suited for disease with minimal involvement of conjunctiva (i.e. aniridia, contact lens induced LASC, etc.) [65].

Living Related Conjunctival Limbal Allograft (lr-CLAL)

This procedure use a patient's living relative as donor of limbal stem cell and conjunctiva. The technique is similar to CLAU, but systemic immunosuppression are required to minimize the risk of rejection. HLA matching and tissue typing help to identify the best donor possibly reducing the rejection risk and the amount of systemic immunosuppression. This technique is indicated in case of bilateral LSCD and, compared to KLAL, it supplies both stem cells and conjunctiva, which is extremely important for patients affected by cicatrizing conjunctivitis (Fig. 2.6).

On the other hand lr-CLAL does not supply 360° of stem cells. Interesting, Holland and al described the Cincinnati procedure, a combined living-related conjunctival limbal allografts and keratolimbal allografts in severe ocular surface failure. This technique provides a significant amount of conjunctiva and an encircling ring of stem cells; it should be considered in case of SJS, cicatricial pemphigoid and chemical injuries with severe conjunctival involvement [66].

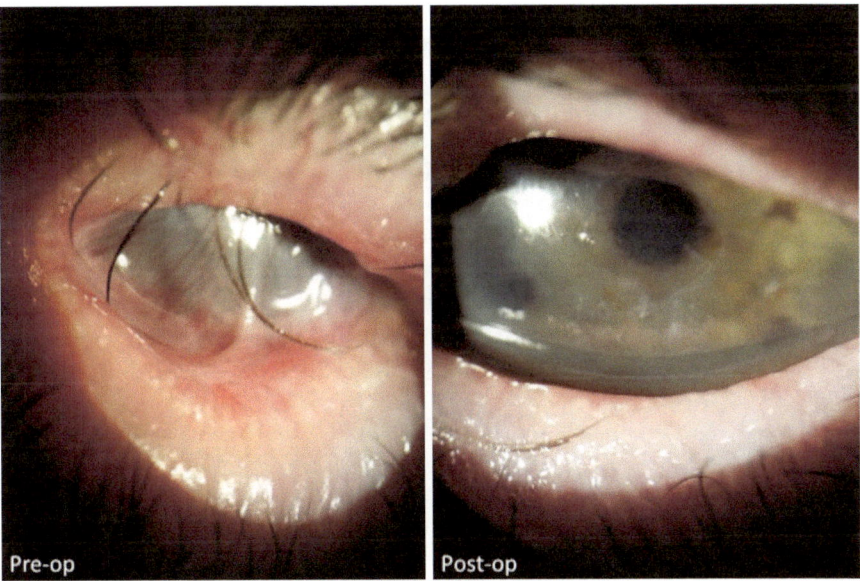

Pre-op

Post-op

**Fig. 2.6** Lr-CLAL in mucous membrane pemphigoid

Ex-Vivo Cultured Graft

Tissue engineering approaches for corneal epithelium reconstruction utilize adult stem cells derived from a small tissue biopsy from either the patient (autologous) or a donor (allogeneic), followed by their ex vivo expansion in culture on a natural scaffold, generating a three-dimensional epithelial constructs for transplantation. Indications are unilateral or partial bilateral stem cell deficiencies.

Currently, cultivated limbal epithelial transplantation (CLET) and cultivated oral mucosal epithelial transplantation (COMET) are the only clinically validated techniques.

These techniques are very expensive, provides a limited number of stem cells, cannot manage conjunctival deficiency, and the literature is lacking of long term results [67, 68].

Keratoprosthesis (K-pro I, K-pro II; OOKP)

Keratoprosthesis is a surgical option for patient with bilateral LSCD that cannot be treated with systemic immunosuppression or who have failed a limbal stem cell allograft.

In patients with a wet ocular surface and good eyelid function a Boston Kpro type I can be used to restore a visual rehabilitation.

Boston Kpro type I is made of a polymethyl methacrylate (PMMA) front plate, a corneal graft and a locking titanium or PMMA back plate. Additional procedures such as lensectomy, glaucoma shunt placement or vitrectomy may be required at the time of surgery [69].

Patients with severe bilateral autoimmune ocular surface disease, such as severe SJS and MMP have a greater risk of extrusion and melting; they can be treated with a Boston Kpro type II, with an osteo-odonto-keratoprosthesis (OOKP).

Boston Kpro type II design is similar to the type I except for an anterior extension to allow implantation through surgically closed eyelid. It is associated with significant complications, long postoperative care and it alters the cosmetic appearance [70].

The OOKP utilizes an autologous canine tooth and adjacent bone as support for a PMMA Kpro and it is a very complex surgical procedure indicated in end-stage blindness [71, 72].

# References

1. Dua HS, Said DG, Messmer EM, Rolando M, Benitez-Del-Castillo JM, Hossain PN, et al. Neurotrophic keratopathy. Prog Retin Eye Res. 2018;66:107–31.
2. Bonini S, Lambiase A, Rama P, Sinigaglia F, Allegretti M, Chao W, et al. Phase II randomized, double-masked, vehicle-controlled trial of recombinant human nerve growth factor for neurotrophic keratitis. Ophthalmology. 2018;125(9):1332–43.

3. Vaddavalli PK, Garg P, Sharma S, Sangwan VS, Rao GN, Thomas R. Role of confocal microscopy in the diagnosis of fungal and acanthamoeba keratitis. Ophthalmology. 2011;118(1):29–35.
4. Inoue T, Ohashi Y. Utility of real-time PCR analysis for appropriate diagnosis for keratitis. Cornea. 2013;32(Suppl 1):S71–6.
5. Eguchi H, Hotta F, Kuwahara T, Imaohji H, Miyazaki C, Hirose M, et al. Diagnostic approach to ocular infections using various techniques from conventional culture to next-generation sequencing analysis. Cornea. 2017;36(Suppl 1):S46–52.
6. Spoerl E, Wollensak G, Seiler T. Increased resistance of crosslinked cornea against enzymatic digestion. Curr Eye Res. 2004;29(1):35–40.
7. Price MO, Price FW. Corneal cross-linking in the treatment of corneal ulcers. Curr Opin Ophthalmol. 2016;27(3):250–5.
8. Austin A, Lietman T, Rose-Nussbaumer J. Update on the management of Infectious keratitis. Ophthalmology. 2017;124(11):1678–89.
9. Richoz O, Gatzioufas Z, Francois P, Schrenzel J, Hafezi F. Impact of fluorescein on the antimicrobial efficacy of photoactivated riboflavin in corneal collagen cross-linking. J Refract Surg. 2013;29(12):842–5.
10. Grzybowski A, Kanclerz P, Myers WG. The use of povidone-iodine in ophthalmology. Curr Opin Ophthalmol. 2018;29(1):19–32.
11. Hsu J, Gerstenblith AT, Garg SJ, Vander JF. Conjunctival flora antibiotic resistance patterns after serial intravitreal injections without postinjection topical antibiotics. Am J Ophthalmol. 2014;157(3):514–8.e1.
12. Isenberg SJ, Apt L, Valenton M, Sharma S, Garg P, Thomas PA, et al. Prospective, randomized clinical trial of povidone-iodine 1.25% solution versus topical antibiotics for treatment of bacterial keratitis. Am J Ophthalmol. 2017;176:244–53.
13. Yamasaki K, Saito F, Ota R, Kilvington S. Antimicrobial efficacy of a novel povidone iodine contact lens disinfection system. Cont Lens Anterior Eye. 2018;41(3):277–81.
14. Cho P, Reyes S, Boost MV. Microbiocidal characterization of a novel povidone-iodine based rigid contact lens disinfecting solution. Cont Lens Anterior Eye. 2018;41(6):542–6.
15. Abidi A, Shukla P, Ahmad A. Lifitegrast: a novel drug for treatment of dry eye disease. J Pharmacol Pharmacother. 2016;7(4):194–8.
16. Chan CC, Prokopich CL. Lifitegrast ophthalmic solution 5.0% for treatment of dry eye disease: overview of clinical trial program. J Pharm Pharm Sci. 2019;22(1):49–56.
17. Cohn GS, Corbett D, Tenen A, Coroneo M, McAlister J, Craig JP, et al. Randomized, controlled, double-masked, multicenter, pilot study evaluating safety and efficacy of intranasal neurostimulation for dry eye disease. Invest Ophthalmol Vis Sci. 2019;60(1):147–53.
18. Arenas E, Esquenazi S, Anwar M, Terry M. Lamellar corneal transplantation. Surv Ophthalmol. 2012;57(6):510–29.
19. McAllum PJ, Segev F, Herzig S, Rootman DS. Deep anterior lamellar keratoplasty for post-LASIK ectasia. Cornea. 2007;26(4):507–11.
20. Ramamurthi S, Cornish KS, Steeples L, Ramaesh K. Deep anterior lamellar keratoplasty on a previously failed full-thickness graft. Cornea. 2009;28(4):456–7.
21. Lake D, Hamada S, Khan S, Daya SM. Deep anterior lamellar keratoplasty over penetrating keratoplasty for host rim thinning and ectasia. Cornea. 2009;28(5):489–92.
22. Singh G, Singh Bhinder H. Evaluation of therapeutic deep anterior lamellar keratoplasty in acute ocular chemical burns. Eur J Ophthalmol. 2008;18(4):517–28.
23. Fogla R, Padmanabhan P. Deep anterior lamellar keratoplasty combined with autologous limbal stem cell transplantation in unilateral severe chemical injury. Cornea. 2005;24(4):421–5.
24. Luengo-Gimeno F, Tan DT, Mehta JS. Evolution of deep anterior lamellar keratoplasty (DALK). Ocul Surf. 2011;9(2):98–110.
25. Bhatt PR, Lim LT, Ramaesh K. Therapeutic deep lamellar keratoplasty for corneal perforations. Eye (Lond). 2007;21(9):1168–73.
26. Sarnicola E, Sarnicola C, Sabatino F, Tosi GM, Perri P, Sarnicola V. Early deep anterior lamellar keratoplasty (DALK) for Acanthamoeba keratitis poorly responsive to medical treatment. Cornea. 2016;35(1):1–5.

27. Sabatino F, Sarnicola E, Sarnicola C, Tosi GM, Perri P, Sarnicola V, et al. Early deep anterior lamellar keratoplasty for fungal keratitis poorly responsive to medical treatment. Eye (Lond). 2017;31:1639–46.
28. Anwar M, Teichmann KD. Big-bubble technique to bare Descemet's membrane in anterior lamellar keratoplasty. J Cataract Refract Surg. 2002;28(3):398–403.
29. Sarnicola E, Sarnicola C, Sabatino F, Tosi GM, Perri P, Sarnicola V. Cannula DALK versus needle DALK for keratoconus. Cornea. 2016;35(12):1508–11.
30. Sarnicola V, Toro P. Blunt cannula for descemetic deep anterior lamellar keratoplasty. Cornea. 2011;30(8):895–8.
31. Fournié P, Malecaze F, Coullet J, Arné JL. Variant of the big bubble technique in deep anterior lamellar keratoplasty. J Cataract Refract Surg. 2007;33(3):371–5.
32. Muftuoglu O, Toro P, Hogan RN, Bowman RW, Cavanagh HD, McCulley JP, et al. Sarnicola air-visco bubble technique in deep anterior lamellar keratoplasty. Cornea. 2013;32(4):527–32.
33. Feizi S, Javadi MA, Jamali H, Mirbabaee F. Deep anterior lamellar keratoplasty in patients with keratoconus: big-bubble technique. Cornea. 2010;29(2):177–82.
34. Sarnicola V, Toro P, Sarnicola C, Sarnicola E, Ruggiero A. Long-term graft survival in deep anterior lamellar keratoplasty. Cornea. 2012;31(6):621–6.
35. Holland EJ, Mannis MJ. Cornea. 4th ed. Amsterdam: Elsevier; 2016.
36. Deng SX, Lee WB, Hammersmith KM, Kuo AN, Li JY, Shen JF, et al. Descemet membrane endothelial keratoplasty: safety and outcomes: a report by the American Academy of Ophthalmology. Ophthalmology. 2018;125(2):295–310.
37. Gorovoy MS. Descemet-stripping automated endothelial keratoplasty. Cornea. 2006;25(8):886–9.
38. Melles GR, Wijdh RH, Nieuwendaal CP. A technique to excise the descemet membrane from a recipient cornea (descemetorhexis). Cornea. 2004;23(3):286–8.
39. Busin M, Albé E. Does thickness matter: ultrathin Descemet stripping automated endothelial keratoplasty. Curr Opin Ophthalmol. 2014;25(4):312–8.
40. Cheung AY, Hou JH, Bedard P, Grimes V, Buckman N, Eslani M, et al. Technique for preparing ultrathin and nanothin descemet stripping automated endothelial keratoplasty tissue. Cornea. 2018;37(5):661–6.
41. Sarnicola V, Millacci C, Sarnicola E, Sarnicola C, Sabatino F, Ruggiero A. Suture pull-through insertion of graft donor in Descemet stripping automated endothelial keratoplasty: results of 4-year follow-up. Taiwan J Ophthalmol. 2015;5(3):114–9.
42. Price FW, Feng MT, Price MO. Evolution of endothelial keratoplasty: where are we headed? Cornea. 2015;34(Suppl 10):S41–7.
43. Melles GR, Lander F, Rietveld FJ. Transplantation of Descemet's membrane carrying viable endothelium through a small scleral incision. Cornea. 2002;21(4):415–8.
44. Dapena I, Moutsouris K, Droutsas K, Ham L, van Dijk K, Melles GR. Standardized "no-touch" technique for descemet membrane endothelial keratoplasty. Arch Ophthalmol. 2011;129(1):88–94.
45. Veldman PB, Dye PK, Holiman JD, Mayko ZM, Sáles CS, Straiko MD, et al. The S-stamp in Descemet membrane endothelial keratoplasty safely eliminates upside-down graft implantation. Ophthalmology. 2016;123(1):161–4.
46. Sarnicola C, Sabatino F, Sarnicola E, Perri P, Cheung AY, Sarnicola V. Cannula-assisted technique to unfold grafts in descemet membrane endothelial keratoplasty. Cornea. 2019;38(3):275–9.
47. Yoeruek E, Bayyoud T, Hofmann J, Bartz-Schmidt KU. Novel maneuver facilitating Descemet membrane unfolding in the anterior chamber. Cornea. 2013;32(3):370–3.
48. Liarakos VS, Dapena I, Ham L, van Dijk K, Melles GR. Intraocular graft unfolding techniques in descemet membrane endothelial keratoplasty. JAMA Ophthalmol. 2013;131(1):29–35.
49. Melles GR, Ong TS, Ververs B, van der Wees J. Descemet membrane endothelial keratoplasty (DMEK). Cornea. 2006;25(8):987–90.
50. Okumura N, Kinoshita S, Koizumi N. The role of Rho kinase inhibitors in corneal endothelial dysfunction. Curr Pharm Des. 2017;23:660–6.

51. Okumura N, Fujii K, Kagami T, Makiko N, Kitahara M, Kinoshita S, et al. Activation of the Rho/Rho kinase signaling pathway is involved in cell death of corneal endothelium. Invest Ophthalmol Vis Sci. 2016;57(15):6843–51.

52. Okumura N, Koizumi N, Ueno M, Sakamoto Y, Takahashi H, Tsuchiya H, et al. ROCK inhibitor converts corneal endothelial cells into a phenotype capable of regenerating in vivo endothelial tissue. Am J Pathol. 2012;181(1):268–77.

53. Okumura N, Okazaki Y, Inoue R, Kakutani K, Nakano S, Kinoshita S, et al. Effect of the Rho-associated kinase inhibitor eye drop (Ripasudil) on corneal endothelial wound healing. Invest Ophthalmol Vis Sci. 2016;57(3):1284–92.

54. Kinoshita S, Koizumi N, Ueno M, Okumura N, Imai K, Tanaka H, et al. Injection of cultured cells with a ROCK inhibitor for bullous keratopathy. N Engl J Med. 2018;378(11):995–1003.

55. Sarnicola C, Farooq AV, Colby K. Fuchs endothelial corneal dystrophy: update on pathogenesis and future directions. Eye Contact Lens. 2019;45(1):1–10.

56. Borboli S, Colby K. Mechanisms of disease: Fuchs' endothelial dystrophy. Ophthalmol Clin N Am. 2002;15(1):17–25.

57. Moloney G, Petsoglou C, Ball M, Kerdraon Y, Höllhumer R, Spiteri N, et al. Descemetorhexis without grafting for Fuchs endothelial dystrophy-supplementation with topical Ripasudil. Cornea. 2017;36(6):642–8.

58. Macsai MS, Shiloach M. Use of topical Rho kinase inhibitors in the treatment of Fuchs dystrophy after descemet stripping only. Cornea. 2019;38(5):529–34.

59. Liang L, Sheha H, Li J, Tseng SC. Limbal stem cell transplantation: new progresses and challenges. Eye (Lond). 2009;23(10):1946–53.

60. Atallah MR, Palioura S, Perez VL, Amescua G. Limbal stem cell transplantation: current perspectives. Clin Ophthalmol. 2016;10:593–602.

61. Kenyon KR, Tseng SC. Limbal autograft transplantation for ocular surface disorders. Ophthalmology. 1989;96(5):709–22; discussion 22-3.

62. Cheung AY, Sarnicola E, Holland EJ. Long-term ocular surface stability in conjunctival limbal autograft donor eyes. Cornea. 2017;36(9):1031–5.

63. Sangwan VS, Basu S, MacNeil S, Balasubramanian D. Simple limbal epithelial transplantation (SLET): a novel surgical technique for the treatment of unilateral limbal stem cell deficiency. Br J Ophthalmol. 2012;96(7):931–4.

64. Amescua G, Atallah M, Nikpoor N, Galor A, Perez VL. Modified simple limbal epithelial transplantation using cryopreserved amniotic membrane for unilateral limbal stem cell deficiency. Am J Ophthalmol. 2014;158(3):469–75.e2.

65. Croasdale CR, Schwartz GS, Malling JV, Holland EJ. Keratolimbal allograft: recommendations for tissue procurement and preparation by eye banks, and standard surgical technique. Cornea. 1999;18(1):52–8.

66. Biber JM, Skeens HM, Neff KD, Holland EJ. The cincinnati procedure: technique and outcomes of combined living-related conjunctival limbal allografts and keratolimbal allografts in severe ocular surface failure. Cornea. 2011;30(7):765–71.

67. Tsai RJ, Li LM, Chen JK. Reconstruction of damaged corneas by transplantation of autologous limbal epithelial cells. N Engl J Med. 2000;343(2):86–93.

68. Satake Y, Higa K, Tsubota K, Shimazaki J. Long-term outcome of cultivated oral mucosal epithelial sheet transplantation in treatment of total limbal stem cell deficiency. Ophthalmology. 2011;118(8):1524–30.

69. Sejpal K, Yu F, Aldave AJ. The Boston keratoprosthesis in the management of corneal limbal stem cell deficiency. Cornea. 2011;30(11):1187–94.

70. Pujari S, Siddique SS, Dohlman CH, Chodosh J. The Boston keratoprosthesis type II: the Massachusetts Eye and Ear Infirmary experience. Cornea. 2011;30(12):1298–303.

71. Strampelll B. Osteo-odontokeratoprosthesis. Ann Ottalmol Clin Ocul. 1963;89:1039–44.

72. Michael R, Charoenrook V, de la Paz MF, Hitzl W, Temprano J, Barraquer RI. Long-term functional and anatomical results of osteo- and osteoodonto-keratoprosthesis. Graefes Arch Clin Exp Ophthalmol. 2008;246(8):1133–7.

# Chapter 3
# Recent Developments in Cataract Surgery

Andrzej Grzybowski and Piotr Kanclerz

## Introduction

Cataract surgery is the most common surgical procedure performed in medicine. In the 2015 over 20 million surgeries were carried out worldwide, of which 3.6 million in the United States of America [1] and 4.2 million in the European Union [2]. The progress in technology enabled cataract surgery to be the safest and most predictable eye surgery. On the other hand, the increase in life expectancy and quality of life result in higher surmises regarding the outcomes. Currently, individuals over 70 years of age might be declared inactive or retired, however, still wish to maintain an active lifestyle, including driving a car and performing sports. Subsequently, there is a demand for techniques that are even more perfect. New encounters include surgeries performed on patients with dementia and other comorbidities related with ageing. The anticipated duration of intraocular lens (IOL) in the eye has significantly increased. Thus physico-chemical characteristics and IOL endurance should allow the lens to keep its' optical properties for up to three decades. The most significant advances in cataract surgery will be briefly discussed within this chapter.

A. Grzybowski (✉)
Department of Ophthalmology, University of Warmia and Mazury, Olsztyn, Poland

Institute for Research in Ophthalmology, Foundation for Ophthalmology Development, Poznan, Poland

P. Kanclerz
Department of Ophthalmology, Hygeia Clinic, Gdańsk, Poland

# Preoperative Considerations

## Preoperative Examinations

Patients undergoing phacoemulsification cataract surgery (PCS) should have a scrupulous ophthalmic evaluation, preferably by the operating ophthalmologist [3]. This allows the surgeon to formulate the treatment plan and establish a relationship with the patient. Biometry might be conducted on the preoperative visit, particularly if intraocular lens (IOL) banking is not available or if a specific IOL type is required.

Routine preoperative non-ophthalmic medical testing is not recommended in patients undergoing low-risk surgery. However, such examinations commonly take place before PCS and other ambulatory procedures [4]. Almost two decades ago Schein et al. presented that performing tests such as electrocardiograms, blood cell count, radiographic examinations, serum chemical analysis or urea nitrogen, creatinine, and glucose, does not increase the safety of cataract surgery [5]. Consecutively, the Cochrane Database of Systematic Reviews confirmed that routine preoperative examinations do not improve the safety of PCS [6]. On the other hand, adverse medical events precipitated by cataract surgery remain a concern, as commonly elderly patients with multiple medical comorbidities undergo surgery [6]. Self-administered health questionnaires could be concerned as a substitute, nevertheless they might be useless in developing countries where some people have ever been to a physician [6].

The problem is not trivial; the unneeded tests and procedures in the United States are appraised to be as high as 30% of all health care expenditures [7]. Up to 97.1% clinicians believe that the frequency of unnecessary tests and procedures is a serious problem [8]. Rationing and elimination of wasteful, non-beneficial interventions was proposed to be ethically mandated [9]. The annual cost of routine preoperative screening before cataract surgery solely in Medicare beneficients was estimated as $45.4 million [4], and it might reach up to $150 million in the whole United States. Interestingly, the patient's probability of undergoing preoperative screening was found to be associated mainly with the ophthalmologist who conducted the preoperative evaluation, rather than his medical characteristics [10].

## Anticoagulants and Cataract Surgery

Preventive antiplatelet use is one of the preventive strategies to decrease mortality due to heart attacks and strokes, which are the leading causes of mortality in the United States. Antiplatelet or anticoagulant medications are commonly used for prevention of venous thromboembolism, in atrial fibrillation or valvular heart disease. It is estimated that one third of adults aged 40 years or older take preventive antiplatelet medications. The use increases with age and reached 54% of those ≥80 years of age [11].

Routine clear corneal incision (CCI) PCS carries a very small risk of clinically significant bleeding [12]. Benzimra et al. reported that the incidence of subconjunctival hemorrhage is increased in patients taking clopidogrel or warfarin compared to controls [13]. In their study patients underwent local anaesthetic block with a sharp needle or subtenon's cannula. It should be underlined that subconjunctival hemorrhage cannot be considered as a potentially life-threatening or sight-threatening complication, but rather a minor complication that should be reported. Furthermore, with the CCI PCS surgeries are commonly performed under topical anesthesia, and such an administration method should be considered without the use of a sharp needle. The review by Grzybowski et al. showed that PCS can be performed safely in high-risk patients, taking both anticoagulants and antiplatelet agents if the procedure is performed by a skilled surgeon, through a CCI and in topical anesthesia [14]. This was further referenced by the American Academy of Ophthalmology Preferred Practice Pattern as a strong recommendation [3].

Importantly, discontinuation of antiplatelet agents or anticoagulants may increase the risk of thrombotic events such as myocardial infarction or stroke in patients undergoing PCS [12]. A scrupulous risk/benefit analysis and patient selection should be performed. For example perioperative circumstances—small pupils, floppy iris syndrome, iris neovascularization, pseudoexfoliation or phacodonesis—may increase the risk for intraocular hemorrhage [12]. In cases requiring IOL suturing or concomitant invasive vitrectomy, particularly in diabetic patients, discontinuation of antiplatelet agents or anticoagulants might be considered [12].

## Methods for Assessing Corneal Power

The corneal power can be assessed with the diagnostic procedures of keratometry and topography/tomography. Keratometry is a measurement of the anterior central corneal curvature and is performed with a manual keratometer, or more commonly automatically. The two basic manual keratometers are the Javal-Schiotz type and the Helmholtz type [15]. Automated keratometry measures the radius of the curvature of the anterior surface of the cornea from four reflected points approximately 3 mm apart. Topography derives from the Greek words "to place" (topo) and "to write" (graphein), which means to describe a place. This is classically related to the study of Earth's surface shape [16]; corneal topography is the study of the shape of the corneal surface [17]. Corneal topographers include the videokeratoscope or Placido-based devices, e. g., Topographic Modeling System (Tomey Corporation, Nagoya, Japan), Keratron (Optikon 2000 S.p.A., Rome, Italy), Zeiss Atlas (Carl Zeiss Meditec AG, Jena, Germany). Tomography derives from the Greek words "to cut or section" (tomos) and "to write" (graphein). In medicine the classic term computed tomography scanning is used for referring to the radiographic technique for imaging a section of an internal solid organ, producing a three-dimensional image. Corneal tomography presents a three-dimensional image of the cornea and is used for the examination of the front and back surfaces of the cornea along with pachymetric mapping. Currently, the corneal tomography might be assessed with:

(1) Scanning slit devices, e. g. Orbscan IIz (Bausch & Lomb, Rochester, NY) (2) The Scheimpflug devices, e.g. Pentacam (OCULUS Optikgeräte GmbH, Wetzlar, Germany), Sirius (CSO, Firenze, Italy), and the Galilei (Ziemer Ophthalmic Systems AG, Port, Switzerland). The latter two have and additional large cone Placido disc incorporated in them. (3) OCT-based devices e.g. Visante (Carl Zeiss Meditec AG, Jena, Germany).

A significant problem in determining the true corneal power is the difficulty to assess the posterior corneal surface. In most keratometric devices the relationship between the anterior and posterior corneal surfaces is fixed and estimated based on an empiric "keratometric index". A recent study by LaHood et al. revealed that the magnitude of anterior and posterior astigmatism is greater when the steep axis of the anterior astigmatism is oriented vertically [18]. Such evaluation leads to overestimation of astigmatism in with-the-rule astigmatism, whereas in eyes with against-the-rule astigmatism it could be underestimated. Therefore, assessing the optical power of the posterior corneal surface, and specifically it's astigmatism with corneal tomography devices could potentially increase the refractive outcome in lens surgery [19]. This issue is particularly important in IOL calculations of eyes that underwent corneal refractive surgery. As in these procedures corneal tissue is removed for refractive purposes changes, similarly the relationship between the front and back surfaces of the cornea is altered, invalidating the use of this standardized index of refraction. Currently, the optical biometers that employ corneal tomography, routinely allow measurement of the posterior corneal astigmatism [18].

It might be concluded that corneal tomography (or topography, when evaluating the posterior corneal surface is not neccessary) should be performed in patients with irregular, abnormally flat or steep corneas, in eyes with significant astigmatism, after previous corneal refractive surgery, or if it is not possible to achieve accurate keratometric measurements [20].

## Devices for Biometry

Primarily ultrasonography, which analyzed the echo delay time, was applied for preoperative biometry. The accuracy of ultrasound biometry was about 100 µm in older devices, and 20 µm in high precision instruments [21, 22]. This issue of accuracy is significant, as an error of 0.1 mm in axial length might result in a spherical equivalent error of 0.3 D [22]. Contact A-mode biometry is an applanation method and requires touching the cornea with an ultrasound probe. Corneal indentation, which alters the measurement results, is a significant disadvantage of this method [23]. In immersion ultrasound biometry a scleral cup filled with a coupling agent is applied, and the probe is immersed in the fluid so it does not depress the cornea.

Optical methods are less invasive, more user- and patient-friendly, less dependent on the examiner, show high accuracy and repeatability [24]. Optical biometry is currently considered as the gold standard and techniques employed in this method are presented in Table 3.1. A disadvantage of optical biometry is unattainability in patients unable to fixate, and in dense cataracts due to light scattering. Similarly, axial lens opacities might alter light transmission and give inaccurate results. Higher wavelength results in improved tissue penetration and higher success rate. For example in the study by Hirnschall et al. 78 of 1226 eyes (6.4%) were not measured successfully with partial coherence interferometry (780 nm), while with swept-source optical coherence tomography (1055 nm) the rate of unsuccessful scans was lower, and expected to reach only 0.5% [25]. In these cases immersion measurements still have a role in contemporary ocular biometry [25]. Currently, performing optical biometry requires a particular device solely for performing the measurements and IOL calculation. However, in future it might be employed in a standard anterior/posterior segment OCT, and such devices are availabe commercially (Fig. 3.1) [26].

**Table 3.1** Techniques employed for optical biometry

| Technology | Light source (wavelength) | Example biometers |
|---|---|---|
| PCI | Blue-light emitting diode (475 nm) | Oculus Pentacam AXL |
| PCI | Semiconductor diode laser (780 nm) | Zeiss IOL Master 500<br>Nidek AL-scan |
| LCOR | Superluminescent diode laser (820 nm) | Haag-Streit Lenstar LS 900<br>Topcon Aladdin/Aladdin LT<br>Ziemer Galilei G6 |
| OCT | Superluminescent diode laser (830 nm) | Optopol Revo NX |
| SS-OCT | Rapidly tuned laser with longer wavelength (1050–1060 nm) | Zeiss IOL Master 700<br>Movu Argos<br>Tomey OA-2000<br>Heidelberg Engineering Anterion |

Abbreviations: *LCOR* low-coherence optical reflectometry, *OCT* optical coherence tomography, *PCI* partial coherence interferometry, *SS-OCT* swept source-OCT

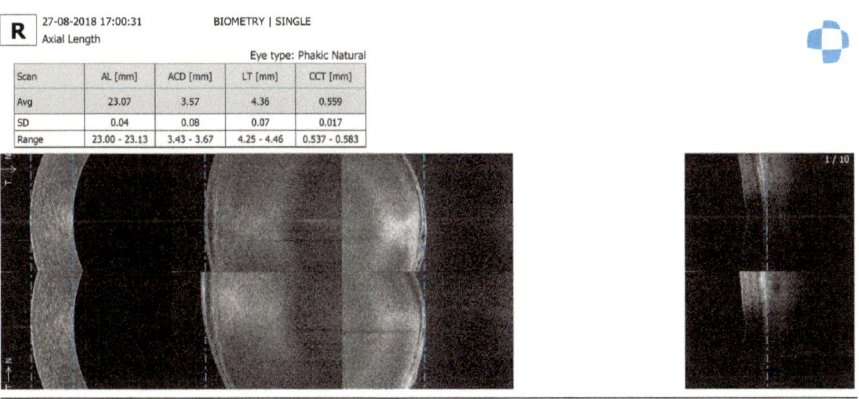

**Fig. 3.1** Biometry of a patient with dense posterior subcapsular cataract in a commercially available optical coherence tomography device (Revo NX, Optopol Technology Sp. z o.o., Zawiercie, Poland). Although the visualization in the lower and temporal part of the macula is hampered (lower parts of the retinal images), axial length measurements can be obtained

## *IOL Calculation Formulas*

The earliest IOL calculation formula was proposed over 50 years ago by Fedorov et al. [27]. First generation formulas were based on a thin-lens paraxial approximation, omitting factors such as lens thickness, corneal thickness or IOL design. Second generation formulas (regression formulas) decoupled eye as an optical system and were purely based on statistical analysis of refractive outcomes. The main improvement of third generation formulas was based on the assumption that the effective lens position is not a constant, but a function of axial length and corneal power. The goal of fourth generation formulas was to develop a universal calculation method giving the best outcome in all eyes despite axial length. Fifth generation formulas consider even more input parameters including gender or race to achieve a higher level of customization [28].

Recently, Koch et al. presented a different classification of IOL calculation formulas using a logical approach [29]. The reason for creating the new classification were difficulties with categorizing new formulas that employ ray tracing or artificial intelligence. The first proposed group is historical/refraction based formula, which include early attempts to calculate IOL power i.e. 18.0 Dpsh + 1.25 × preoperative spherical equivalent. Regression formulas, such as SRK or SRK II, do not rely on theoretical optics, but on analysis of previous data. The most numerous are vergence formulas. They rely on Gaussian optic and the assumption that the image vergence is equal to the sum of object and lens vergence. Certain formulas with the variables required for IOL calculation are presented in Table 3.2.

**Table 3.2** IOL calculation formulas

| Formula | Generation[*] | Logical approach classification | AL | K | ACD | LT | WTW | RxPre | Age |
|---|---|---|---|---|---|---|---|---|---|
| | | | \multicolumn{7}{Variables required} | | | | | | |
| SRK-I, Binkhorst I | 1st | V | X | X | | | | | |
| SRK-II, Binkhorst II | 2nd | V | X | X | | | | | |
| Holladay 1 | 3rd | V | X | X | | | | | |
| SRK/T | 3rd | V | X | X | | | | | |
| Hoffer Q | 3rd | V | X | X | | | | | |
| Holladay 2 | 4th | V | X | X | X | X | X | X | X |
| Olsen | 4th | V | X | X | X | X | X | | |
| Haigis | * | V | X | X | X | | | | |
| Hill-RBF | * | AI | X | X | X | X | X | | |
| Barrett Universal II | * | V | X | X | X | X | X | X | |

Abbreviations: *AI* artificial intelligence formulas, *AL* axial length, *K* keratometry, *ACD* anterior chamber depth, *LT* Lens thickness, *RxPre* preoperative refraction, *WTW* horizontal corneal white-to-white diameter, *V* vergence formulas
*Within the traditional classification it is difficult to categorize new IOL calculation formulas

Similarly to regression-based, artificial intelligence formulas use huge databases and a sophisticated statistical model to find relationship between not evident approaches; these include the Clarke neuronal network or Hill-RBF formula (radial basis function) [29, 30]. Another approach for improving the accuracy of IOL calculation is the application of ray-tracing analysis. Ray-tracing is method for calculation of every single ray passing through the optical system, and the refraction of rays at each optical surface is calculated using Snell's law. A map of corneal power achieved in topography or tomography can be transformed into an array of individual measurements representing a polygonal shape. Ray-tracing is employed to analyze the optical properties of every element of the eye in order to establish the performance of the entire optical system. Particularly in eyes after refractive surgery it might help to solve the issue of higher-order aberrations of the cornea by selecting a particular design of an IOL. Software applied for IOL calculation include Okulix or Phacooptics (Olsen).

When choosing the formula for IOL calculation the performance depending on the axial length of the eye should be taken into account (Table 3.3). The Haigis can be considered as the first choice for most routine cases [31]. It possesses rather small postoperative median absolute error and can be used with eyes of all axial lengths. For eyes under 22 mm in axial length the Hoffer Q formula should be applied for comparative assessment. The SRK-T formula manifests a lower predictive accuracy in short eyes; for that reason it should be employed for comparative purposes only in eyes over 22 mm of axial length. The Holladay I formula might be the second choice for eyes with axial length of 22–26 mm. The Holladay II takes into account the disparities in the anterior segment by adding the corneal white-to-white diameter and lens thickness, and might facilitate estimating the effective lens position. It shows benefits in eyes under 22 mm of axial length.

A notable percentage of patients undergoing PCS demonstrate corneal astigmatism. In a study by Hoffmann more than 36% of eyes had astigmatism 1 D or greater, while over 8% over 2 D or more [32]. For toric IOLs calculations manufacturers commonly provide an online calculator which employs the formerly presented formulae, but has incorporated IOL models and constants (e.g. Alcon, Bausch and Lomb, Johnson & Johnson Vision, Sifi). Also the Berdahl and Hardten calculator should be mentioned, as it allows to assess if the residual astigmatism after surgery is a result of toric IOL misalignment [33].

Table 3.3 The preferred IOL calculation formula based on the axial length of the eye

| Axial length | <22 mm | 22–24.5 mm | 24.5–26 mm | >26 mm | All lengths |
|---|---|---|---|---|---|
| 1st choice formula | Hoffer Q, Haigis | SRK-T, Haigis | SRK-T, Haigis | SRK-T, Haigis | Barrett Universal II, Hill-RBF |
| 2nd choice formula | Holladay II | Holladay | Holladay | – | |

## Benchmarking

Achieving an accurate refractive target is desired in contemporary PCS. Employing optical biometry and proper IOL calculation formulas allows achieving ≤0.5 D of the refractive target in 79.1% of eyes, while ≤1.0 D in 97.2% of cases [34]. Interestingly, the interocular axial length difference influences the refractive outcome. The odds ratio (OR) of having a refractive outcome >0.5 D is 1.4, 1.6 and 1.8, for interocular axial length difference of 0.2, 0.4 and 0.6 mm, respectively [34]. If the interocular axial length differences is 0.2 mm or more it would be advised to remeasure with the same device or, if possible, use another device to confirm the axial length [35]. Myopic patients have a lower chance of achieving the refractive target than non-myopic individuals (OR 1.9) [34].

Han and McGhee emphasized that in the current patient-focussed climate it becomes difficult to establish a clear definition of a complication in contemporary cataract surgery [36]. Thirty years ago a postoperative best correct visual acuity of 6/12 (20/40) might have been considered as a good outcome. Currently, in the era of postoperative visual acuity of 6/6 (20/20) and ±0.5 D of emmetropia, such a result could be considered a complication. With proper preoperative assessment and allocation of high-risk phacoemulsification procedures to experienced surgeons it is possible to reduce the rate of intraoperative complications by 40% and the rate of posterior capsule tear from 2.6 to 0.6% [37]. Within the Auckland Cataract Study the proposed stratification system risk factors for intraoperative complications included cataracts with no fundus view, pseudoexfoliation, phacodonesis, oral alpha-receptor antagonist intake, high ametropia, posterior capsule cataract or plaque or corneal scarring [37]. Moreover, it was proposed that patients after prior vitrectomy or with only one eye should be operated by experienced surgeons only.

## IOL Types

IOLs were introduced by Sir Harold Ridley, and the first successful IOL implantation was performed in the 1950 [38]. IOLs can be divided based on the material they are made of. Silicone lenses composed of polyorganosiloxane materials, with high refractive indices, were the first available foldable IOLs. Acrylic lenses can be made of rigid polymethyl methacrylate (PMMA), foldable hydrophilic or hydrophobic acrylic materials [39]. Addition of a blue-light filtering chromofore or UV-protection is employed in some IOL models.

The IOL design basically mirrors the intended location of IOL implantation. Posterior chamber lenses can be placed in the capsular bag, in the ciliary sulcus, or fixated to the iris. Single-piece IOLs may be open loop or overall plate lenses (Fig. 3.2a, b). Three-piece IOLs have haptic components made of PMMA, polypropylene, polyimide or polyvinylidene fluoride (Fig. 3.2c). In general, IOLs placed in the sulcus should have rounded optic edge and thinner haptics to prevent irritating the posterior part of iris, larger size of more than 13–14 mm (depending on the size

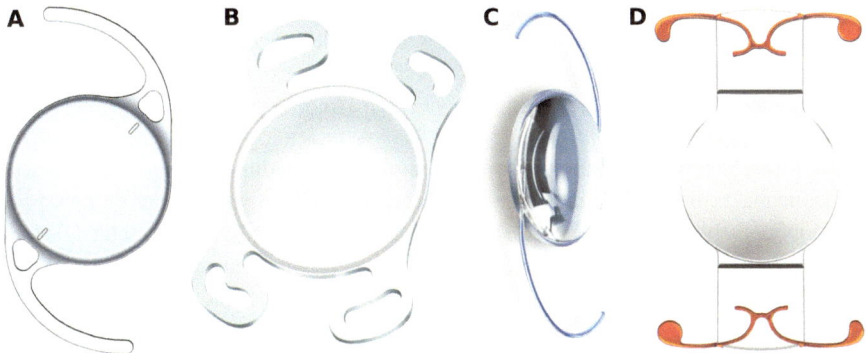

**Fig. 3.2** IOL designs. (**a**) A single-piece hydrophobic acrylic toric IOL (Bausch+Lomb EnVista Toric). (**b**) A single-piece hydrophilic acrylic IOL for micro-incisional cataract surgery—designed for a 1.8 mm incision size (Bausch + Lomb Akreos AO60). (**c**) A three-piece IOL with silicone optic anda haptics made of polymethylmethacrylate (Bausch + Lomb SofPort). (**d**) An accommodating IOL designed for in-the-bag implantation (Bausch + Lomb Crystalens AO)

of the eye) and a three-piece design. Sulcus placement of standard one-piece IOLs should be avoided as it increases the risk of postoperative complications, including pigment dispersion, uveitis–glaucoma–hyphema syndrome, and recurrent vitreous hemorrhages. On the other hand, IOLs implanted in the capsular bag should have a squared, truncated posterior optic edge to prevent lens epithelial cell migration and posterior capsule opacification [40]. Anterior chamber IOLs can be placed in the anterior chamber angle (open-loop design is preferred) or fixated to the iris (iris-claw IOLs).

Based on the optical properties IOLs can be divided into monofocal IOLs or multifocal/accommodating IOLs. Both monofocal and multifocal IOLs might have a spherical power, or toric in order to compensate astigmatism. The positive spherical aberration of the cornea can be compensated by aspheric design IOLs, having negative or zero spherical aberration to improve the patient's quality of vision. In order to achieve multifocality or an extended depth-of-field different optical principles are employed. A diffractive IOL generates multifocality making use of light interference and is independent of pupil size. It incorporates a pattern consisting of a series of annular concentric grooves less than one micron in depth, which are engraved around the optical axis on either the front or the back surface of a lens (the echelette technology). The refractive design allows to achieve depth of focus with light refraction on the IOL surfaces based on Snell's law. The optical power decreases continuously from the center to the periphery of the lens creating an infinite number of focal points and is derived from the smooth hyperbolic shape of its optics. The performance of refractive design IOLs is dependent on pupil size and IOL centration. Other optical concepts such as the pinhole effect [41] or light sword optical element [42] might be employed. Accommodating IOLs may change their curvature, or have a fixed-power presenting axial shift in order to restore accommodation (Fig. 3.2d) [43].

Ametropia following cataract surgery can be treated by performing a corneal refractive enhancement. Secondary piggyback IOLs are designed for secondary implantation in the ciliary sulcus to correct pseudophakic ametropias or pseudophakic lack of accommodation. Another potential option for avoiding pseudophakic ametropia is implantation of Light Adjustable Lens (LAL). A technology developed by Calhoun Vision Inc. involves implantation of a three-piece light-adjustable silicone IOL with silicone macrometrs containing an ultraviolet (UV) light-activated photo initiator [44]. Postoperatively, the IOL power can be adjusted by exposure to a customizable UV light profile resulting in polymerization of the IOL macromers. Clinical studies confirmed the safety of this technology to corneal endothelial cells [45] and to the retina [46].

## Glaucoma and Cataract Surgery

Cataract surgery alone results in a modest reduction of intraocular pressure [47, 48]. The reduction is proportional to preoperative IOP and ranges from 8.5 mmHg in eyes with preoperative IOP of 23–29 mmHg to 1.7 mmHg in eyes with IOP 5–14 mmHg [49]. The decrease in IOP is attributed to the increase in anterior chamber depth, flattening of the iris diaphragm, and subsequent extension of the trabecular meshwork. These changes are particularly advantageous in patients with angle-closure glaucoma. In open-angle glaucoma although IOP parameters improve after cataract surgery, glaucomatous visual field decay does not slow compared to rates measured during the progression of cataract [50]. Another option that should be considered in glaucoma patients is conjunction of PCS with endoscopic cyclophotocoagulation, trabecular micro-bypass stent, ab interno trabeculectomy, and canaloplasty [51]. These procedures are associated with a lower risk of surgical complications, however, are less effective than trabeculectomy.

Many antiglaucoma agents were reported to cause pseudophakic cystoid macular edema (PCME). Particularly prostaglandins—often the first line of treatment for IOP lowering—were believed to increase the risk of PCME [52, 53]. Miyake et al. presented findings suggesting that the preservatives used in these pharmaceutical cause increases synthesis of prostaglandins, intensifies postoperative inflammation and results PCME [54]. Nevertheless, more recently no association between prostaglandin analogue administration and PCME was reported [55]. It might be concluded that there is no evidence to discontinue antiglaucoma medications during cataract surgery and the risk associated with IOP elevation might be greater than disadvantages associated with their use.

## AMD and Cataract Surgery

The Beaver Dam Eye Study presented that having undergone PCS before baseline examination was associated with age-related maculopathy and the exudative age-related macular degeneration [56]. Some newer studies confirmed cataract surgery as being a risk factor for AMD [57–59], while other reported conflicting results [60–63]. The Cochrane Database for Systematic Reviews revealed that it is not possible to draw reliable conclusions from the available data as to whether cataract surgery is beneficial or harmful in people with AMD after 12 months [64]. It was concluded that in general cataract surgery provides short-term improvement in best corrected visual acuity in AMD patients compared to patients with no surgery. It is unclear whether the timing of surgery has an effect on long-term outcomes in AMD [64]. As *in vivo* studies demonstrated that blue light (430 nm wavelength) is harmful to retinal pigment epithelium cells, some authors believe that the protective effect of UV-blocking and blue-blocking IOLs might be greater than solely UV-blocking IOLs [65]. Nevertheless, the application of blue-blocking IOLs in not based on clinical evidence, as there are no studies truly confirming significant photoprotection [66].

Visual rehabilitation is necessary in patients with advanced AMD. Usually spectacles, magnifying glasses or electronic devices are used as visual aids. For several years specially designed intraocular implants have become an appealing alternative to extraocular aids. The possible options include implantable macular telescope, an IOL-VIP System, Lipshitz macular implant (for capsular bag or sulcus fixation), Fresnel Prism IOL, iolAMD or Scharioth Macula Lens [67]. However, the results so far were variable, and the available studies focused mainly on short-term outcomes [68].

Importantly, cataract surgery after previous intravitreal therapy is associated with a higher likelihood of posterior capsule rupture (PVR); 10 or more previous injections is associated with a 2.59 higher likelihood of PCR [69].

## Combined Surgeries (Efficacy vs Safety)

The efficacy and safety of combined phacoemulsification and vitrectomy was reported in several surgical indications, including macular hole, macular pucker, and in diabetic patients. A combined procedure eliminates the need for two operations and enables faster visual rehabilitation. Another rationale for this approach is that vitrectomy itself is known to induce cataract. For example, in a study by Jackson et al. 51.8% of phakic patients after vitrectomy with gas tamponade developed cataract requiring PCS in the following 6 months [70]. Lens opacification is associated with increased retrolental oxygen levels, particularly in extended vitrectomy with surgical posterior vitreous detachment and anterior vitreous removal [71]. The increased risk of intraoperative complications during PCS in vitrectomized eyes is well known, and might be associated with lens touch during vitrectomy, zonular dehiscence or intraoperative miosis [72–75]. The absence of vitreous support might also result in increased anterior depth and a disparity between fluid inflow and outflow during phacoemulsification or irrigation/aspiration [76–78].

Combined phacoemulsification with intraocular lens implantation and keratoplasty is known as the triple procedure. It is a safe and effective approach in patients with coexisting cataract and corneal pathologies [79]. A significant problem in the triple procedure is an unacceptable postoperative refractive error. It is a concern both in penetrating keratoplasty (where some suggest PCS after suture removal due to the refractive change associated with their removal) and lamellar keratoplasties. In deep anterior lamellar keratoplasty a large proportion of the stroma is replaced giving uncertainty of postoperative refraction, while in endothelial keratoplasties the cornea is preoperatively swollen due to endothelial dysfunction altering its optical power.

In cases of visually significant cataract and co-existent glaucoma, combined surgery (phacotrabeculectomy) can be considered. Filtration surgery presents a high risk of intraoperative bleeding, in contrary to PCS alone [80]. With that, there is evidence that long-term IOP is lowered by combined glaucoma and cataract surgery, however, giving a smaller effect than trabeculectomy alone [81, 82]. This might be possibly due to inflammation related to phacoemulsification. On the other hand, some studies presented that PCS performed after trabeculectomy might reduce the function of a filtering bleb in some eyes [83, 84]. In patients with angle-closure glaucoma, PCS alone might be an effective treatment [85]. Interestingly, combined cataract surgery (with corneal, glaucoma or vitreoretinal procedures) has a higher incidence of acute postoperative endophthalmitis than stand-alone PCS (0.149% vs. 0.102%, respectively).

## Settings (Ambulatory or Hospitalization, Operating Theater or in Office)

Currently, almost all cataract surgeries are performed in outpatient settings. These include a hospital-based outpatient departments or a standalone ambulatory surgical centers. The Cochrane Database for Systematic Reviews found cost savings associated with same-day discharge cataract surgery versus in-patient cataract surgery, however, the evidence regarding postoperative complications was inconclusive because the effect estimates were imprecise [86]. Some patients may still require an operative room or in-patient setting, intravenous sedation or general anaesthesia, and particularly complex cataract cases, or in individuals with severe comorbidities.

Recently, safety and effectiveness of PCS performed in an office-based minor procedure room in a series of 21,501 eyes was presented [87]; it was efficient for surgeon, as well as comfortable for the patient [85]. Another study conferred the safety of outpatient cataract surgery without presence or a dedicated access to anaesthetic service [88]. The monitoring was limited to blood pressure and plethysmography pre- and intraoperatively. Although office-based surgery is presently not reimbursed by Medicare, such relocation of the procedure might occur in future as it is cost-effective.

## Anesthesia (Topical vs Peribulbar vs Retrobulbar vs General)

The majority of cataract surgeries are performed under local anesthesia. General anesthesia should be considered in pediatric patients and for adults having difficulties with cooperation during surgery due to head tremor, deafness, mental retardation, neck or back problems, claustrophobia.

Retrobulbar anesthesia is performed by injecting the anesthetic drug to the intraconal space behind the eye [89]. In peribulbar anesthesia the drug is injected to the extraconal space, and diffuses between the intra- and extracone space to achieve anesthetic effect. Peribulbar and retrobulbar anaesthesia for cataract surgery show similar akinesia and pain control in cataract surgery [90]. However, the need for additional injections of local anaesthetic is greater with peribulbar anaesthesia. Another option is sub-Tenon anesthesia which involves creating a conjunctival buttonhole, blunt dissection of the Tenon's space and introduction of anesthetic to the subtenonian space.

Topical anesthesia may be preferred in phacoemulsification due to lower complication rates. Nevertheless, PCS under topical anesthesia may not be a completely painless procedure [91]. In these cases another option is additional intracameral anesthetic administration during the surgery.

## *Difficult Cases: Increased Risk of Complications*

Preoperative definition which eyes poses a potential risk of complications is critical, as in these eyes proper planning of the surgery is the key to success. Anatomic difficulties including deep set eyes or a protruding brow might impede surgical manipulations and proper instrument fitting it the operative field. Another group of challenges are high ametropias. Small hyperopic eyes make it difficult to perform intraocular manipulations, have increased chance of irid injury, cyclodialysis or fluid misdirection syndrome [92]. In deep myopic eyes the nucleus can be very large and the anterior chamber very deep. These patients also have a lower risk of accurate IOL power prediction [34]. Corneal opacities or scarring impede proper visualization of the operative field, which is particularly important during the capsulotomy [93]. Hard, dense or hypermature cataracts might be difficult to remove with phacoemulsification, and in these cases extracapsular extraction might be required. Eyes with pseudoexfoliation, with subluxated or dislocated lens (due to very mature lens, trauma, of Marfan's syndrome) have an increased chance of zonular dialysis, and might require supplementary means to fixate the lens. Eyes with small pupils, bound down pupil, floppy iris syndrome or a posterior pole cataract present an increased risk for intraoperative complications. General health problems including chronic obstructive pulmonary disease or dementia might impede proper patient positioning and cooperation [92].

The National Institute for Health and Care Excellence recommends that one IOL should be in the theater, an additional identical one should be in stock, and an alternative IOL (anterior chamber (AC)-IOL, sulcus IOL or iris-claw IOL) in case the lens needs to be changed if there are complications during surgery [20]. Additional accessories such as pupil expansion rings, iris hooks or capsular tension rings should be in stock.

## Bilateral Operation

The principle of immediate sequential bilateral cataract surgery (ISBCS) is to treat each eye as an individual and autonomous surgery during the same session in the operating theater. Each eye requires a change of draping, gloves, gowns and instruments [94]. Some authors recommend that instruments should come from disparate sterilization cycles, while viscoelastics or irrigation fluids from different companies or, at least, have different lots [95]. With these precautions employed, the greatest potential risk of ISBCS—bilateral endophthalmitis—has never been reported.

ISBCS is comparable with delayed sequential bilateral cataract surgery (when the second eye is operated on days to weeks later) in long-term patient satisfaction, visual acuity and complication rates [96]. A significant advantage of ISBCS is faster visual rehabilitation [97]. This approach is also cost-effective: it requires fewer hospital visits, allows faster return to work and only one pair of glasses. ISBCS is an ideal solution for patients requiring general anaesthesia, in order to eliminate the risks associated with a second intervention [98].

An argument commonly picked up by its opponents is the problem of anisometropia. In delayed sequential cataract surgery it is possible to adjust the IOL power of the second eye based on the postoperative results of the surgery. Nevertheless, with the advances of optical biometry, and due to the fact after simultaneous surgery, the errors are minor and symmetrical, ISBCS does not cause anisometropia.

## Intraoperative Considerations

### Intracapsular vs Extracapsular Cataract Extraction

Intracapsular cataract extraction (ICCE) involves removal of the opaque lens with the capsule in one piece. Samuel Sharp (1709–1778) was he first to perform intracapsular cataract extraction (ICCE). His report was presented to the Royal Society of London and subsequently published in the Philosophical Transactions [99]. A significant problem encountered during ICCE was zonular resistance, which needed to be overcome while releasing the lens. This was augmented with the development of the *erisophake*—a special cup with suction apparatus introduced into the anterior chamber—in order to hold firmly the lens with its capsule [100]. Alpha chymotrypsin could have been applied for enzymatic zonulolysis to augment lens liberation [101, 102]. Krwawicz proposed utilizing low temperatures with a *cryoextractor* which firmly attached to the lens capsule and subcapsular masses [103]. Cryoextraction cataract surgery led to a substantial progress in ophthalmology by reducing the number of complications, particularly capsule rupture, and resulted in achieving better outcome compared to other methods. Nevertheless, disadvantages of ICCE included large incision size and relatively high rate complication rate including vitreous loss, retinal detachment, endothelial cell damage or cystoid macular edema [104]. Another problem in ICCE is the lack of the lense capsule, which limits the possible options for IOL implantation.

Extracapsular cataract extraction (ECCE) involves removing the opaque lens, while leaving it's elastic capsule. Jacques Daviel (1693–1762) is believed to be the first to perform ECCE and presented this method in 1752 to the French Academy of Surgery [105]. Sushruta (600 BCE) might be considered as the a precursor of ECCE, however, he only described a paracentesis, and some extraocular evacuation of cortical masses, but not a large enough incision which could enable the extraction of the entire lens, as it is usually required in a classic ECCE [106]. Currently, most cataract surgeries attempt to preserve the lens capsule. The modification of ECCE, manual small incision cataract surgery (MSICS) is the most commonly employed form of ECCE, particularly in the developing world [107]. The principal feature of MSICS is hydrodissection and hydrodelineation of lens lamella, followed by hydroexpression of core nucleus into the anterior chamber [108]. An advantage of the procedure is that is does not require an ophthalmic viscoelastic device nor complex instrumentation. The Cochrane Database for Systematic Reviews presented that the number of complications in both MSICS and phacoemulsification are low [109]. Another conclusion was that removing cataract by phacoemulsification may result in better uncorrected visual acuity in the short term (up to 3 months after surgery) compared to MSICS, but similar best-corrected visual acuity. MSICS is faster, less expensive and less technology-dependent than phacoemulsification. It may be a convenient option in eyes with mature cataract in the developing world [110].

The main difference between ICCE and ECCE (particularly with preserved intact capsule) is the complication rate. ICCE presents more wound-related complications due to larger incision size than ECCE. With that, due to breaking the anterior hyaloid membrane, ICCE more commonly induces posterior vitreous detachments, macular edema and macular holes [111]. Primarily ICCE gained popularity in the twentieth century as, particularly with the cryoextractor, it was easy to completely remove the lens. Later on, due to higher complication rates of ICCE than ECCE, it was completely replaced by extracapsular methods.

## Phacoemulsification

A critical advancement in cataract surgery was introduction of phacoemulsification by Charles Kelman in 1967 [112]. As it was possible to divide and remove the lens within the eye, this portended the upcoming of the "small-incision cataract surgery". Phacoemulsification allows exceptional anterior chamber control as the incision is significantly reduced in size and is tightly sealed around the handpiece. IOP can be held within normal range with improved anterior chamber maintenance, reducing the likelihood of suprachoroidal or expulsive hemorrhage [113]. The decrease in wound size supports omission of corneal suturing, leading to less induced astigmatism and faster visual recovery. Finally, it is possible to significantly reduce the complication rates. Disadvantages of phacoemulsification include a steep learning curve, high reliability on the phacoemulsification unit and cost related to purchasing and maintaining it. The size of the IOLs for some time impeded the decrease in incision diameter, as is was necessary to extend the initial cut in order to implant an IOL [38].

## Femtosecond Laser-Assisted Cataract Surgery (FLACS)

Femtosecond lasers employ infrared light of the wavelength of 1053 nm and operate at high energy levels and very short, femtosecond range, pulses. The initial results of using femtosecond lasers for cataract surgery were presented in 2009 [114]. FLACS has raised a lot of hope as a mean to improve cataract surgery. The reported benefits included increased precision of the anterior capsulotomy, improved wound architecture and reduced ultrasound power during phacoemulsification (leading to a lower endothelial cell loss and collateral tissue damage). FLACS was proposed as a safe alternative for patients with Fuchs endothelial corneal dystrophy [115]. Nevertheless, in a recent study it was presented that FLACS does not lower the rate of corneal decompensation in eyes with mild to moderate Fuchs dystrophy [116].

Disadvantages of FLACS include mainly the price of the surgery, and that it is not cost-effective [117]. Another issue is the prevalence of PCME, which was shown to be higher in FLACS than in conventional PCS. This might be attributed to increased aqueous humor prostaglandin levels, possible due to increased surgical trauma caused by the laser to ocular tissue [118]. The main trigger for prostaglandin release was anterior capsulotomy [119], and the application of topical NSAIDs preoperatively could prevent this increase [120]. Another drawback is the potential of FLACS-specific intraoperative complications, such as anterior radial tears, capsular tags, suction break or pupillary constriction. The Cochrane Database for Systematic Reviews did not determine the superiority of laser-assisted cataract surgery compared to standard manual phacoemulsification [121].

## Micro-incisional Cataract Surgery (MICS)

MICS is a modification of a standard cataract surgery with the approach of a minimally invasive procedure. Coaxial or biaxial methods are employed, although with the smallest possible incision. MICS with the final incision of 1.6–1.8 mm for IOL implantation is believed to improve the visual and surgical outcome, and reduce the risk of associated complications [122]. In a biaxial procedure the steepest corneal meridian is marked and two incisions are executed 90° apart from each other. Currently, 19 G (1/1.1 mm) and 21 G (0.7 mm) instrumentation is employed for MICS. A relatively wider incisions should be made to enable unhampered manipulations within the AC: a 1.2 mm internally and 1.4 mm externally for 19 G tools, and 1-mm for 21 G. One of the incisions should be located in the positive meridian of the cornea—it will be enlarged for IOL implantation. Another approach is to create another, third incision for IOL implantation in the positive meridian shortly before IOL introduction into the eye. As a result of small incision size the continuous curvilinear capsulorhexis has to be carried out with a bent capsulotomy needle or 23-gauge vitrectomy-style micro-incisional capsulorhexis forceps. Cortical cleaving hydrodissection should be performed in two distal quadrants. Particularly in refractive lens exchange the use of specially designed symmetrical prechoppers such as Alió-Scimitar MICS (Katena Inc., Denville, NJ) might yield cutting the nucleus in half without placing any asymmetrical pressure on the zonules, and using high values of fluidics [123].

Following emulsification of the nuclear segments, the cortical material remaining in the capsular bag is removed with irrigation/aspiration. Separation of irrigation and aspiration in two independent handpieces prevents generating vortex currents at the end of the phaco-tip. Another advantage of the bimanual technique is the feasibility to remove the sub-incisional cortex without switching handpieces. It is worth highlighting that MICS presents outstanding AC stability. One of the reasons is that the irrigation handpiece is constantly within the AC. As well, the impermeability of two smaller incisions is greater than with a larger incision. Accordingly, the incidence of intraocular hypotony and the risk of AC collapse or posterior vitreous detachment during surgery declines considerably.

The value of MICS is that it can be performed with most phacoemulsification platforms. The parameters favour fluidics with high levels of irrigation/aspiration pressure, rather than phaco power. As a consequence of fast reaction and great flexibility, a Venturi pump system may be recommended. Standard infusion tools could be insufficient regarding hydrodynamics, hence particular MICS high-inflow tools should be employed. The major disadvantage of bimanual phacoemulsification lies in the current limitations of the IOL technology.

## *Wound Construction*

Currently cataract surgery employs CCI or scleral incisions, and their classification is presented in Table 3.4. Superiorly placed scleral tunnel incisions are used mainly in MSICS and by beginning cataract surgeons. Scleral incisions induce significantly less astigmatic change compared to CCI, which constitutes a significant advantage of this approach [124]. Creating a scleral incision is more challenging and time consuming compared to a CCI, and peribulbar or retrobulbar anesthesia is required. Proper tunnel incision architecture, at least 1–2 mm into the clear cornea, has self-sealing wound properties. Disadvantages of scleral incisions is occasional requirement of cautery, as the conjunctiva is highly vascular. If the initial groove is too superficial, a thin scleral flap will be prone to tearing or lacerations. If the initial groove is too deep, the anterior chamber might be penetrated too early. When the corneal part of the tunnel is performed too anteriorly, the visualisation will be hampered due to striae when the phaco tip is tilted down. Ballooning of the conjunctiva might impede access to the tunnell and require an additional cut.

**Table 3.4** Classification of scleral and corneal tunnel incisions

| Scleral tunnel incisions | | |
|---|---|---|
| **Conjunctival flap architecture** | Limbal-based flap | |
| | Fornix-based flap | |
| **Based on scleral groove shape** | Smile incision | Following the limbus |
| | Straight incision | Straight line |
| | Frown incision | Curve opposite to the limbus |
| | Blumental side cut | Straight line with sides receding from limbus |
| | Chevron 'v' incision | V-incision, sides receding from the limbus |
| **Corneal tunnel incisions** | | |
| **Based on external incision location** | Clear corneal incision | Entry anterior to conjunctival insertion |
| | Limbal corneal incision | Entry through the conjunctiva and limbus |
| | Scleral corneal incision | Entry posterior to the limbus |
| **Based on architecture** | Single plane | No groove |
| | Shallow groove | Below 400 μm |
| | Deep groove | Over 400 μm |

Primarily CCIs were criticized because of presumed increased risk of endophthalmitis due to uncertain sealability and poor wound healing (Fig. 3.3). Thus CCIs were indicated only in patients with pre-existing filtering blebs, taking anticoagulants [125], with blood coagulation disorders or cicatrizing diseases i.e., ocular cicatricial pemphigoid or Stevens-Johnson syndrome. Afterwards, as CCI can be performed under topical anesthesia, they became more and more commonly used. In general, regional blocks presented increased risk of complications compared to topical anesthesia. Other advantages of CCIs include ease of approach to the incision site, preservation of options for future filtering surgeries, increased stability in refractive results (neutralization of the forces from lid blink and gravity), no need for bridle sutures and the location of the lateral canthal angle under the incision which facilitates drainage. A disadvantage of CCI is the induction of astigmatism. In general, the main incision should be located in the steep meridian of the cornea, particularly if the corneal astigmatism is higher than 0.50 cylindrical diopter. Interestingly, the CCI-induced astigmatism significantly differences among surgeons. In a study conducted by Ernest et al. all of the surgeons have performed CCIs in the same manner and using identical surgical tools, the surgically induced astigmatism differed double-fold (mean induced astigmatism from 0.38 to 0.88 D depending on surgeon) [126]. Furthermore, the location of the incision influences the size of astigmatism. Incisions performed in the nasal quadrant induce significantly higher astigmatism than the temporal ones [127, 128]. Although clear corneal and scleral incisions might engender complications by nature of their architecture and location, some complications are unique to CCI. If the conjunctiva is unintentionally incised at the time of creating a CCI, ballooning

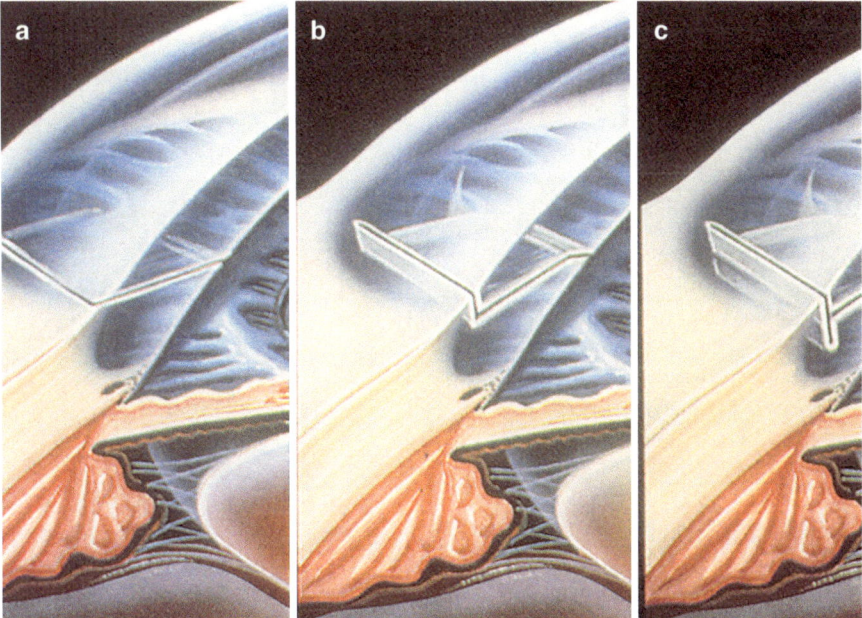

**Fig. 3.3** Artist's interpretation of cross-section view of clear corneal incisions. (**a**) A single plane incision. (**b**) The modified incision by making a shallow, perpendicular groove before incising the cornea. (**c**) A deepened perpendicular groove, which was believed to lead to greater stability

of the conjunctiva can develop which may compromise visualization of anterior structures. If this develops, the use of a suction catheter is usually required by the assistant to aid in visualization. Early entry into the anterior chamber might result in an incision of insufficient length to be self sealing, increased tendency for iris prolapse, and requires placing a suture at the conclusion of the procedure. Late entry may result in a long corneal tunnel, so that the phacoemulsification tip would create striae in the cornea and hamper visualization of the anterior chamber. Manipulation of the phacoemulsification handpiece intraoperatively may result in tearing of the roof of the CCI, particularly at the edges, compromising the ability to self-seal, or occasionally resulting in minor detachment or scrolling of Descemet's membrane. Incisional burns similarly compromise self-sealability, result in corneal edema and severe induced astigmatism [129]. In addition, manipulations in the proximity of the wound can cause epithelial abrasion.

## Intraoperative Complications

The overall complication rates in PCS are presented in Table 3.5. PCR is the most common a potentially serious complication of PCS. It is associated with the risk of dropped nucleus, vitreous loss, difficulties in placement of the IOL, and postoperative complications such as retinal detachment or PCME. Risk indicators for PCR are

**Table 3.5** Intraoperative cataract surgery complication rates in selected studies

| | CND dataset (n = 55,567) (%) [130] | UKHS dataset (n = 20,070) (%) [130] |
|---|---|---|
| Posterior capsule rupture with or without vitreous loss | 1.41 | 0.53 |
| Iris damage from phaco | 0.55 | 0.06 |
| Zonular dialysis | 0.46 | 0.1 |
| IOL complications (decentration, IOL in the vitreous, lens exchange required) | 0.36 | 0.05 |
| Phaco wound burn | 0.25 | 0.0 |
| Nuclear fragment into the vitreous/dropped nucleus | 0.18 | 0.03 |
| Corneal epithelial abrasion | 0.17 | 0.12 |
| Vitreous in the anterior chamber | 0.17 | 0.08 |
| Choroidal/suprachoroidal haemorrhage | 0.07 | 0.0 |
| Hyphema | 0.07 | 0.0 |

Abbreviations: *IOL* intraocular lens, *UKSH* United Kingdom Specialist Hospitals, *CND* United Kingdom Cataract National Dataset

brunescent/white cataract (adjusted odds ratio (AOR) 2.99), pseudoexfoliation syndrome/phacodonesis (AOR 2.92), no fundus view during surgery (AOR 2.46), diabetic retinopathy (AOR 1.63), doxazosin intake (AOR 1.51), axial length equal or greater than 26.0 mm (AOR 1.47), small pupil size (AOR 1.45) as well as inability to lie flat (AOR 1.27), presence of glaucoma (AOR 1.3) and surgery performed by trainees (AOR 3.73, when comparing to senior house officer) [131]. The cause of PCR usually involves touching the posterior capsule with surgical instruments, and may occur at any stage of the surgery. Particularly patients with congenital posterior polar cataract are at risk of PCR, and in these cases hydrodelineation rather than hydrodissection should be performed [132].

When dealing with PCR it is critical to remove the vitreous from the wound and anterior chamber [20]. This should be employed with a vitreous cutter in order to minimize any traction on the retina. All the lens fragments and soft lens matter should be removed, both from the posterior chamber and vitreous cavity. As visualization of the vitreous body might be difficult, the use of triamcinolone for staining is recommended.

A small pupil makes PCS technically challenging, and usually a stepwise approach for pupil dilation is recommended. If poor dilation is surmised, mydriasis might be achieved preoperative application of atropine, which is strongest mydriatic agent. In these cases atropine sulfate 1% is applied three times for 1–3 days before surgery. Additionally, intracameral sympathomimetics agents (e.g. epinephrine in a 1:2500 dilution) might be administered intraoperatively [133]. The mydriatic effect might be also achieved with intracameral preservative-free lidocaine 1% [134, 135]. Lidocaine might be combined with sympathomimetics and/or tropicamide. Such a preparation for intracameral administration is available commercially (Mydrane, Thea Pharmaceuticals, Clermont-Ferrand, France). In moderate to severe cases the use of iris expansion rings or iris hooks might be necessary.

Intraoperative floppy iris syndrome (IFIS) is a condition that significantly increases the risk of complications. IFIS is associated with a higher rate of surgical complications, especially when the condition is not recognized or anticipated [136]. The relationship between IFIS and the systemic use of α-blockers, particularly tamsulosin, was reported almost 10 years ago [137]. Importantly, discontinuation of tamsulosin prior to PCS does not decrease the severity of IFIS [138]. IFIS can be prevented and treated by maintaining proper mydriasis and restraining the iris from prolapsing during cataract surgery [139]. Proper wound construction is critical, and the tunnel should be slightly longer and more anteriorly-situated than in normal cases. Lower vacuum and aspiration would be recommended for surgery and repeated injections of a viscoelastic agent.

Pseudoexfoliation syndrome (XFS) is an age-related disorder in which abnormal fibrillar extracellular material is produced and accumulates in several ocular tissues. No symptoms are usually associated with XFS, however, individuals have a risk of increased IOP, glaucoma, and poor pupil dilation. With that, it was reported that XFS cases might manifest zonular instability [140]. Thus, XFS eyes present an increased risk of dropping the nucleus or nucleus fragment, zonular dialysis, phacodonesis or lens sublutaxion.

## Retained Lens Fragments and Nucleus Luxation

Retained lens material is a rare complication of PCS, however, was reported in up to 0.8% of patients having undergone resident performed PCS [141]. The presence of retained lens fragments may result in postoperative inflammation, secondary glaucoma, corneal edema, PCME or rhegmatogenous retinal detachment. As these complication might result in long-term visual impairment, proper management plays a great role in the final visual outcome.

Small amounts of cortical material may become absorbed without surgery. In cases with large cortical parts or fragments of the nucleus, such material should be removed with pars plana vitrectomy (PPV). Small pieces of the nucleus can be removed with a vitrectomy handpiece alone, while harder nuclear material should be removed with a phacoemulsification instrument within the posterior segment [142]. Treatment is theoretically possible during the same surgery with conversion from PCS to pars plana vitrectomy while the patient is still draped. However, such treatment has some disadvantages. Firstly, the anesthesia for vitrectomy and cataract surgery is different. Some studies identified a substantially increased risk of intraoperative bleeding during PPV, thus discontinuation of antiplatelet agents or anticoagulants could be considered for vitrectomy (but is not usually done in PCS) [12]. In some countries it is infrequent for cataract surgeons to perform PPV. A vitreoretinal surgeon might not be available immediately at the same setting, and even if so he might be reluctant to perform immediate surgery in a patients with whom he does not have a professional relationship. Not all phacoemulsification devices are enabled to perform PPV or phacofragmentation, and endoillumination might be required in these cases. Importantly, efforts to retrieve lens fragments without proper posterior segment instrumentation might result in complex retinal detachment and should be discouraged [143].

If performing immediate PPV is not possible, it is advocated to remove lens fragments from the anterior chamber and capsular bag, place the IOL (into the capsular bag, or alternatively to the sulcus or anterior chamber) and suture the corneal incision [144]. Subsequently, it is postulated that PPV should be performed up to 7 days after PCS [145]. Histopathologic investigations of vitreous specimens obtained during PPV revealed that lens-induced inflammation increases with time that retained lens material remains in the eye [146]. No macrophages, phacolytic cells, neutrophils and multinucleated giant cells were present if vitrectomy was performed with 3 days after PCS. Clinically, a delayed interval between PCS and PPV results in higher retinal detachment rate [147], poorer visual outcome, and a higher risk of developing persistent glaucoma [145]. Contrarily, some other studies did not find an association between time of intervention and final outcome [148, 149]. In a publication by Scott et al. 44% of patients had a final visual acuity of 20/40 and worse, and the main cause of visual impairment was cystoid macular edema [148].

## Posterior Capsulotomy

Performing a primary surgical capsulotomy is an option for eyes having a high risk of developing significant posterior capsule opacification (PCO). This should be considered in pediatric cataracts and particularly in patients under 6 years of age [150], as well as in adults undergoing combined vitrectomy and cataract surgery [151]. Similarly, posterior capsulotomy might be performed in eyes having a dense PCO discovered intraoperatively [152]. Posterior capsulotomy is also postulated in refractive lens exchange in young patients, however, no long-term studies confirmed the safety in this cohort [153]. Opening the posterior capsule might be supplemented with vitreous staining with preservative-free triamcinolone acetonide and anterior vitrectomy.

## Dropless Cataract Surgery

As topical antibiotics are difficult to instill and their effect is dependent on patient compliance, dropless cataract surgery might be a viable option [154]. In a study by An et al. 92.6% of patients after PCS demonstrated improper eye drop administration technique, including missing the eye, instilling an incorrect amount of drops, contaminating the bottle, or failing to wash hands before instillation [155]. Consequences of poor compliance can affect both the patient (in cases of complications) and the society (by development of antibiotic resistance). TriMoxi (Imprimis Pharmaceuticals) is a single use suspension containing 15 mg/mL of triamcinolone and 1 mg/mL of moxifloxacin. Another formulation, TriMoxiVanc, adds 10 mg/mL of vancomycin to the compound. At the conclusion of surgery 0.2 mL of the suspension is introduced into the posterior chamber through a transzonular injection. A disadvantage of this approach is the reduction of "the wow factor", as the visible drug affects the vision for up to 3–7 days after surgery. Over time, a dropless approach might become universally preferred over topical post-cataract prophylaxis.

## Postoperative Complications

### Postoperative Follow Ups

The timing of postoperative examinations should be adjusted to ensure the expeditious recognition and management of complications in order to optimize the final outcome of surgery. The frequency of postoperative complications in recent studies is presented in Table 3.6.

Several reviews were conducted to assess the value of early postoperative examinations after PCS, not finding an increase in patient safety associated with postoperative day 1 (POD1) [158, 162]. Deferment of the postoperative review was suggested in low-risk patients. A closer follow-up was recommended in patients with glaucoma

**Table 3.6** Prevalence of postoperative complications in selected cataract surgery studies

| | Greenberg et al. 2011 [156] (n = 45,082) | Syed et al. 2015 [130] (n = 20,070) | Jaycock et al. 2009 [157] (n = 16,731) |
|---|---|---|---|
| Posterior capsule opacification | **4.2%** | 0.34% | **1.22%** |
| Cystoid macular edema | **3.3%** | 0.22% | **1.62%** |
| Retained soft lens matter | **1.7%** | 0.19% | 0.45% |
| Raised IOP (>21 mmHg) | N/A | 0.31% | **2.57%** |
| Retinal tear or detachment | **1.0%** | 0.03% | N/A |
| IOL decentration/dislocation/ exchange | 0.9% | N/A | 0.22% |
| Vitreous hemorrhage | 0.4% | 0.01% | N/A |
| Hyphema | 0.2% | N/A | 0.07% |
| Hypopyon/endophthalmitis | 0.2% | 0.04% | N/A |
| Iris prolapse/iris to wound | N/A | 0.04% | 0.16% |
| Vitreous to section | N/A | 0.09% | 0.39% |
| Vitreous in the AC | N/A | N/A | 0.17% |
| Wound leak | N/A | 0.02% | 0.14% |
| Choroidal effusion/ hemorrhage | 0.1% | N/A | 0.13% |
| TASS | N/A | 0.1% | N/A |

Complications with the prevalence rate of 1% or more are presented in bold. Abbreviations: *AC* anterior chamber, *IOL* intraocular lens, *IOP* intraocular pressure, *N/A* not available, *TASS* toxic anterior segment syndrome in order to evaluate postoperative IOP spikes, in eyes with intraoperative complications, posterior synechiae, chronic/recurrent uveits), or in patients operated on by less-experienced surgeons. Tan et al. suggested that the POD1 hospital visit may be safely managed by way of a nurse-administered telephone questionnaire with patient contentment achieved and the liberation of clinic resources ensured [159]. In their study, only one of 238 patients reported a poor general condition, blurred vision, and pain, and was asked to return for a clinic review on POD1. Tufail and associates compared the complications seen with same-day discharge surgery (with a review occurring at 4–6 h postoperatively) with those seen with in-patient surgery (with a POD1 review) and found that the most common complications in both groups were IOP rise, corneal edema, and wound leaks [160]. Only one patient in each group, with an iris prolapse, required attending to the department. It was concluded that there were no additional risks related to same-day discharge surgery.

With that in mind, Eloranta et al. suggested that a postoperative check-up visit might not be required in the majority of cases [161]. In the year 2006, a follow-up visit was advised to occur 1 month after surgery, while in 2009 patients were informed that such an postoperative complications in recent appointment is not necessary. Contacting the department was advised if they experienced pain, vision deterioration, or ocular discharge. Only patients with intraoperative complications or comorbidities influencing postoperative recovery were selected for a follow-up visit. In the postoperative period, 4.2% of patients in 2006, and 3.9% of patients in 2009 contacted the hospital because of symptoms. Referral was necessary in only 0.5% of patients in the 2006 cohort, and 0.3% of patients in the 2009 cohort, while a surgical or medical intervention was needed by only one-third of the referred individuals. It was concluded that the lack of a 1-month check-up did not influence patient's safety, however, in cases with intraoperative problems, comorbidities influencing recovery, or postoperative symptoms, the patients should be seen at a low threshold [162]. Moreover, eliminating POD1 follow-up could result in significant health care savings without an increased risk to the patient.

The American Academy of Ophthalmology recommends that a POD1 visit should be done in functionally monocular patients, following intraoperative complications, or in those at a high risk of immediate postoperative complications such as IOP spike. In patients without these risks the follow-up visit should be scheduled within 48 h [3]. According to the Royal College of Ophthalmologists, POD1 review is no longer in widespread use in the United Kingdom (UK). Such an examination is recommended only in complicated surgeries, in eyes with co-existing diseases (e.g., glaucoma, uveitis), or in patients with only one eye [163]. Upon discharge, comprehensive information to identify potential complications should be provided with a postoperative appointment date confirmed and the required medications dispensed.

## Pseudophakic Cystoid Macular Edema (PCME)

PCME is one of the most common complication of PCS resulting in long-term vision impairment (Fig. 3.4). PCME usually develops 1–6 weeks after cataract surgery. It is postulated that physical trauma related to surgical manipulations within

**Fig. 3.4** Optical coherence tomography of a patient with pseudophakic cystoid macular edema

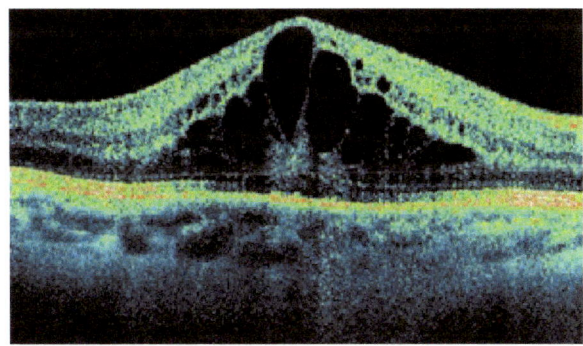

**Table 3.7** Risk factors for pseudophakic cystoid macular edema in eyes undergoing cataract surgery

| Risk factor | | Relative risk (95% CI) |
|---|---|---|
| Diabetes | No signs of retinopathy | 1.8 (1.36–2.36) |
| | Presence of diabetic retinopathy | 6.23 (5.12–7.58) |
| | Presence of proliferative diabetic retinopathy | 10.34 (5.13–20.85) |
| Epiretinal membrane | | 5.60 (3.45–9.07) |
| Retinal vein occlusion | | 4.47 (2.6–5.92) |
| Previous retinal detachment repair | | 3.93 (2.60–5.92) |
| Uveitis | | 2.88 (1.50–5.51) |
| Posterior capsule tear with or without vitreous loss | | 2.61 (1.57–4.34) |

**Source**: Chu CJ, Johnston RL, Buscombe C, et al. Risk Factors and Incidence of Macular Edema after Cataract Surgery: A Database Study of 81984 Eyes. Ophthalmology. 2016;123(2):316–323

the anterior chamber induces an inflammatory response. The release of arachidonic acid from uveal tissue results in production of leukotrienes (via the lipoxygenase pathway) and/or prostaglandins (via the cyclooxygenase pathway). These mediators of inflammation diffuse posteriorly and ensue the disruption of the blood–aqueous barrier. This results in increased permeability and accumulation of the extravascular fluid within the retina. Reduced fluid reabsorption within the macula may be partially explained by the absence of blood vessels within the foveal avascular zone. Histological studies showed dilatation of retinal capillaries and gathering of serous fluid in the outer plexiform and inner nuclear layers of the retina [164].

The risk factors of developing PCME are presented in Table 3.7. Based on the current literature intensive use of potent corticosteroids with adequate intraocular penetration remain the mainstay of PCME prophylaxis in uncomplicated cataract surgery, while it is unclear if nonsteroidal anti-inflammatory drugs (NSAIDs) can offer additional benefit [165]. Postoperative topical treatment is usually applied for 2–4 weeks after PCS [166, 167]. In patients with risk factors for PCME development an additional subconjunctival injection of triamcinolone acetonide may prevent PCME development.

When assessing treatment options one should remember that PCME has a tendency to resolve spontaneously [168]. With topical treatment it can be estimated that about 54% of PCME cases completely resolve, while a decrease in macular thickness is be observed in 80% of eyes within 6 weeks [169]. Higher baseline visual acuity was found to be associated with successful treatment and PCME resolution [169], the outcomes may also be worse in patients with hypertension [170]. For PCME a step-wise approach is recommended, a topical strong steroid optionally supplemented with some NSAIDs, subsequently a posterior sub-Tenon or retrobulbar steroid, and finally, intravitreal steroid treatment or a steroid drug delivery system. Intravitreal anti-vascular endothelial growth factor agents may be considered in patients unresponsive to steroid therapy and/or at risk of elevated intraocular pressure.

## Posterior Capsule Opacification (PCO)

PCO is a relatively common complication reported in up to 50% of patients after PCS in a 5 year observation period [171]. In refractive lens exchange for high myopia PCO rates are even higher with 77.89% of patients requiring neodymium:YAG (Nd:YAG) laser capsulotomy in a 7-year follow-up [172, 173].

Advances in surgical techniques, IOL materials and designs have been employed in order to reduce the PCO rate [174, 175]. One example is an increase of biocompatibility determined by the relationship of the IOL with remaining lens epithelial cells within the capsular bag to inhibit their proliferation, migration, and epithelial-to-mesenchymal transition. The truncated, square edge of the acrylic IOLs causes a blockage of epithelial cells at the optic edge, preventing ingrowth over the posterior capsule [176]. However, a complete elimination of PCO has not been achieved yet, and with recent improvements the overall incidence of PCO was reported as less than 10% in a 5 year follow-up [177]. The annual volume of cataract surgery is still increasing. Currently, Nd:YAG laser capsulotomy is accepted as a standard and effective treatment for PCO. Importantly, although cataract surgery itself is a risk factor for postoperative retinal detachment, Nd:YAG capsulotomy does not increase this risk [178].

## Endophthalmitis and Toxic Anterior Segment Syndrome (TASS)

Postoperative endophthalmitis (POE) is the most severe complication of cataract surgery (Fig. 3.5). Although rare, infectious POE is a severe intraocular infection that can result in devastating loss of vision or even loss of the eye [179]. Recent reports confirmed low incidence of POE, under 0.1% [180]. POE usually develops 4–7 days after surgery; however, if caused by high-virulence microorganisms it might occur 1 day after surgery [181, 182]. Symptoms include eye redness, pain, ocular discharge and blurred vision, while lid swelling can be found in up to one-third of cases [182].

TASS is a sterile anterior segment inflammatory response related to an ingress of toxic substances (Fig. 3.6) [183]. Several outbreaks of TASS were reported in recently [184–186]. TASS typically presents within 12–48 h after surgery, however, recent

**Fig. 3.5** Postoperative
endophthalmitis is the
most severe complication
of cataract surgery

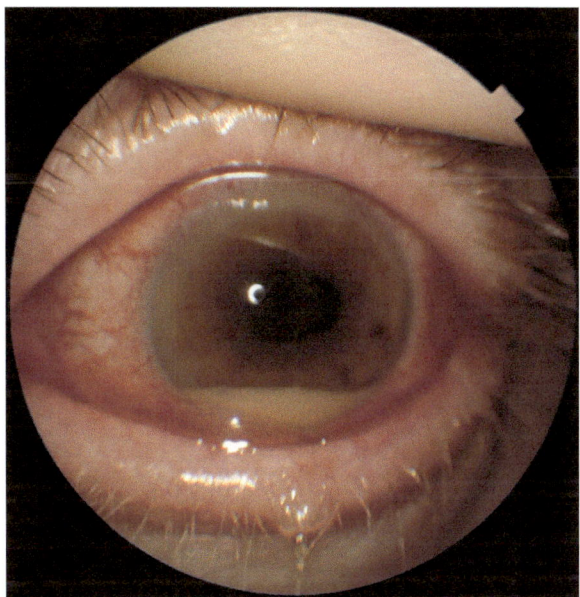

**Fig. 3.6** Toxic anterior
segment syndrome

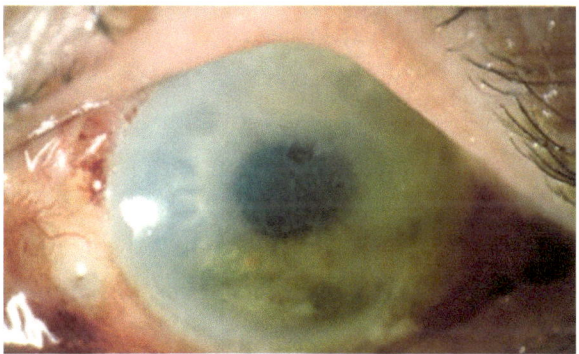

studies noted onset 38–137 days after surgery [184, 187]. TASS is characterized by
anterior chamber inflammation and other symptoms such as conjunctival injection/
chemosis, hypopyon or anterior vitreous opacities may be present. Endothelial cell
damage in TASS might lead to diffuse corneal edema, however, the incidence of corneal edema in TASS in large series was reported as 15.6–19.1% [184, 185].

Symptoms of endophthalmitis and TASS are presented in Table 3.8. Distinguishing
between these two conditions is critical, as the management is different. POE treatment includes administration of intravitreal antibiotics with vitreous tapping and/or
vitrectomy [179]. In contrary, TASS usually resolves with topical steroid treatment.

Antibiotics may be used before, during or after surgery in order to decrease the
rates of endophthalmitis. Due to low endophthalmitis rates after cataract surgery it
is difficult to verify prophylactic algorithms [189]. Thus, indirect risk measures are

**Table 3.8** Symptoms of endophthalmitis and TASS

| Symptom | | Prevalence in endophthalmitis [188] | Prevalence in TASS [185] |
|---|---|---|---|
| Red eye | | **82.1%** | 39.8% |
| Pain | | **74.3%** | 9.5% |
| Lid swelling | | 34.5% | – |
| Hypopyon | Hypopyon | **85.7%** | 10.6% |
| | Cells | – | **97.2%** |
| | Flare | – | **63.0%** |
| Red reflex present | | 32.0% | – |
| Vitreous opacities | | – | 21.6% |
| Keratic precipitates | | – | 21.6% |
| Corneal edema | | – | 15.6% |
| Days from cataract surgery to presentation: median (range) | | 6 (1–63) | 13.1 (1–88) |

frequently employed. There are wide variations in prevention practices around the world [190]. Nevertheless, aseptic technique with application of povidone-iodine remains the only technique supported by level I evidence to reduce the incidence of endophthalmitis [191]. Intracameral administration of antibiotics is based on recommendations of the European Society of Cataract and Refractive Surgeons (ESCRS) study [192]. In their randomized controlled trial involving 16,603 cataract surgeries the reported rate of proven POE was 0.025% in patients receiving levofloxacin drops and intracameral cefuroxime, 0.049% in intracameral cefuroxime with no antibiotic drops, 0.173% in patients receiving solely topical levofloxacin, and 0.247% in those receiving no antibiotic. Despite the criticism regarding the methodology of ESCRS Study, the results confirmed by many later retrospective case series showing 2–5 fold protection against endophthalmitis with the intracameral antibiotic use. However, all of these studies were based on endophthalmitis rate greater than 0.05%. Thus, it is not clear if it is possible to achieve similar results in cases with lower endophthalmitis rate. On the other hand, some recent studies showed that it is possible to achieve very low endophthalmitis rate with only topical antibiotics [191]. Recent investigations underline the importance antisepsis with povidone-iodine for POE prophylaxis, while the evidence for using topical antibiotics, when intracameral agents are applied, is not compelling [189, 193].

## Intraocular Pressure (IOP) Spikes

The incidence of postoperative IOP increase to 28 mmHg and above was noted in up to 46.4% in populations of high-risk patients [194]. IOP usually peaks at 3–7 h after surgery and remains increased during the first 24 h postoperatively. Such an early IOP elevation is a result of surgical trauma and consecutive prostaglandin release with consecutive anterior chamber inflammation [195]. Although the increase generally does not influence the long-term quality of vision, IOP spikes are potentially more dangerous in patients with preexisting optic nerve damage i.e., in glaucoma or atherosclerosis-related ischemia [196]. Occasionally, an individual with the pressure of 40–50 mmHg will experience pain or nausea, which will prompt disappointment with the surgery or result a phone call to the surgeon in the middle of the night.

It is estimated that up to 9.8% of patients manifest an IOP increase by 10 mmHg. Risk factors for postoperative IOP spikes include residual viscoelastic material [197–199], resident performed surgery [200–203], glaucoma [194, 204, 205], pseudoexfoliation syndrome [47], axial length above 25 mm [206], tamsulosin intake [207], topical steroid application in steroid responders [208]. Patients with higher baseline IOP were found to have a more pronounced IOP increase [209].

Several topical IOP lowering agents were appraised in order to prevent the occurrence of early IOP increase. Nevertheless, no protocol has completely eliminated IOP spikes. We would recommend applying a combination of dorzolamide/timolol and brimonidine topically in high-risk patients, particularly with preexisting optic nerve damage. When the IOP is exceedingly elevated side-port paracentesis might be conducted with, or without, supplemental antiglaucoma medications [194]. Usually a 25-gauge needle is used to depress the posterior lip of the side-port incision.

## Late Postoperative IOL Opacifications

Long-term alterations found in IOL materials include mainly glistening and IOL calcification. Glistenings are small (1.0–20.0 μm) fluid-filled microvacuoles which appear within the IOL optic when it is placed in an aqueous environment (Fig. 3.7). Subsurface nanoglistenings (SSNGs) are fluid filled gaps, measuring <200 nm in size and situated up to 120 microns from the surface of the optic of the IOL

**Fig. 3.7** Light photomicrograph of a hydrophobic acrylic IOL explanted because of error in power calculation. The presence of microvacuoles (glistenings) can be seen, within the optic substance of the lens (original magnification ×200). Courtesy: Liliana Werner, MD, PhD, University of Utah

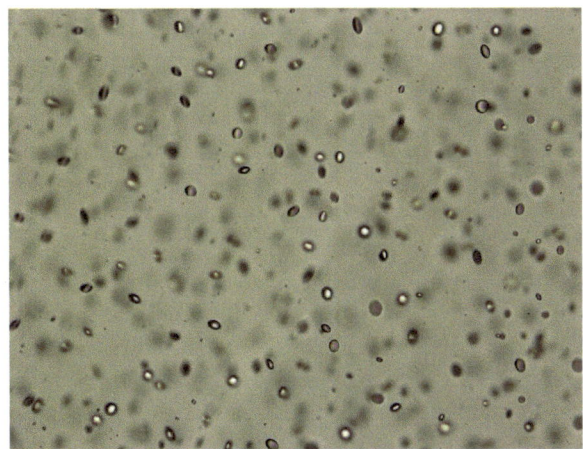

**Fig. 3.8** Gross photograph (macroscopic dark-field image with a 90-degree off-axis illumination; hydrated) of a hydrophobic acrylic IOL removed from a cadaver eye (bottom) and a control IOL of the same model (top). The IOL on the bottom shows an overall white discoloration or haze resulting from the presence of subsurface nanoglistenings ("whitening"). Some microvacuoles (glistenings) can also be seen within the optic substance of the lens. Courtesy: Liliana Werner, MD, PhD, University of Utah

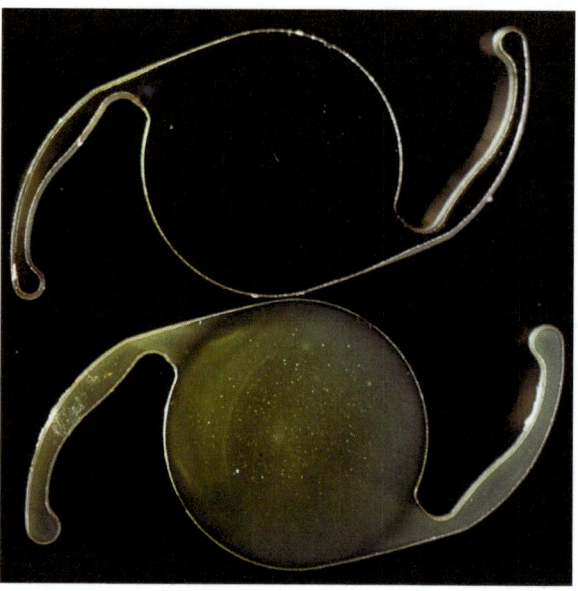

(Fig. 3.8). Both glistenings and SSNG's have been reported in most types of IOL material and only heparin-surface-modified PMMA lenses do not manifest glistenings. Glistening is most common in hydrophobic acrylic materials, and IOL models differ in their resistance to glistening [210]. It has been argued that the optical quality of an acrylic foldable intraocular lens is not significantly affected by the glistenings usually seen in the clinical setting, as glistenings usually does not adversely affect the light transmittance, power performance of an IOL and the visual acuity [211, 212]. With that, numerous glistenings are needed to cause significant straylight elevation or decrease high spatial frequency contrast sensitivity [213]. However, recent studies reported that commonly glistenings and SSNG's increase retinal straylight and decrease contrast sensitivity also under no glare conditions, tending to impair subjective visual performance [213–216]. It was also proposed that glistenings might impair driving ability and lead to driving accidents [217, 218]. One should remember that glistening increases with time after IOL implantation, so with the increased life expectancy and performing surgery in younger patients with less advanced cataract, it might represent a significant problem in IOLs that have already been implanted [219]. Glistening has also been reported in paediatric patients [220, 221], and in these cases there might be a concern for visual function in children with IOL implants over their 80-year lifespan.

Calcification is more common in hydrophilic acrylic IOLs than in hydrophobic or silicone IOLs (Fig. 3.9). Calcification deposits present as clusters o nanocrystallites (500–600 μm) or dense formations (10–70 μm) situated on the surface of the IOL [222]. Calcification might occur due to environmental circumstances, disruption of the blood-aqueous barrier and changes in the aqueous ambience. However, in some cases no medical or surgical trigger could be determined, and the incidence of calcification was supposedly related to manufacturing issues [223]. Importantly,

**Fig. 3.9** Light
photomicrograph of a
MemoryLens IOL
(CibaVision) explanted
because of calcification.
Original magnification ×40.
Courtesy: Liliana Werner,
MD, PhD, University of
Utah

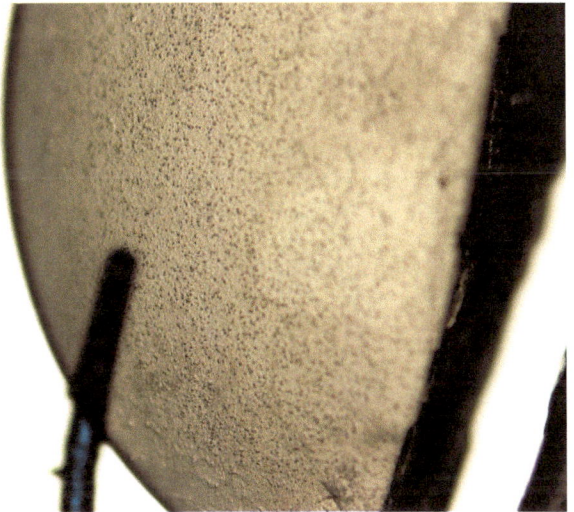

**Fig. 3.9** Light photomicrograph of a MemoryLens IOL (CibaVision) explanted because of calcification. Original magnification ×40. Courtesy: Liliana Werner, MD, PhD, University of Utah

the advancement of IOL opacification commonly is a progressive process, which can develop many years after primary IOL implantation. In several cases calcification results in a decrease in visual acuity and the need for IOL explantation.

## Aphakia Management

There is a wide range of methods used for correcting aphakia. Aphakic glasses and contact lenses have historically been a common way to correct aphakia. These methods, however, have their downsides. Glasses are often heavy and can cause distortion of the image at the edge of the lens. Due to anisometropia glasses cannot be used to correct unilateral aphakia. Contact lenses might be difficult to apply, and extended wear has risks [224].

Surgical options for correcting aphakia in eyes with a present lens capsule include placing the IOL in the bag or in the sulcus. For a small anterior capsule rim tear, small posterior capsule tear or longstanding traumatic tear with fibrosis it is commonly possible to place a lens in the capsule. In eyes with a posterior capsule rupture or zonular dehiscence placing a three-piece IOL with angulated haptics into the sulcus should be considered [225]. One-piece IOLs should not be used for sulcus placement, as they might lead pigment dispersion, uveitis–glaucoma–hyphema syndrome, and recurrent vitreous hemorrhage. Importantly, when placing an IOL anteriorly to the capsular bag it is necessary to slightly reduce the power of the IOL compared to in-the-bag implantation, usually by −0.5 D. In these cases optic capture with the capsulorhexis might be considered. If lacking optic capture, the overall haptic diameter should be sufficiently long to avoid lateral subluxation within the sulcus space. Another option for severe zonular dehiscence is suturing a Cionni capsular tension ring to the sclera.

In eyes with no capsular support inserting an anterior chamber IOL can be considered, as well as iris or scleral fixation. Anterior chamber IOLs primarily had a bad reputation due to development possible development of symptoms such as uveitis, glaucoma or hyphema. With open-loop haptics such complications have been currently minimized, however, a deep anterior chamber is still required. Another option in eyes with a healthy iris and deep anterior chamber is iris fixation. Commonly the iris-claw IOL is placed in the anterior chamber, although fixing such an IOL behind the iris is also possible [226]. In scleral fixation the IOL haptics are fixated to the sclera by a suture, by glue or in a scleral tunnel; such an approach might be required in eyes with poor endothelium or with major loss of the iris. A disadvantage of scleral-fixation methods is the difficulty of the procedure and generating more trauma compared to other procedures. Recently, Yamane et al. proposed a flanged IOL fixation technique [227]. It is based on using diathermy to create a flange from haptics of certain three-piece IOLs, and subsequently pushing them back into scleral tunnels. An advantage of this technique is its simplicity and that it is minimally invasive.

## Conclusions

Modern cataract surgery has become a refractive procedure. Intraoperative and postoperative complications are infrequent. Certain comorbidities increase the complication rate and in these cases preventive measures should be employed. Femtosecond laser-assisted cataract surgery does not provide significant benefits for the patient, particularly if considering the additional costs.

**Acknowledgements** Dr. Grzybowski reports grants, personal fees and non-financial support from Bayer; grants, non-financial support from Novartis; non-financial support from Alcon, personal fees and non-financial support from Valeant, grants and non-financial support from Allergan, grants and non-financial support from Pfizer, grants, and financial support from Santen. Dr. Kanclerz reports non-financial support from Visim. No conflicting relationship exists for any author.

## References

1. Lindstrom R. Thoughts on cataract surgery: 2015. https://www.reviewofophthalmology.com/article/thoughts-on%2D%2Dcataract-surgery-2015. Accessed 22 Oct 2018.
2. Surgical operations and procedures statistics—statistics explained. https://ec.europa.eu/eurostat/statistics-explained/index.php/Surgical_operations_and_procedures_statistics. Accessed 22 Oct 2018.
3. Olson RJ, Braga-Mele R, Chen SH, et al. Cataract in the adult eye preferred practice pattern®. Ophthalmology. 2017;124(2):P1–P119.
4. Chen CL, Clay TH, McLeod S, Chang H-YP, Gelb AW, Dudley RA. A revised estimate of costs associated with routine preoperative testing in medicare cataract patients with a procedure-specific indicator. JAMA Ophthalmol. 2018;136(3):231–8.

5. Schein OD, Katz J, Bass EB, et al. The value of routine preoperative medical testing before cataract surgery. N Engl J Med. 2000;342(3):168–75.
6. Keay L, Lindsley K, Tielsch J, Katz J, Schein O. Routine preoperative medical testing for cataract surgery. Cochrane Database Syst Rev. 2012;(3):CD007293.
7. Grzybowski A, Kanclerz P. Less might be more: are disposable gloves and gowns necessary for cataract surgery? Acta Ophthalmol. 2018;96(7):e896–7. https://doi.org/10.1111/aos.13686.
8. Grover M, McLemore R, Tilburt J. Clinicians report difficulty limiting low-value services in daily practice. J Prim Care Community Health. 2016;7(2):135–8.
9. Brody H. From an ethics of rationing to an ethics of waste avoidance. N Engl J Med. 2012;366(21):1949–51.
10. Chen CL, Lin GA, Bardach NS, et al. Preoperative medical testing in medicare patients undergoing cataract surgery. N Engl J Med. 2015;372(16):1530–8.
11. Gu Q, Dillon CF, Eberhardt MS, Wright JD, Burt VL. Preventive aspirin and other antiplatelet medication use among U.S. adults aged ≥ 40 years: data from the National Health and Nutrition Examination Survey, 2011-2012. Public Health Rep. 2015;130(6):643–54.
12. Grzybowski A, Kupidura-Majewski K, Kupidura P. Controversies in anticoagulant therapy in vitreo-retinal surgery. Curr Pharm Des. 2015;21(32):4661–6.
13. Benzimra JD, Johnston RL, Jaycock P, et al. The Cataract National Dataset electronic multicentre audit of 55 567 operations: antiplatelet and anticoagulant medications. Eye. 2008;23(1):10–6.
14. Grzybowski A, Ascaso FJ, Kupidura-Majewski K, Packer M. Continuation of anticoagulant and antiplatelet therapy during phacoemulsification cataract surgery. Curr Opin Ophthalmol. 2015;26(1):28–33.
15. Visnjić MB, Zrinsćak O, Barisić F, Iveković R, Laus KN, Mandić Z. Astigmatism and diagnostic procedures. Acta Clin Croat. 2012;51(2):285–8.
16. Ambrósio R Jr, Belin MW. Imaging of the cornea: topography vs tomography. J Refract Surg. 2010;26(11):847–9.
17. Nayak BK, Dharwadkar S. Corneal topography and tomography. J Clin Ophthalmol Res. 2015;3(1):45.
18. LaHood BR, Goggin M. Measurement of posterior corneal astigmatism by the IOLMaster 700. J Refract Surg. 2018;34(5):331–6.
19. Rydström E, Westin O, Koskela T, Behndig A. Posterior corneal astigmatism in refractive lens exchange surgery. Acta Ophthalmol. 2016;94(3):295–300.
20. NICE Guideline 77: cataracts in adults: management. https://nice.org.uk/guidance/ng77. Published 26 Oct 2018. Accessed 26 Sept 2018.
21. Haigis W, Lege B, Miller N, Schneider B. Comparison of immersion ultrasound biometry and partial coherence interferometry for intraocular lens calculation according to Haigis. Graefes Arch Clin Exp Ophthalmol. 2000;238(9):765–73.
22. Olsen T. The accuracy of ultrasonic determination of axial length in pseudophakic eyes. Acta Ophthalmol. 1989;67(2):141–4.
23. Rajan MS, Keilhorn I, Bell JA. Partial coherence laser interferometry vs conventional ultrasound biometry in intraocular lens power calculations. Eye. 2002;16(5):552–6.
24. Chakrabarti A, Nazm N. Update on optical biometry and intraocular lens power calculation. TNOA J Ophthalm Sci Res. 2017;55(3):196.
25. Hirnschall N, Varsits R, Doeller B, Findl O. Enhanced penetration for axial length measurement of eyes with dense cataracts using swept source optical coherence tomography: a consecutive observational study. Ophthalmol Ther. 2018;7(1):119–24.
26. Kanclerz P. Optical biometry in a commercially available anterior and posterior segment optical coherence tomography device. Clin Exp Optom. 2019. https://doi.org/10.1111/cxo.12880.
27. Fedorov SN, Kolinko AI, Kolinko AI. [A method of calculating the optical power of the intraocular lens]. Vestn Oftalmol. 1967;80(4):27–31.
28. Siddiqui AA, Devgan U. Mastering lens calculations: new formulas and comparisons. Current Ophthalmology Reports. 2018;6(4):233–6. https://doi.org/10.1007/s40135-018-0186-z.

29. Koch DD, Hill W, Abulafia A, Wang L. Pursuing perfection in intraocular lens calculations: I. Logical approach for classifying IOL calculation formulas. J Cataract Refract Surg. 2017;43(6):717–8.
30. Clarke GP, Burmeister J. Comparison of intraocular lens computations using a neural network versus the Holladay formula. J Cataract Refract Surg. 1997;23(10):1585–9.
31. Alió JL, Grzybowski A, Romaniuk D. Refractive lens exchange in modern practice: when and when not to do it? Eye Vis (Lond). 2014;1:10.
32. Hoffmann PC, Hütz WW. Analysis of biometry and prevalence data for corneal astigmatism in 23 239 eyes. J Cataract Refract Surg. 2010;36(9):1479–85.
33. Potvin R, Berdahl J, Hardten D, Kramer B. Toric intraocular lens orientation and residual refractive astigmatism: an analysis. Clin Ophthalmol. 2016;10:1829–36.
34. Kansal V, Schlenker M, Ahmed IIK. Interocular axial length and corneal power differences as predictors of postoperative refractive outcomes after cataract surgery. Ophthalmology. 2018;125(7):972–81.
35. Oetting TA. Predicting refractive success in the age of more precise measurements. Ophthalmology. 2018;125(7):982–3.
36. Han JV, McGhee CN. When is a complication a complication in contemporary cataract surgery? Clin Exp Ophthalmol. 2018;46(1):7–10.
37. Han JV, Patel DV, Wallace HB, Kim BZ, Sherwin T, McGhee CN. Auckland Cataract Study III: refining preoperative assessment with cataract risk stratification to reduce intraoperative complications. Am J Ophthalmol. 2019;197:114–20. https://doi.org/10.1016/j.ajo.2018.09.026.
38. Ridley H. Intra-ocular acrylic lenses; a recent development in the surgery of cataract. Br J Ophthalmol. 1952;36(3):113–22.
39. Nguyen J, Werner L. Intraocular lenses for cataract surgery. In: Kolb H, Fernandez E, Nelson R, editors. Webvision: the organization of the retina and visual system. Salt Lake City: University of Utah Health Sciences Center; 2017.
40. Ollerton A, Werner L, Strenk S, et al. Pathologic comparison of asymmetric or sulcus fixation of 3-piece intraocular lenses with square versus round anterior optic edges. Ophthalmology. 2013;120(8):1580–7.
41. Grabner G, Ang RE, Vilupuru S. The small-aperture IC-8 intraocular lens: a new concept for added depth of focus in cataract patients. Am J Ophthalmol. 2015;160(6):1176–1184.e1.
42. Mira-Agudelo A, Torres-Sepúlveda W, Barrera JF, et al. Compensation of presbyopia with the light sword lens. Invest Ophthalmol Vis Sci. 2016;57(15):6870–7.
43. Alio JL, Simonov A, Plaza-Puche AB, et al. Visual outcomes and accommodative response of the lumina accommodative intraocular lens. Am J Ophthalmol. 2016;164:37–48.
44. Mamalis N. Adjustable intraocular lens technology. J Cataract Refract Surg. 2014;40(7):1059–60.
45. Werner L, Yeh O, Haymore J, Haugen B, Romaniv N, Mamalis N. Corneal endothelial safety with the irradiation system for light-adjustable intraocular lenses. J Cataract Refract Surg. 2007;33(5):873–8.
46. Hengerer FH, Müller M, Dick HB, Conrad-Hengerer I. Clinical evaluation of macular thickness changes in cataract surgery using a light-adjustable intraocular lens. J Refract Surg. 2016;32(4):250–4.
47. Pohjalainen T, Vesti E, Uusitalo RJ, Laatikainen L. Intraocular pressure after phacoemulsification and intraocular lens implantation in nonglaucomatous eyes with and without exfoliation. J Cataract Refract Surg. 2001;27(3):426–31.
48. Shingleton BJ, Gamell LS, O'Donoghue MW, Baylus SL, King R. Long-term changes in intraocular pressure after clear corneal phacoemulsification: normal patients versus glaucoma suspect and glaucoma patients. J Cataract Refract Surg. 1999;25(7):885–90.
49. Poley BJ, Lindstrom RL, Samuelson TW, Schulze R Jr. Intraocular pressure reduction after phacoemulsification with intraocular lens implantation in glaucomatous and nonglaucomatous eyes: evaluation of a causal relationship between the natural lens and open-angle glaucoma. J Cataract Refract Surg. 2009;35(11):1946–55.

50. Kim JH, Rabiolo A, Morales E, et al. Cataract surgery and rate of visual field progression in primary open-angle glaucoma. Am J Ophthalmol. 2019;201:19–30. https://doi.org/10.1016/j.ajo.2019.01.019.
51. Budenz DL, Gedde SJ. New options for combined cataract and glaucoma surgery. Curr Opin Ophthalmol. 2014;25(2):141–7.
52. Wand M, Gaudio AR, Bruce Shields M. Latanoprost and cystoid macular edema in high-risk aphakic or pseudophakic eyes. J Cataract Refract Surg. 2001;27(9):1397–401.
53. Lima MC, Paranhos A Jr, Salim S, et al. Visually significant cystoid macular edema in pseudophakic and aphakic patients with glaucoma receiving latanoprost. J Glaucoma. 2000;9(4):317–21.
54. Miyake K, Ibaraki N, Goto Y, et al. ESCRS Binkhorst lecture 2002: pseudophakic preservative maculopathy. J Cataract Refract Surg. 2003;29(9):1800–10.
55. Henderson BA, Kim JY, Ament CS, Ferrufino-Ponce ZK, Grabowska A, Cremers SL. Clinical pseudophakic cystoid macular edema. J Cataract Refract Surg. 2007;33(9):1550–8.
56. Klein R, Klein BEK, Wong TY, Tomany SC, Cruickshanks KJ. The association of cataract and cataract surgery with the long-term incidence of age-related maculopathy: the Beaver Dam eye study. Arch Ophthalmol. 2002;120(11):1551–8.
57. Cugati S, Mitchell P, Rochtchina E, Tan AG, Smith W, Wang JJ. Cataract surgery and the 10-year incidence of age-related maculopathy: the Blue Mountains Eye Study. Ophthalmology. 2006;113(11):2020–5.
58. Wang JJ, Klein R, Smith W, Klein BEK, Tomany S, Mitchell P. Cataract surgery and the 5-year incidence of late-stage age-related maculopathy: pooled findings from the Beaver Dam and Blue Mountains eye studies. Ophthalmology. 2003;110(10):1960–7.
59. Ho L, Boekhoorn SS, Liana, et al. Cataract surgery and the risk of aging macula disorder: the Rotterdam study. Invest Ophthalmol Vis Sci. 2008;49(11):4795–800.
60. Buch H, Vinding T, La Cour M, Jensen GB, Prause JU, Nielsen NV. Risk factors for age-related maculopathy in a 14-year follow-up study: the Copenhagen City Eye Study. Acta Ophthalmol Scand. 2005;83(4):409–18.
61. Chew EY, Sperduto RD, Milton RC, et al. Risk of advanced age-related macular degeneration after cataract surgery in the Age-Related Eye Disease Study: AREDS report 25. Ophthalmology. 2009;116(2):297–303.
62. Age-Related Eye Disease Study 2 Research Group, Huynh N, Nicholson BP, et al. Visual acuity after cataract surgery in patients with age-related macular degeneration: age-related eye disease study 2 report number 5. Ophthalmology. 2014;121(6):1229–36.
63. Dong LM, Stark WJ, Jefferys JL, et al. Progression of age-related macular degeneration after cataract surgery. Arch Ophthalmol. 2009;127(11):1412–9.
64. Casparis H, Lindsley K, Kuo IC, Sikder S, Bressler NM. Surgery for cataracts in people with age-related macular degeneration. Cochrane Database Syst Rev. 2017;(2):CD006757.
65. Kernt M, Walch A, Neubauer AS, et al. Filtering blue light reduces light-induced oxidative stress, senescence and accumulation of extracellular matrix proteins in human retinal pigment epithelium cells. Clin Exp Ophthalmol. 2012;40(1):e87–97.
66. Mainster MA, Turner PL. Blue-blocking IOLs decrease photoreception without providing significant photoprotection. Surv Ophthalmol. 2010;55(3):272–89.
67. Grzybowski A, Wasinska-Borowiec W, Alio JL, Amat-Peral P, Tabernero J. Intraocular lenses in age-related macular degeneration. Graefes Arch Clin Exp Ophthalmol. 2017;255(9):1687–96.
68. Grzybowski A, Wasińska-Borowiec W. Fresnel prism intraocular lens and scharioth macula lens. Surv Ophthalmol. 2018;63(1):132.
69. Lee AY, Day AC, Egan C et al. Previous Intravitreal Therapy is Associated with Increased Risk of Posterior Capsule Rupture during Cataract Surgery. Ophthalmology 2016;123(6):1252–6.
70. Jackson TL, Donachie PHJ, Sparrow JM, Johnston RL. United Kingdom National Ophthalmology Database study of vitreoretinal surgery: report 2, macular hole. Ophthalmology. 2013;120(3):629–34.

71. Yee KMP, Tan S, Lesnik Oberstein SY, et al. Incidence of cataract surgery after vitrectomy for vitreous opacities. Ophthalmol Retina. 2017;1(2):154–7.
72. Biró Z, Kovacs B. Results of cataract surgery in previously vitrectomized eyes. J Cataract Refract Surg. 2002;28(6):1003–6.
73. Elhousseini Z, Lee E, Williamson TH. Incidence of lens touch during pars plana vitrectomy and outcomes from subsequent cataract surgery. Retina. 2016;36(4):825–9.
74. Smiddy WE, Stark WJ, Michels RG, Edward Maumenee A, Terry AC, Glaser BM. Cataract extraction after vitrectomy. Ophthalmology. 1987;94(5):483–7.
75. McDermott ML, Puklin JE, Abrams GW, Eliott D. Phacoemulsification for cataract following pars plana vitrectomy. Ophthalmic Surg Lasers. 1997;28(7):558–64.
76. Grusha YO, Masket S, Miller KM. Phacoemulsification and lens implantation after pars plana vitrectomy. Ophthalmology. 1998;105(2):287–94.
77. Lacalle VD, Gárate FJO, Alday NM, Garrido JAL, Agesta JA. Phacoemulsification cataract surgery in vitrectomized eyes. J Cataract Refract Surg. 1998;24(6):806–9.
78. Tandogan T, Khoramnia R, Auffarth GU, Koss MJ, Choi CY. In vivo imaging of intraocular fluidics in vitrectomized swine eyes using a digital fluoroscopy system. J Ophthalmol. 2016;2016:9695165.
79. Javadi M-A, Feizi S, Moein H-R. Simultaneous penetrating keratoplasty and cataract surgery. J Ophthalmic Vis Res. 2013;8(1):39–46.
80. Kiire CA, Mukherjee R, Ruparelia N, Keeling D, Prendergast B, Norris JH. Managing anti-platelet and anticoagulant drugs in patients undergoing elective ophthalmic surgery. Br J Ophthalmol. 2014;98(10):1320–4.
81. Friedman DS, Jampel HD, Lubomski LH, et al. Surgical strategies for coexisting glaucoma and cataract: an evidence-based update. Ophthalmology. 2002;109(10):1902–13.
82. Zhang ML, Hirunyachote P, Jampel H. Combined surgery versus cataract surgery alone for eyes with cataract and glaucoma. Cochrane Database Syst Rev. 2015;(7):CD008671.
83. Longo A, Uva MG, Reibaldi A, Avitabile T, Reibaldi M. Long-term effect of phacoemulsification on trabeculectomy function. Eye. 2015;29(10):1347–52.
84. Nguyen DQ, Niyadurupola N, Tapp RJ, O'Connell RA, Coote MA, Crowston JG. Effect of phacoemulsification on trabeculectomy function. Clin Exp Ophthalmol. 2014;42(5):433–9.
85. Creuzot-Garcher CP, Mariet AS, Benzenine E, et al. Is combined cataract surgery associated with acute postoperative endophthalmitis? A nationwide study from 2005 to 2014. Br J Ophthalmol. 2019;103(4):534–8.
86. Lawrence D, Fedorowicz Z, van Zuuren EJ. Day care versus in-patient surgery for age-related cataract. Cochrane Database Syst Rev. 2015;(11):CD004242.
87. Ianchulev T, Litoff D, Ellinger D, Stiverson K, Packer M. Office-based cataract surgery: population health outcomes study of more than 21 000 cases in the United States. Ophthalmology. 2016;123(4):723–8.
88. Koolwijk J, Fick M, Selles C, et al. Outpatient cataract surgery: incident and procedural risk analysis do not support current clinical ophthalmology guidelines. Ophthalmology. 2015;122(2):281–7.
89. Baeza M, Martinez-Toldos JJ. Anesthesia. In: Martinez-Toldos JJ, Hoyos JE, editors. Step by step: vitrectomy. JP Medical Ltd; 2013. p. 28–42.
90. Alhassan MB, Kyari F, Ejere HOD. Peribulbar versus retrobulbar anaesthesia for cataract surgery. Cochrane Database Syst Rev. 2015;(7):CD004083.
91. Apil A, Kartal B, Ekinci M, et al. Topical anesthesia for cataract surgery: the patients' perspective. Pain Res Treat. 2014;2014:827659.
92. Grzybowski A, Kanclerz P. Acute and chronic fluid misdirection syndrome: pathophysiology and treatment. Graefes Arch Clin Exp Ophthalmol. 2018;256(1):135–54.
93. Gogate P, Wood M. Recognising "high-risk" eyes before cataract surgery. Community Eye Health. 2008;21(65):12–4.
94. Grzybowski A, Wasinska-Borowiec W, Claoué C. Pros and cons of immediately sequential bilateral cataract surgery (ISBCS). Saudi J Ophthalmol. 2016;30(4):244–9.

95. Arshinoff SA, Partner D, York Finch Eye Associates, et al. Immediately sequential bilateral cataract surgery—a global perspective. US Ophthalm Rev. 2015;8(1):14.
96. Singh R, Dohlman TH, Sun G. Immediately sequential bilateral cataract surgery: advantages and disadvantages. Curr Opin Ophthalmol. 2017;28(1):81–6.
97. Nassiri N, Nassiri N, Sadeghi Yarandi SH, Rahnavardi M. Immediate vs delayed sequential cataract surgery: a comparative study. Eye. 2009;23(1):89–95.
98. Grzybowski A, Krzyżanowska-Berkowska P. Immediate sequential bilateral cataract surgery: who might benefit from the procedure? J Cataract Refract Surg. 2013;39(7):1119–20.
99. Sharp S. A description of a new method of opening the cornea, in order to extract the crystalline humour; By Mr. Samuel Sharp, Surgeon to Guy's Hospital, and F. R. S. Philos Trans R Soc Lond. 1753;48:161–3.
100. Barraquer J, Boberg-Ans J. Cataract surgery. Br J Ophthalmol. 1959;43(2):69–77.
101. Hill HF, Barraquer J. Some aspects of the use of enzymatic zonulolysis∗. Am J Ophthalmol. 1962;54(1):89–95.
102. Smith H. The Barraquer operation for cataract. Br J Ophthalmol. 1921;5(12):552–3.
103. Krwawicz T. Intracapsular extraction of intumescent cataract by application of low temperature. Br J Ophthalmol. 1961;45(4):279–83.
104. Cataract surgery with intracapsular cataract extraction and spectacles. Surv Ophthalmol. 2000;45:S45–52.
105. Lois M. Mémoires de L'Académie Royale de Chirurgie. Paris: Théophile Barrois Lejeune; 1787.
106. Grzybowski A, Ascaso FJ. Sushruta in 600 B.C. introduced extraocular expulsion of lens material. Acta Ophthalmol. 2014;92(2):194–7.
107. Haldipurkar SS, Shikari HT, Gokhale V. Wound construction in manual small incision cataract surgery. Indian J Ophthalmol. 2009;57(1):9–13.
108. Blumenthal M, Ashkenazi I, Assia E, Cahane M. Small-incision manual extracapsular cataract extraction using selective hydrodissection. Ophthalmic Surg. 1992;23(10):699–701.
109. Riaz Y, de Silva SR, Evans JR. Manual small incision cataract surgery (MSICS) with posterior chamber intraocular lens versus phacoemulsification with posterior chamber intraocular lens for age-related cataract. Cochrane Database Syst Rev. 2013;(10):CD008813.
110. Venkatesh R, Tan CSH, Sengupta S, Ravindran RD, Krishnan KT, Chang DF. Phacoemulsification versus manual small-incision cataract surgery for white cataract. J Cataract Refract Surg. 2010;36(11):1849–54.
111. McDonnell PJ, Patel A, Green WR. Comparison of intracapsular and extracapsular cataract surgery. Ophthalmology. 1985;92(9):1208–25.
112. Kelman CD. Phaco-emulsification and aspiration. Am J Ophthalmol. 1967;64(1):23–35.
113. Linebarger EJ, Hardten DR, Shah GK, Lindstrom RL. Phacoemulsification and modern cataract surgery. Surv Ophthalmol. 1999;44(2):123–47.
114. Nagy Z, Takacs A, Filkorn T, Sarayba M. Initial clinical evaluation of an intraocular femtosecond laser in cataract surgery. J Refract Surg. 2009;25(12):1053–60.
115. Fan W, Yan H, Zhang G. Femtosecond laser-assisted cataract surgery in Fuchs endothelial corneal dystrophy: long-term outcomes. J Cataract Refract Surg. 2018;44(7):864–70.
116. Zhu DC, Shah P, Feuer WJ, Shi W, Koo EH. Outcomes of conventional phacoemulsification versus femtosecond laser-assisted cataract surgery in eyes with Fuchs endothelial corneal dystrophy. J Cataract Refract Surg. 2018;44(5):534–40.
117. Abell RG, Vote BJ. Cost-effectiveness of femtosecond laser-assisted cataract surgery versus phacoemulsification cataract surgery. Ophthalmology. 2014;121(1):10–6.
118. Ewe SYP, Oakley CL, Abell RG, Allen PL, Vote BJ. Cystoid macular edema after femtosecond laser-assisted versus phacoemulsification cataract surgery. J Cataract Refract Surg. 2015;41(11):2373–8.
119. Schultz T, Joachim SC, Stellbogen M, Dick HB. Prostaglandin release during femtosecond laser-assisted cataract surgery: main inducer. J Refract Surg. 2015;31(2):78–81.

120. Jun JH, Yoo Y-S, Lim SA, Joo C-K. Effects of topical ketorolac tromethamine 0.45% on intraoperative miosis and prostaglandin E release during femtosecond laser-assisted cataract surgery. J Cataract Refract Surg. 2017;43(4):492–7.
121. Day AC, Gore DM, Bunce C, Evans JR. Laser-assisted cataract surgery versus standard ultrasound phacoemulsification cataract surgery. Cochrane Database Syst Rev. 2016;(7):CD010735.
122. Alió JL, Klonowski P, El Kady B. Microincisional lens surgery. In: Essentials in ophthalmology. p. 11–26.
123. Alio JL, Grzybowski A, El Aswad A, Romaniuk D. Refractive lens exchange. Surv Ophthalmol. 2014;59(6):579–98.
124. Olsen T, Dam-Johansen M, Bek T, Hjortdal JO. Corneal versus scleral tunnel incision in cataract surgery: a randomized study. J Cataract Refract Surg. 1997;23(3):337–41.
125. Park HJ, Kwon YH, Weitzman M, Caprioli J. Temporal corneal phacoemulsification in patients with filtered glaucoma. Arch Ophthalmol. 1997;115(11):1375–80.
126. Ernest P, Hill W, Potvin R. Minimizing surgically induced astigmatism at the time of cataract surgery using a square posterior limbal incision. J Ophthalmol. 2011;2011:243170.
127. Yoon JH, Kim K-H, Lee JY, Nam DH. Surgically induced astigmatism after 3.0 mm temporal and nasal clear corneal incisions in bilateral cataract surgery. Indian J Ophthalmol. 2014;62(6):753.
128. Pakravan M, Nikkhah H, Yazdani S, Shahabi C, Sedigh-Rahimabadi M. Astigmatic outcomes of temporal versus nasal clear corneal phacoemulsification. J Ophthalmic Vis Res. 2009;4(2):79–83.
129. Sugar A, Schertzer RM. Clinical course of phacoemulsification wound burns. J Cataract Refract Surg. 1999;25(5):688–92.
130. Syed ZA, Moayedi J, Mohamedi M, et al. Cataract surgery outcomes at a UK independent sector treatment centre. Br J Ophthalmol. 2015;99(11):1460–5.
131. Chan E, Mahroo OAR, Spalton DJ. Complications of cataract surgery. Clin Exp Optom. 2010;93(6):379–89.
132. Osher RH, Yu BC, Koch DD. Posterior polar cataracts: a predisposition to intraoperative posterior capsular rupture. J Cataract Refract Surg. 1990;16(2):157–62.
133. Masket S, Belani S. Combined preoperative topical atropine sulfate 1% and intracameral nonpreserved epinephrine hydrochloride 1:4000 [corrected] for management of intraoperative floppy-iris syndrome. J Cataract Refract Surg. 2007;33(4):580–2.
134. Nikeghbali A, Falavarjani KG, Kheirkhah A. Pupil dilation with intracameral lidocaine during phacoemulsification: benefits for the patient and surgeon. Indian J Ophthalmol. 2008;56(1):63–4.
135. Nikeghbali A, Falavarjani KG, Kheirkhah A, Bakhtiari P, Kashkouli MB. Pupil dilation with intracameral lidocaine during phacoemulsification. J Cataract Refract Surg. 2007;33(1):101–3.
136. Chang DF, Braga-Mele R, Mamalis N, et al. ASCRS White Paper: clinical review of intraoperative floppy-iris syndrome. J Cataract Refract Surg. 2008;34(12):2153–62.
137. Palea S, Chang DF, Rekik M, Regnier A, Lluel P. Comparative effect of alfuzosin and tamsulosin on the contractile response of isolated rabbit prostatic and iris dilator smooth muscles. J Cataract Refract Surg. 2008;34(3):489–96.
138. Chang DF, Osher RH, Wang L, Koch DD. Prospective multicenter evaluation of cataract surgery in patients taking tamsulosin (Flomax). Ophthalmology. 2007;114(5):957–64.
139. Flach AJ. Intraoperative floppy iris syndrome: pathophysiology, prevention, and treatment. Trans Am Ophthalmol Soc. 2009;107:234–9.
140. Schlötzer-Schrehardt U, Naumann GO. A histopathologic study of zonular instability in pseudoexfoliation syndrome. Am J Ophthalmol. 1994;118(6):730–43.
141. Schwartz SG, Holz ER, Mieler WF, Kuhl DP. Retained lens fragments in resident-performed cataract extractions. CLAO J. 2002;28(1):44–7.

142. Garg SJ, Lane RG. Pars plana torsional phacoemulsification for removal of retained lens material during pars plana vitrectomy. Retina. 2011;31(4):804–5.
143. Stewart MW. Managing retained lens fragments: raising the bar. Am J Ophthalmol. 2009;147(4):569–70.
144. Stewart MW. Management of retained lens fragments: can we improve? Am J Ophthalmol. 2007;144(3):445–6.
145. Ho LY, Doft BH, Wang L, Bunker CH. Clinical predictors and outcomes of pars plana vitrectomy for retained lens material after cataract extraction. Am J Ophthalmol. 2009;147(4):587–594.e1.
146. Wilkinson CP, Green WR. Vitrectomy for retained lens material after cataract extraction: the relationship between histopathologic findings and the time of vitreous surgery. Ophthalmology. 2001;108(9):1633–7.
147. Merani R, Hunyor AP, Playfair TJ, et al. Pars plana vitrectomy for the management of retained lens material after cataract surgery. Am J Ophthalmol. 2007;144(3):364–70.
148. Scott IU, Flynn HW Jr, Smiddy WE, et al. Clinical features and outcomes of pars plana vitrectomy in patients with retained lens fragments. Ophthalmology. 2003;110(8):1567–72.
149. Peck T, Park J, Bajwa A, Shildkrot Y. Timing of vitrectomy for retained lens fragments after cataract surgery. Int Ophthalmol. 2018;38(6):2699–707. https://doi.org/10.1007/s10792-017-0719-8.
150. Gupta R, Ram J, Sukhija J, Singh R. Outcome of paediatric cataract surgery with primary posterior capsulotomy and anterior vitrectomy using intra-operative preservative-free triamcinolone acetonide. Acta Ophthalmol. 2014;92(5):e358–61.
151. Sato S, Inoue M, Kobayashi S, Watanabe Y, Kadonosono K. Primary posterior capsulotomy using a 25-gauge vitreous cutter in vitrectomy combined with cataract surgery. J Cataract Refract Surg. 2010;36(1):2–5.
152. Al-Nashar HY, Khalil AS. Primary posterior capsulotomy in adults with posterior capsule opacification. J Cataract Refract Surg. 2016;42(11):1615–9.
153. Mohamed TA, Soliman W, El Sebaity DM, Fathalla AM. Refractive lens exchange combined with primary posterior vitrectorhexis in highly myopic patients. J Ophthalmol. 2017;2017:7826735.
154. Lindstrom RL, Galloway MS, Grzybowski A, Liegner JT. Dropless cataract surgery: an overview. Curr Pharm Des. 2017;23(4):558–64.
155. An JA, Kasner O, Samek DA, Lévesque V. Evaluation of eyedrop administration by inexperienced patients after cataract surgery. J Cataract Refract Surg. 2014;40(11):1857–61.
156. Greenberg PB, Tseng VL, Wu W-C, et al. Prevalence and predictors of ocular complications associated with cataract surgery in United States veterans. Ophthalmology. 2011;118(3):507–14.
157. Jaycock P, Johnston RL, Taylor H, et al. The Cataract National Dataset electronic multi-centre audit of 55 567 operations: updating benchmark standards of care in the United Kingdom and internationally. Eye. 2007;23(1):38–49.
158. Kessel L, Andresen J, Erngaard D, Flesner P, Tendal B, Hjortdal J. Safety of deferring review after uneventful cataract surgery until 2 weeks postoperatively. J Cataract Refract Surg. 2015;41(12):2755–64.
159. Tan P, Foo FY, Teoh SC, Wong HT. Evaluation of the use of a nurse-administered telephone questionnaire for post-operative cataract surgery review. Int J Health Care Qual Assur. 2014;27(4):347–54.
160. Tufail A, Foss AJ, Hamilton AM. Is the first day postoperative review necessary after cataract extraction? Br J Ophthalmol. 1995;79(7):646–8.
161. Eloranta H, Falck A. Is an ophthalmic check-up needed after uneventful cataract surgery? A large retrospective comparative cohort study of Finnish patients. Acta Ophthalmol. 2017;95(7):665–70. https://doi.org/10.1111/aos.13373.
162. Grzybowski A, Kanclerz P. Do we need day-1 postoperative follow-up after cataract surgery. Graefes Arch Clin Exp Ophthalmol. 2019;257(5):855–61.

163. The Royal College of Ophthalmologists. Commissioning guide: cataract surgery. https://www.rcophth.ac.uk/wp-content/uploads/2015/03/Commissioning-Guide-Cataract-Surgery-Final-February-2015.pdf. Published Feb 2015. Accessed 20 Oct 2017.
164. Tsangaridou M-A, Grzybowski A, Gundlach E, Pleyer U. Controversies in NSAIDs use in cataract surgery. Curr Pharm Des. 2015;21(32):4707–17.
165. Grzybowski A, Adamiec-Mroczek J. Topical nonsteroidal anti-inflammatory drugs for cystoid macular edema prevention in patients with diabetic retinopathy. Am J Ophthalmol. 2017;181:xiv–vi.
166. Modi SS, Lehmann RP, Walters TR, et al. Once-daily nepafenac ophthalmic suspension 0.3% to prevent and treat ocular inflammation and pain after cataract surgery: phase 3 study. J Cataract Refract Surg. 2014;40(2):203–11.
167. Singh R, Alpern L, Jaffe GJ, et al. Evaluation of nepafenac in prevention of macular edema following cataract surgery in patients with diabetic retinopathy. Clin Ophthalmol. 2012;6:1259–69.
168. Grzybowski A, Kanclerz P. Pseudophakic macular edema in primary open-angle glaucoma: a prospective study using spectral-domain optical coherence tomography. Am J Ophthalmol. 2017;181:181.
169. Sengupta S, Vasavada D, Pan U, Sindal M. Factors predicting response of pseudophakic cystoid macular edema to topical steroids and nepafenac. Indian J Ophthalmol. 2018;66(6):827–30.
170. Kakkassery V, Schultz T, Wunderlich MI, Schargus M, Dick HB, Rehrmann J. Evaluation of predictive factors for successful intravitreal dexamethasone in pseudophakic cystoid macular edema. J Ophthalmol. 2017;2017:4625730.
171. Apple DJ, Solomon KD, Tetz MR, et al. Posterior capsule opacification. Surv Ophthalmol. 1992;37(2):73–116.
172. Colin J, Robinet A, Cochener B. Retinal detachment after clear lens extraction for high myopia: seven-year follow-up. Ophthalmology. 1999;106(12):2281–4; discussion 2285.
173. Fernández-Vega L, Alfonso JF, Villacampa T. Clear lens extraction for the correction of high myopia. Ophthalmology. 2003;110(12):2349–54.
174. Awasthi N, Guo S, Wagner BJ. Posterior capsular opacification: a problem reduced but not yet eradicated. Arch Ophthalmol. 2009;127(4):555–62.
175. Werner L. Biocompatibility of intraocular lens materials. Curr Opin Ophthalmol. 2008;19(1):41–9.
176. Olsen G, Olson RJ. Update on a long-term, prospective study of capsulotomy and retinal detachment rates after cataract surgery. J Cataract Refract Surg. 2000;26(7):1017–21.
177. Pandey SK, Apple DJ, Werner L, Maloof AJ, Milverton EJ. Posterior capsule opacification: a review of the aetiopathogenesis, experimental and clinical studies and factors for prevention. Indian J Ophthalmol. 2004;52(2):99–112.
178. Grzybowski A, Kanclerz P. Does Nd:YAG capsulotomy increase the risk of retinal detachment? Asia Pac J Ophthalmol (Phila). 2018;7(5):339–44. https://doi.org/10.22608/APO.2018275.
179. Grzybowski A, Turczynowska M, Kuhn F. The treatment of postoperative endophthalmitis: should we still follow the endophthalmitis vitrectomy study more than two decades after its publication? Acta Ophthalmol. 2018;96(5):e651–4.
180. Inoue T, Uno T, Usui N, et al. Incidence of endophthalmitis and the perioperative practices of cataract surgery in Japan: Japanese Prospective Multicenter Study for Postoperative Endophthalmitis after Cataract Surgery. Jpn J Ophthalmol. 2018;62(1):24–30.
181. Flynn HW, Batra NR, Schwartz SG, Grzybowski A. Differential diagnosis of endophthalmitis. In: Flynn HW, Batra NR, Schwartz SG, Grzybowski A, editors. Endophthalmitis in clinical practice. Cham: Springer International Publishing AG; 2018. p. 19–40.
182. Endophthalmitis Vitrectomy Study Group. Results of the endophthalmitis vitrectomy study. Arch Ophthalmol. 1995;113(12):1479–96.

183. Arslan OS, Tunc Z, Ucar D, et al. Histologic findings of corneal buttons in decompensated corneas with toxic anterior segment syndrome after cataract surgery. Cornea. 2013;32(10):1387–90.
184. Suzuki T, Ohashi Y, Oshika T, et al. Outbreak of late-onset toxic anterior segment syndrome after implantation of one-piece intraocular lenses. Am J Ophthalmol. 2015;159(5):934–939. e2.
185. Oshika T, Eguchi S, Goto H, Ohashi Y. Outbreak of subacute-onset toxic anterior segment syndrome associated with single-piece acrylic intraocular lenses. Ophthalmology. 2017;124(4):519–23.
186. Sorenson AL, Sorenson RL, Evans DJ. Toxic anterior segment syndrome caused by autoclave reservoir wall biofilms and their residual toxins. J Cataract Refract Surg. 2016;42(11):1602–14.
187. Miyake G, Ota I, Miyake K, Zako M, Iwaki M, Shibuya A. Late-onset toxic anterior segment syndrome. J Cataract Refract Surg. 2015;41(3):666–9.
188. Results of the endophthalmitis vitrectomy study. Arch Ophthalmol. 1995;113(12):1479.
189. Grzybowski A, Kuklo P, Pieczynski J, Beiko G. A review of preoperative manoeuvres for prophylaxis of endophthalmitis in intraocular surgery: topical application of antibiotics, disinfectants, or both? Curr Opin Ophthalmol. 2016;27(1):9–23.
190. Kuklo P, Grzybowski A, Schwartz SG, Flynn HW, Pathengay A. Hot topics in perioperative antibiotics for cataract surgery. Curr Pharm Des. 2017;23(4):551–7.
191. George NK, Stewart MW. The routine use of intracameral antibiotics to prevent endophthalmitis after cataract surgery: how good is the evidence? Ophthalmol Therapy. 2018;7(2):233–45. https://doi.org/10.1007/s40123-018-0138-6.
192. Endophthalmitis Study Group, European Society of Cataract & Refractive Surgeons. Prophylaxis of postoperative endophthalmitis following cataract surgery: results of the ESCRS multicenter study and identification of risk factors. J Cataract Refract Surg. 2007;33(6):978–88.
193. Grzybowski A, Kanclerz P, Myers WG. The use of povidone-iodine in ophthalmology. Curr Opin Ophthalmol. 2018;29(1):19–32.
194. Ahmed IIK, Kranemann C, Chipman M, Malam F. Revisiting early postoperative follow-up after phacoemulsification. J Cataract Refract Surg. 2002;28(1):100–8.
195. Laurell CG, Wickström K, Zetterström C, Lundgren B. Inflammatory response after endocapsular phacoemulsification or conventional extracapsular lens extraction in the rabbit eye. Acta Ophthalmol Scand. 1997;75(4):401–4.
196. Grzybowski A, Kanclerz P. Early postoperative intraocular pressure elevation following cataract surgery. Curr Opin Ophthalmol. 2019;30(1):56–62.
197. Oshika T, Okamoto F, Kaji Y, et al. Retention and removal of a new viscous dispersive ophthalmic viscosurgical device during cataract surgery in animal eyes. Br J Ophthalmol. 2006;90(4):485–7.
198. Kohnen T, von Ehr M, Schütte E, Koch DD. Evaluation of intraocular pressure with Healon and Healon GV in sutureless cataract surgery with foldable lens implantation. J Cataract Refract Surg. 1996;22(2):227–37.
199. Rainer G, Menapace R, Findl O, Petternel V, Kiss B, Georgopoulos M. Effect of topical brimonidine on intraocular pressure after small incision cataract surgery. J Cataract Refract Surg. 2001;27(8):1227–31.
200. Bömer TG, Lagrèze WD, Funk J. Intraocular pressure rise after phacoemulsification with posterior chamber lens implantation: effect of prophylactic medication, wound closure, and surgeon's experience. Br J Ophthalmol. 1995;79(9):809–13.
201. Jarstad JS, Jarstad AR, Chung GW, Tester RA, Day LE. Immediate postoperative intraocular pressure adjustment reduces risk of cystoid macular edema after uncomplicated micro incision coaxial phacoemulsification cataract surgery. Korean J Ophthalmol. 2017;31(1):39–43.
202. Rhee DJ, Deramo VA, Connolly BP, Blecher MH. Intraocular pressure trends after supranormal pressurization to aid closure of sutureless cataract wounds. J Cataract Refract Surg. 1999;25(4):546–9.

203. Elfersy AJ, Prinzi RA, Peracha ZH, et al. IOP elevation after cataract surgery: results for residents and senior staff at henry ford health system. J Glaucoma. 2016;25(10):802–6.
204. Yasutani H, Hayashi K, Hayashi H, Hayashi F. Intraocular pressure rise after phacoemulsification surgery in glaucoma patients. J Cataract Refract Surg. 2004;30(6):1219–24.
205. Slabaugh MA, Bojikian KD, Moore DB, Chen PP. Risk factors for acute postoperative intraocular pressure elevation after phacoemulsification in glaucoma patients. J Cataract Refract Surg. 2014;40(4):538–44.
206. Cho YK. Early intraocular pressure and anterior chamber depth changes after phacoemulsification and intraocular lens implantation in nonglaucomatous eyes. Comparison of groups stratified by axial length. J Cataract Refract Surg. 2008;34(7):1104–9.
207. Bonnell LN, SooHoo JR, Seibold LK, et al. One-day postoperative intraocular pressure spikes after phacoemulsification cataract surgery in patients taking tamsulosin. J Cataract Refract Surg. 2016;42(12):1753–8.
208. Chang DF, Tan JJ, Tripodis Y. Risk factors for steroid response among cataract patients. J Cataract Refract Surg. 2011;37(4):675–81.
209. O'Brien PD, Ho SL, Fitzpatrick P, Power W. Risk factors for a postoperative intraocular pressure spike after phacoemulsification. Can J Ophthalmol. 2007;42(1):51–5.
210. Łabuz G, Knebel D, Auffarth GU, et al. Glistening formation and light scattering in six hydrophobic-acrylic intraocular lenses. Am J Ophthalmol. 2018;196:112–20. https://doi.org/10.1016/j.ajo.2018.08.032.
211. Colin J, Orignac I, Touboul D. Glistenings in a large series of hydrophobic acrylic intraocular lenses. J Cataract Refract Surg. 2009;35(12):2121–6.
212. Łabuz G, Reus NJ, van den Berg TJTP. Straylight from glistenings in intraocular lenses: in vitro study. J Cataract Refract Surg. 2017;43(1):102–8.
213. van der Mooren M, Franssen L, Piers P. Effects of glistenings in intraocular lenses. Biomed Opt Express. 2013;4(8):1294–304.
214. Matsushima H, Nagata M, Katsuki Y, et al. Decreased visual acuity resulting from glistening and sub-surface nano-glistening formation in intraocular lenses: a retrospective analysis of 5 cases. Saudi J Ophthalmol. 2015;29(4):259–63.
215. Beiko GH, Grzybowski A. Glistenings in hydrophobic acrylic intraocular lenses do affect visual function. Clin Ophthalmol. 2013;7:2271–4.
216. Luo F, Bao X, Qin Y, Hou M, Wu M. Subjective visual performance and objective optical quality with intraocular lens glistening and surface light scattering. J Refract Surg. 2018;34(6):372–8.
217. Beiko GH. A pilot study to determine if intraocular lens choice at the time of cataract surgery has an impact on patient-reported driving habits. Clin Ophthalmol. 2015;9:1573–9.
218. Beiko GH, Gostimir M, Haj-Ahmad L. A comparison of mesopic visual acuity and objective visual quality following cataract surgery with hydrophobic acrylic intraocular lenses. Clin Ophthalmol. 2017;11:641–6.
219. Schweitzer C, Orignac I, Praud D, Chatoux O, Colin J. Glistening in glaucomatous eyes: visual performances and risk factors. Acta Ophthalmol. 2014;92(6):529–34.
220. Müllner-Eidenböck A, Amon M, Moser E, et al. Morphological and functional results of AcrySof intraocular lens implantation in children: prospective randomized study of age-related surgical management. J Cataract Refract Surg. 2003;29(2):285–93.
221. Hidaka Y, Negishi K, Matsushima H, et al. [A case of impaired vision due to glistening and whitening of hydrophobic acrylic intraocular lens]. Rinsho Ganka. 2013;67:199–202.
222. Gartaganis SP, Prahs P, Lazari ED, Gartaganis PS, Helbig H, Koutsoukos PG. Calcification of hydrophilic acrylic intraocular lenses with a hydrophobic surface: laboratory analysis of 6 cases. Am J Ophthalmol. 2016;168:68–77.
223. Gurabardhi M, Häberle H, Aurich H, Werner L, Pham D-T. Serial intraocular lens opacifications of different designs from the same manufacturer: clinical and light microscopic results of 71 explant cases. J Cataract Refract Surg. 2018;44(11):1326–32.
224. Mathers WD, Fraunfelder FW, Rich LF. Risk of Lasik surgery vs contact lenses. Arch Ophthalmol. 2006;124(10):1510–1.

225. Grzybowski A, Kanclerz P. Clarifying the methods of fixation of intraocular lenses. Clin Anat. 2017;31(1):2–3.
226. De Silva SR, Arun K, Anandan M, Glover N, Patel CK, Rosen P. Iris-claw intraocular lenses to correct aphakia in the absence of capsule support. J Cataract Refract Surg. 2011;37(9):1667–72.
227. Yamane S, Sato S, Maruyama-Inoue M, Kadonosono K. Flanged intrascleral intraocular lens fixation with double-needle technique. Ophthalmology. 2017;124(8):1136–42.

# Chapter 4
# Recent Developments in Glaucoma

Nathan M. Kerr and Keith Barton

## Introduction

Glaucoma is one of the most commonly encountered ophthalmic conditions, affecting over 60 million people worldwide [1]. It is the leading cause of irreversible blindness and is responsible for bilateral blindness in over eight million people globally [1]. Because the condition is often asymptomatic in the early stages, over 50% of cases are undiagnosed [2]. Due to an ageing population the prevalence of glaucoma is expected to increase substantially over the coming decades [3]. The goal of management is to prevent vision loss from glaucoma in a patient's lifetime and to maintain or enhance quality of life.

The past 5 years have seen significant advances in imaging, visual field testing, and therapeutics for glaucoma. The objective of this chapter is to provide ophthalmologists with an update on the developments in the field of glaucoma. It focuses on clinically-relevant aspects including novel imaging techniques, new pharmacological approaches, and the latest in surgical treatment.

N. M. Kerr
Royal Victorian Eye and Ear Hospital, Melbourne, VIC, Australia

Centre for Eye Research Australia, Melbourne, VIC, Australia

K. Barton (✉)
Moorfields Eye Hospital, London, UK

UCL Institute of Ophthalmology, London, UK
e-mail: keith@keithbarton.co.uk

© Springer Nature Switzerland AG 2020
A. Grzybowski (ed.), *Current Concepts in Ophthalmology*,
https://doi.org/10.1007/978-3-030-25389-9_4

## Recent Developments in Imaging

Optical coherence tomography (OCT) is now the most widely adopted imaging modality for the management of glaucoma. New parameters, imaging protocols, and modalities are further enhancing the ability to diagnose and monitor glaucoma. Major developments in recent years include the introduction of three-dimensional OCT scanning, swept-source OCT, OCT angiography, and adaptive optics.

## *Three-Dimensional Optical Coherence Tomography*

The adoption of optical coherence tomography (OCT) has enabled highly-accurate quantitative assessment of the optic nerve head and surrounding retinal structures to assist in the diagnosis and monitoring of glaucoma. Traditional parameters include assessment of optic disc area, rim area, cup-to-disc ratio, and two-dimensional measurement of the thickness of the peripapillary retinal nerve fiber layer (RNFL) and ganglion cell-inner plexiform layer (GC-IPL). These parameters have been shown to have good reproducibility and the ability to distinguish between glaucomatous and non-glaucomatous eyes [4]. The detection of RNFL damage is helpful in the early detection of glaucoma, frequently preceding the development of visual field loss [5]. However, two-dimensional parameters are susceptible to artifacts that may adversely affect their diagnostic ability [6, 7]. This is especially problematic where there are variations in optic disc size, optic nerve head tilt, peripapillary atrophy, and myopia [8]. These imaging artifacts or inaccuracies may cause erroneous RNFL measurements that may lead to inaccurate assessments [7]. The introduction of three-dimensional volume scans enable high-density sampling of nerve tissue and 3D reconstruction of the neuroretinal rim anatomy which may assist in the diagnosis and monitoring of glaucoma [9].

Three-dimensional scanning of RNFL and ganglion cell layer (GCL) volumes permits the assessment of new parameters such as the minimum distance band (MDB) [10]. The MDB is the shortest distance between the internal limiting membrane (ILM) and the optic disc margin, defined as the termination of the retinal pigment epithelium (RPE)/Bruch's membrane (BM) [11]. The MDB has several advantages over standard neuroretinal rim parameters. The RPE/BM termination is an objective, consistent, and easily-identifiable anatomic landmark on OCT compared to traditional parameters that define the optic disc margin based on the clinical optic disc margin [9]. Additionally MDB measurements are perpendicular to the course of retinal ganglion cell (RGC) axons, therefore they take into account the variable orientation of RGC axons as they approach the optic nerve head [9]. MDB has been validated as a marker for glaucoma and has been shown to have good diagnostic performance compared to two-dimensional RNFL measurements [9]. Shieh et al. showed that 3D MDB neuroretinal rim thickness measurements had uniformly equal or better diagnostic performance for glaucoma in all quadrants and was significantly better in the nasal region compared to 2D RNFL thickness measurements [9]. Similarly, Tsikata et al. found that 3D MDB had a higher diagnostic capability for glaucoma than RNFL thickness in the inferonasal, superonasal, and nasal sectors as assessed by the area under the receiver operating characteristic (AUROC) curves [12].

## Wide-Field Swept-Source Optical Coherence Tomography

Traditionally, multiple scans are required to capture an OCT image. However, a recently introduced technology called swept-source OCT (SS-OCT) uses a swept laser to capture wide-angle, high-quality images of the optic nerve and macula in a single scan [13]. This technology may provide better image quality and be less affected by media opacities [14]. Wide-field scanning has been shown to be effective at discriminating between healthy and glaucomatous eyes with a diagnostic accuracy comparable to spectral-domain OCT (SD-OCT) [15–17]. For the detection of early glaucoma, SS-OCT has demonstrated superior diagnostic ability over conventional criteria analyzing peripapillary RNFL and ganglion cell layers [18]. Like 3D OCT, SS-OCT may also be less susceptible to artifacts and centering errors [15]. In addition, a tunable wavelength of operation enables imaging of deep ocular structures such as the lamina cribrosa [19]. The lamina cribrosa has long been presumed to be the primary site of axonal injury in glaucoma [20]. It is believed that posterior bowing of the lamina cribrosa may cause mechanical and/or an ischaemic insult to RGC axons [21]. Using SS-OCT, Kim et al. showed greater posterior displacement of the lamina cribrosa in eyes with primary open angle glaucoma compared to age-matched healthy eyes [19]. SS-OCT may therefore assist in our understanding of the mechanisms involved in glaucoma pathogenesis.

## Optical Coherence Tomography Angiography

Optical coherence tomography angiography (OCT-A) is a new technology that allows non-invasive visualization of the microcirculation of the eye without the use of contrast dye. The technique takes advantage of improvements in OCT image resolution and scanning speed and is gaining popularity in the assessment of retinal vascular diseases. By comparing sequential scans at the same location, OCT-A is able to detect change which are attributed to erythrocyte movement in perfused vessels [22]. The technique offers several advantages over traditional angiography including the ability to simultaneously assess the retinal and choroidal circulations, quantitative assessment of the microcirculation, and three-dimensional assessment of both microvasculature structure and function while avoiding the need for invasive dye injections. Because of the possible role of reduced optic nerve head perfusion and vascular dysregulation in glaucoma [23], OCT-A is being investigated as a tool to help elucidate the pathophysiology of the disease as well as assist clinicians in glaucoma detection and monitoring [24].

Optical coherence tomography angiography provides quantitative information on both blood vessel structure, reported as blood vessel density and foveal avascular zone area, as well as microvasculature function using flow index, a dimensionless parameter between 0 and 1. The measurements have been shown to have high within-visit repeatability and between-visit reproducibility [25, 26]. Differences between healthy and glaucomatous eyes have been observed with respect to vessel density, foveal avascular area, and reduced blood flow index. In patients with ocular hypertension, normal tension glaucoma, and primary open angle glaucoma reductions in vessel density and size of the foveal avascular zone have been reported [27–30]. These changes are associated with a reduction in optic disc flow and correlate with the degree of visual field defect [25]. Jia et al. found a 25% reduction in optic disc flow between healthy and glaucomatous eyes and this reduction correlated strongly with visual field pattern standard deviation (PSD) [25]. Similarly, Liu et al. and Yarmohammadi et al. found significant correlations between flow index and visual field PSD in glaucomatous eyes [26, 31]. The data suggest an association not only with the degree of visual field defect but also the location of the field defect [32]. In a separate study, Yarmohammadi et al. examined vessel density in eyes with visual field defects in a single hemifield and found that vessel density was lowest in the affected hemiretina [32]. Interestingly, reduced vessel density was also noted in the perimetrically intact hemiretina suggesting that microvasculature changes may precede visual field loss [32]. Changes in OCT-A parameters also correlate with the location of RNFL thinning. Mansoori et al. found a reduction in capillary density in eyes with early glaucoma and that capillary density was lowest in areas with focal RNFL defects [33]. This finding is consistent with other studies showing capillary dropout in areas of RNFL thinning [25, 29, 34].

Several studies have investigated the diagnostic performance of OCT-A for glaucoma detection. Using optic disc flow and a cut-off value of 0.1515, Jia et al. reported a sensitivity and specificity of 100% in their study population [25]. The same group then evaluated the ability of peripapillary flow index and vessel density to discriminate between healthy and glaucomatous eyes using AUROC curves and found values of 0.982 and 0.938 respectively [26]. The performance of OCT-A appears to depend on the stage of glaucoma [35]. Wang et al. investigated the correlation between OCT-A parameters and glaucoma severity and found that both vessel density and flow index performed best in advanced glaucoma [35].

There is some emerging data on the effect of IOP reduction on OCT-A parameters [36–38]. In patients with very high IOP who achieved a >50% reduction in IOP with medical therapy there was a significant increase in OCT-A parameters [37]. However, another study found no statistically significant difference in OCT-A parameters in the peripapillary or macular regions following glaucoma filtration surgery, despite an average IOP reduction of 44.2% [36]. Lastly, in patients presenting with acute angle closure, statistically significant changes in OCT-A parameters have been observed following treatment and normalization of IOP [38].

Optical coherence angiography is not without limitations. Currently, there is a lack of comparability between machines and studies due to an absence of standardized measurement protocols. Also, image quality is highly dependent on fixation and patient co-operation. Further longitudinal studies are needed to determine whether OCT-A findings can predict or detect glaucoma progression. Nonetheless, OCT-A remains a promising technology for elucidating the physiology of glaucoma and evaluating structure and function in this disease.

## Adaptive Optics

Adaptive optics (AO) is not an imaging modality, but rather a technology used in combination with existing imaging modalities to improve their performance [39]. Initially developed to reduce ocular aberrations from ground-based telescopes, it has been used in conjunction with fundus cameras, scanning laser ophthalmoscopes, and most recently OCT to provide unprecedented resolution and the ability to visualize structures at the cellular level in real time. Representing a major advance in optical technology, AO uses a wavefront sensor that measures aberrations in ocular optics and a deformable mirror or spatial light modulator to compensate for these aberrations in vivo [40].

Because RNFL loss is one of the earliest detectable changes in glaucoma, often preceding changes at the optic nerve head or visual field loss [41], there has been particular interest in using AO to detect RNFL changes allowing for earlier detection, more precise diagnosis, and improved detection of progression in glaucoma [39]. Several groups have used AO to visualize RNFL bundles and the gaps between them [42–45]. Kocaoglu et al. proved that it was possible to measure the dimensions of RNFL bundles in five health subjects [42]. This work was extended by Takayama et al. who demonstrated reduced RNFL bundle dimensions in glaucomatous eyes and that these abnormalities were associated with visual field defects [43]. Showing the promise for early detection, Chen et al. demonstrated changes in RNFL bundles on AO that were difficult, if not impossible, to discern with current OCT technology [44]. Most recently, Hood et al. followed six eyes of five patients with deep glaucomatous visual field defects using adaptive optics scanning light ophthalmoscopy (AO-SLO) and showed progressive changes in RNFL bundles, demonstrating the potential for AO to be used for monitoring glaucoma progression [46].

To date, it has been difficult to visualize individual RGCs with OA. This is because RGCs are nearly transparent, an important attribute to allow light to pass through them and reach photoreceptor cells. In spite of this property, one group has been able to image the individual somas of neurons within RGCs using confocal AO-SLO and showed progressive changes in RNFL bundles, demonstrating the potential for A in both monkeys and humans [47]. This capability to noninvasively image RGC layer neurons in the living eye without fluorescent labels may one day allow for insights into the pathogenesis of glaucoma and a better diagnostic tool [47].

## Recent Developments in Visual Field Testing

Visual field testing is essential in the detection and monitoring of glaucoma. Recent advances in thresholding algorithms, testing frequency, and new portable perimetry devices are showing potential to improve visual field testing in clinical practice.

### *Testing Strategies and Novel Thresholding Algorithms*

Currently, 24-2 visual fields are the most commonly used method for investigating visual field defects in glaucoma. However, there is an increasing appreciation that damage at the macula can be detected in even early stages of glaucoma [48]. The macula has the highest density of RGCs [49] and thinning of the ganglion cell complex is seen early in the glaucomatous process [50]. In a recent study of patients with early glaucoma, 16 of 26 eyes (61.5%) classified as normal on 24-2 tests were classified as abnormal on 10-2 visual fields [51]. In patients with ocular hypertension, 28 of 79 eyes (35.4%) classified as normal on 24-2 tests were classified as abnormal on 10-2 visual fields [51]. It is therefore apparent that central visual field damage on the 10-2 test may be missed with the 24-2 strategy alone [51]. These findings suggest that in the future it may be necessary to include 10-2 visual field testing to reliably detect central visual field defects. However, further work is required before this becomes the new standard of care.

In addition, novel thresholding strategies are being investigated that incorporate spatial and structural information to improve the speed and precision of visual field testing. Chong et al. introduced a perimetric algorithm that uses spatial information regarding the location of a field defect to improve the characterization of field loss without increasing testing times [52]. Using a computer simulation, Chong et al. reported improved accuracy and precision in testing regions surrounding scotoma edges [52]. The same group then validated the performance of the new algorithm, called Gradient-Oriented Automated Natural Neighbor Approach; (GOANNA) in humans and found results in agreement with earlier simulation studies [53]. Using an alternative approach, Rubinstein et al. introduced a perimetric algorithm (Spatially Weighted Likelihoods in Zippy Estimation by Sequential Testing; SWeLZ) that uses spatial information on every presentation to alter visual field estimates, to reduce test times without affecting output precision or accuracy [54]. Both of these strategies have the potential for significant time savings in clinical settings but require validation in larger scale clinical trials.

Another approach to improve thresholding procedures is to incorporate structural information into the testing process [55]. An example of this approach is demonstrated by Ganeshrao et al. who developed a perimetric test strategy called Structure Estimation of Minimum Uncertainty (SEMU), that uses structural information to drive stimulus choices [56]. One method of accelerating testing times is to make an estimate of sensitivity at a location before any stimuli are shown, and then carefully test around this estimate [56]. SEMU utilizes this approach and predicts sensitivity at a location based on OCT data. Using a computer simulation, the authors tested the performance of SEMU for three different profiles of patient reliability and found reduced testing times while maintaining accuracy and precision [56]. This and other strategies require formal validation before being introduced into routine clinical practice but show progress toward a patient-tailored approach to improve perimetric procedures.

## Impact of Testing Frequency

Detecting visual field progression is a significant challenge in clinical practice. The ability to detect progression depends on many factors including the rate of progression, testing frequency, and level of reliability/measurement variability. It is especially important in the early follow-up period to establish a sufficient baseline to rule out rapid progression [57]. Chauhan et al. calculated that to detect rapid progression (defined as −2 dB/year) the time to detect change with 80% power is 5 years with annual examinations, 2.5 years with two examinations per year, and 1.7 years if examinations are performed three times per year [57]. More recently, Wu et al. examined the impact of testing frequency on the ability to detect progression [58]. Assuming a best-practice scenario with two baselines tests and a requirement to replicate progression on one confirmatory test, they estimated rapid visual progression could be detected with 80% power after 3.3 years, 2.4 years, or 2.1 years when testing was performed once, twice, and three times a year [58]. Based on the diminishing returns from twice to three-times-a-year testing, they concluded that twice yearly testing was a reasonable compromise for achieving sufficient power whilst minimizing treatment burden [58].

## Novel Methods of Assessing Visual Fields

Traditional perimetry requires the patient to maintain fixation throughout the duration of the test. Failure to maintain fixation can lead to poor reliability and unreliable fields. A relatively new method of testing visual fields is fundus-tracked perimetry or microperimetry where the fundus is tracked using a retinal imaging system and stimuli are projected at specific retinal locations. Early perimeters evaluated only the central macular region while newer machines now permit testing of the central 30° radius. The performance of microperimetry has been compared with the Humphrey Visual Field Analyzer in eyes with glaucoma and the sensitivities obtained with microperimetry have been found to be repeatable and comparable to conventional perimetry [59–61]. Another advantage is that microperimetry can be combined with retinal imaging to provide stronger structure-function associations.

Recent advances in smartphone and tablet technology have seen significant improvements in display resolution, dynamic range, and accurate calibration [62]. These devices are portable, do not require a continuous power supply, and are relatively inexpensive allowing them to be used for home or community-based visual field testing, even in remote areas [62]. The potential applications for portable perimetry include targeted screening in high-risk populations, especially where access to healthcare is limited, or for home monitoring between office visits in patients with a diagnosis of glaucoma. Johnson et al. have evaluated the use of a free tablet-based perimetry application in Nepal and found the procedure to be portable, fast, and effective for detecting moderate to advanced field loss [63]. The average testing time was just over 3 min however improvements are underway to reduce testing time, improve performance, and add head/eye tracking [63]. The performance of this tablet perimeter has been compared against the Humphrey Field Analyzer and the results show strong correlation as well as comparable test-retest reliability [64]. The system has also been used in a study investigating whether home-based perimetry can increase test frequency and allow for detection of rapid progression more quickly than conventional perimetry [63]. Using a computer simulation, tablet-based perimetry detected rapid visual field loss after 0.9 years with a sensitivity of 80% compared to 2.5 years for 6-monthly clinic-based testing [63]. These results suggest that home-based perimetry may be a viable strategy to increase testing frequency and allow for more timely detection of rapid visual field progression [63].

## Recent Developments in Medical Therapy

The mainstay of glaucoma treatment has been medical therapy with eye drops. However, multiple medications may be required [65], adherence is a major challenge especially if adjunctive therapy is required [66], instillation can be difficult [67], and medical therapy alone may not always be sufficient in preventing progression [68]. There is therefore great excitement to see the introduction of novel pharmacotherapy agents and alternative drug delivery systems that aim to effectively lower IOP, reduce the need for frequent eye drop administration, and that are well tolerated.

### Rho Kinase Inhibitors

Rho kinase (ROCK) inhibitors are an entirely new class of glaucoma medications. These medications work by relaxing the trabecular meshwork through inhibition of the actin cytoskeleton contractile tone of smooth muscle [69, 70]. This results in increased aqueous outflow, thereby lowering IOP. In addition, animal studies suggest secondary effects which may be beneficial in glaucoma including improved blood flow to the optic nerve [71], neuroprotection of retinal ganglion cells [72], and inhibition of bleb scarring following glaucoma filtration surgery [73].

The most well-studied ROCK inhibitors are ripasudil and netarsudil. Ripasudil has been shown to significantly lower IOP in phase I and II human clinical trials [74, 75]. The medication has a good safety profile with the most common side effect being mild hyperaemia, occurring in approximately 50% of patients [74, 75]. Transient corneal guttae-like findings have been seen and are believed to be due to protrusion formation along intracellular borders caused by the reduction actomyosin contractility in corneal endothelial cells [76]. These are not believed to adversely affect vision [76]. In an open-label study of patients with ocular hypertension or glaucoma, 51 of 388 patients had to discontinue the medication due to blepharitis or allergic conjunctivitis symptoms [77]. Monotherapy with ripasudil 0.4% reduced IOP by an average of 3.7 mmHg at 52 weeks [77]. The medication has also been shown to be effective as an adjunctive agent when combined with either a beta-blocker or prostaglandin analogue [78].

Netarsudil is both a ROCK inhibitor and norepinephrine transporter (NET) inhibitor [79]. This medication is believed to lower IOP by the triple action of reducing aqueous production, increasing trabecular outflow, and decreasing episcleral venous pressure [80]. The medication has been found to be effective and well-tolerated for the treatment of patients with ocular hypertension and open-angle glaucoma in two large randomized, double-masked phase 3 trials (ROCKET-1 and ROCKET-2) [81]. Like other ROCK inhibitors, the most common side effect was conjunctival hyperaemia (occurring in 50–89% of study participants) [79, 81]. In a double-masked, randomized study of netarsudil versus latanoprost in patients with elevated IOP, netarsudil was less effective than latanoprost by approximately 1 mmHg [82]. However, the fixed combination of netarsudil and latanoprost was found to be statistically superior in terms of IOP-lowering than its individual active components at the same concentrations [83].

## *Latanoprostene Bunod*

Latanoprostene bunod is a nitrous oxide-donating prostaglandin agonist that lowers IOP by increasing both trabecular and uveoscleral outflow [84]. The release of nitric oxide relaxes the trabecular meshwork, increasing aqueous outflow [85]. In a randomized, controlled trial comparing latanoprostene bunod and latanoprost 0.005% in patients with ocular hypertension and open-angle glaucoma (VOYAGER study), latanoprostene bunod achieved significantly greater reductions in diurnal IOP while having comparable side effects to latanoprost [86]. The levels of hyperaemia were similar in both treatment arms [86]. In larger subsequent randomized, double-masked, multi-center controlled trials comparing latanoprostene bunod and timolol (APOLLO and LUNAR studies) there was a significantly greater reduction in IOP with latanoprostene bunod than timolol [87, 88].

## Alternative Drug Delivery Systems

Recently, a number of alternative drug delivery systems have been developed that aim to reduce the need for daily medical therapy; helping address problems with glaucoma eye drop administration and adherence. These devices aim to provide a slow and controlled release of glaucoma medication to provide effective control of IOP.

### Travoprost Punctum Plug

The travoprost punctum plug (OTX-TP) is a novel sustained-release delivery system that releases travoprost from a hydrogel punctum plug placed in the superior or inferior canaliculus [89]. The active medication is contained within microspheres which degrade via hydrolysis when they come in contact with the tear film, thereby releasing the medication [89]. In an unmasked, single-arm study the OTX-TP reduced IOP by 24% at day 10 and 15.6% at day 30. The device was tolerated by most patients and side effects were uncommon [89]. Longer duration studies are planned.

### Bimatoprost Ocular Ring

The bimatoprost ocular ring is a simple and novel sustained-release device that is applied topically to the ocular surface by a physician and allows continuous drug delivery for up to 6 months [90]. In a phase II doubled-masked randomized controlled trial, patients with ocular hypertension or open-angle glaucoma were randomized to the bimatoprost ocular insert and artificial tears or a placebo implant and timolol twice daily [90]. The bimatoprost ring was non-inferior to timolol at 9 months, however the study was underpowered for the observed treatment effect [90]. The ring was well-tolerated and adverse events were comparable to topical bimatoprost or timolol exposure [90]. In a 13-month open-label extension study, the ring remained in position without physician intervention in 95% of patients and >97% of participants reported that the ring was comfortable or tolerable [91]. At 13 months the average IOP reduction was 4 mmHg with rescue medical therapy required in 13 of 63 participants [91]. The overall safety profile was very good [91].

### Bimatoprost Sustained-Release (SR) Intracameral Implant

The bimatoprost sustained-release (SR) implant is a biodegradable implant designed to be implanted into the anterior chamber [92]. The implant provides a slow release of bimatoprost overtime and is designed to reduce barriers to adherence and minimize the incidence of adverse effects associated with topical bimatoprost administration [93]. In a prospective, 24-month, phase I/II study bimatoprost SR provided rapid and sustained IOP lowering with a mean IOP reduction of 9.5 mmHg at week

16 for the 20 μg implant [94]. This compared with a reduction of 8.4 mmHg in fellow eyes treated with topical bimatoprost [94]. A single administration controlled IOP in the majority of patients for up to 6 months [94]. Rescue medical therapy was required in 9% of eyes through week 16 and 29% of eyes by month 6 [94]. Adverse events were uncommon and usually occurred within 2 days after implantation [94]. The most frequent adverse event was conjunctival hyperaemia which occurred in 6.7% of bimatoprost SR eyes and 17.3% of topically treated eyes [94].

### iDose

The iDose is a titanium implant which is secured in the anterior chamber during a micro-invasive procedure [95]. The implant is designed to elute therapeutic levels of travoprost in a continuous and controlled fashion [95]. Once depleted, the device can be removed and replaced [95]. In a multicenter, randomized, doubled-masked phase II trial the iDose achieved sustained IOP reductions of approximately 30% in a 12-month interim cohort of patients [95]. The safety profile was favorable with no adverse events of hyperaemia in the iDose group [95].

## Recent Developments in Glaucoma Laser and Surgery

Recent landmark studies have enhanced our understanding about laser iridotomy, clear lens extraction, trabeculectomy, and tube surgery in the management of glaucoma.

## *Laser Iridotomy*

Laser peripheral iridotomy is frequently used to prevent or treat angle closure glaucoma. This procedure is generally safe but may be complicated by visual disturbances or dysphotopsias [96]. In a recent randomized prospective paired eye trial, Vera et al. found that temporal placement of the laser iridotomy was less likely to result in linear dysphotopsia than superior placement [97]. The authors suggested that the ideal location for laser iridotomy was the temporal iris [97]. However, a larger multi-center randomized trial in India found that the incidence of visual dysphotopsia was unaffected by iridotomy location, size, or amount of energy used [98]. In this study, the onset of new dysphotopsia occurred in 8.4% of patients undergoing nasal/temporal iridotomy compared to 9.5% of patients where the iridotomy was placed superiorly [98]. Given data suggesting similar safety with regard to location and dysphotopsia symptoms, it may therefore be advisable to place the iridotomy in a crypt or superiorly which has been shown to cause less pain and discomfort [97].

## *Clear Lens Extraction for Angle-Closure Glaucoma*

An alternative approach to the management of angle-closure glaucoma is surgical lens extraction [99]. A landmark trial has recently evaluated the efficacy, safety, and cost-effectiveness of clear lens extraction compared to laser peripheral iridotomy and topical medical treatment as first-line treatment in people with newly diagnosed primary angle closure (PAC) with an IOP of ≥30 mmHg or primary angle-closure glaucoma (PACG) [100]. It was found that clear lens extraction resulted in greater reduction in IOP, less need for glaucoma medications, and higher quality life scores than laser iridotomy [100]. Furthermore, initial lens extraction was more cost-effective than standard of care with laser iridotomy [100]. Based on these results, the authors suggest that clear lens extraction should be considered as first-line treatment for newly diagnosed PACG or PAC where IOP is 30 mmHg or greater [100].

## *Primary Trabeculectomy or Tube Surgery for Medically Uncontrolled Glaucoma*

In eyes with glaucoma refractory to medical therapy, glaucoma surgery is frequently required. The most commonly performed operations are trabeculectomy and tube shunt surgery [101]. Previously, tube shunt surgery was found to have a higher success rate compared to trabeculectomy at 5 years in eyes with prior trabeculectomy and/or cataract surgery [102]. Recently, a landmark study compared the efficacy and safety of tube shunt surgery and trabeculectomy in eyes without prior ocular surgery [103].

In the Primary Tube Versus Trabeculectomy (PTVT) study patients with medically uncontrolled glaucoma and no previous incisional surgery were randomized to treatment with a 350-mm$^2$ Baerveldt glaucoma implant or trabeculectomy with mitomycin C (0.4 mg/mL for 2 min). The trabeculectomy arm was found to have a lower probability of failure (7.9% vs. 17.3%), lower IOP (12.4 ± 4.4 mmHg vs. 13.8 ± 4.1 mmHg), and less need for glaucoma medications (0.9 ± 1.4 vs. 2.1 ± 1.4) compared to tube surgery at 1 year [103]. There was no significant difference in the rates of intraoperative complications [103]. However, the frequency of serious complications producing vision loss or requiring reoperation was lower for tube shunt surgery [103].

## *Minimally Invasive Glaucoma Surgery*

New minimally invasive glaucoma procedures that aim to lower intraocular pressure with a better safety profile and faster recovery than conventional glaucoma surgery are being increasingly used in clinical practice. Recently there have been a number of major developments in this space.

The iStent inject received approval from the Food and Drug Administration (FDA) in 2018 for use in mild to moderate open-angle glaucoma in patients undergoing cataract surgery [104]. The iStent inject trabecular micro-bypass system consists of two titanium stents approximately 0.23 mm × 0.36 mm that are implanted into the trabecular meshwork using a preloaded auto-injection system through a single corneal entry [104]. The FDA approval was based on a pivotal iStent inject US IDE pivotal study, a prospective randomized, multi-center clinical trial including 505 participants who were randomized to receive the iStent inject with cataract surgery or cataract surgery alone [104]. At 2 years, 75.8% of patients in the iStent inject group had a 20% or greater reduction in unmedicated diurnal IOP compared with 61.9% in the cataract surgery-only group [104]. The safety profile was similar between the two arms of the study.

Another development in minimally invasive glaucoma surgery (MIGS) is the Hydrus Microstent. The Hydrus is placed in Schlemm's canal and helps restore aqueous outflow by bypassing the trabecular meshwork, dilating Schlemm's canal, and allowing access to a number of collector channels over a 90-degree span. In 2018, the Hydrus also received FDA approval to treat patients with mild to moderate primary open-angle glaucoma in conjunction with cataract surgery [105]. The approval was based on the landmark HORIZON trail which included 556 people with mild to moderate glaucoma undergoing cataract surgery. Patients were randomized to receive cataract surgery with the Hydrus Microstent or cataract surgery alone. In the Hydrus group, 77.2% of patients achieved a 20% of greater reduction in unmedicated IOP compared to 57.8% in the cataract surgery alone group at 2 years [105]. Patients who received the Hydrus were twice as likely to be medication-free compared to those who underwent cataract surgery alone [106]. An international multi-center randomized trial comparing the effectiveness of the Hydrus Microstent to two Glaukos iStents in standalone glaucoma, the COMPARE study, is underway [107].

In 2018 the CyPass Micro-Stent was voluntarily withdrawn from sale by the manufacturer due to safety concerns about endothelial cell loss. This voluntary recall has since been updated to a Class 1 recall by the FDA [108]. The CyPass Micro-Stent is a MIGS device that was implanted into the supraciliary space to increase aqueous outflow via the uveoscleral pathway. It was approved based on the results of the COMPASS trial which showed a significant and sustained 2-year reduction in IOP and glaucoma medication use in mild to moderate open-angle glaucoma when performed with cataract surgery [109]. No safety concerns were identified at 2 years with endothelial cell loss being similar between patients who underwent cataract surgery with the CyPass and those who underwent cataract surgery alone [109]. A subset of patients from the COMPASS trial were followed for an additional 3 years in the COMPASS-XT study and based on these results the CyPass was withdrawn from the market. The COMPASS-XT study found that at 5 years there was a higher rate of endothelial cell loss with cataract surgery and CyPass insertion compared to cataract surgery alone [110]. At 5 years, endothelial cell loss was 20.5% in the CyPass group compared to 10.1% in the cataract surgery arm [110]. The rate of endothelial cell loss was found to relate to the depth of insertion. Where the CyPass was implanted with no retention rings visible on gonioscopy the rate of endothelial cell loss was 1.39% per year, where 1 ring was visible the rate was 2.74% per year, however where 2 or more rings were visible the rate increased to 6.96% per year [110]. Surgeons have been advised to cease implanting the CyPass Micro-Stent and to periodically monitor endothelial cell density using specular microscopy where available [110]. The manufacturer is partnering with the FDA and other regulators to explore labelling changes that would support the reintroduction of the CyPass Micro-Stent in the future [111].

Subconjunctival filtration has traditionally delivered the greatest levels of IOP reduction. Trabeculectomy, while effective in reducing IOP, requires extensive dissection, sclerostomy, and suturing which can lead to unpredictability and complications such as bleb leak, hypotony, suprachoroidal haemorrhage, and a reduction in vision [112, 113]. Two new MIGS devices aim to take advantage of the power of subconjunctival filtration while achieving a good safety profile and short surgical time. The XEN is a flexible gelatin implant, 6-mm long, with a 45 μm internal diameter lumen, which is inserted via an ab interno approach from the anterior chamber to the subconjunctival space [114]. The length and diameter of the implant were chosen based on the Hagen-Poiseuille equation to provide sufficient resistance to aqueous outflow to minimize hypotony [114]. The XEN eliminates the need for conjunctival dissection, cutting a scleral flap, sclerosotomy, and iridectomy. The XEN was approved by the FDA in 2016 based on a pivotal trial in patients with refractory glaucoma. In this study, the XEN reduced IOP from a mean medicated baseline of $25.1 \pm 3.7$ mmHg to $15.9 \pm 5.2$ mmHg at 12 months [115]. Glaucoma medication use decreased from a mean of $3.5 \pm 1.0$ to $1.7 \pm 1.5$ medications over the same period [115]. The effectiveness and safety of the XEN has been compared with trabeculectomy in a retrospective interventional cohort study [112]. The baseline characteristics were similar in both groups and there was no detectable difference in the risk of failure and safety profiles between standalone XEN insertion and trabeculectomy with MMC [112].

The latest subconjunctival MIGS device to be introduced is the InnFocus MicroShunt. This device is 8.5 mm long with a 70 μm lumen and is inserted via an ab externo approach [116]. Like the XEN, the MicroShunt avoids the need for a scleral flap, sclerostomy, iridectomy, and post-operative suturelysis, resulting in a short surgical time and predictable post-operative recovery [117]. The device is manufactured from an inert biocompatible material called poly(styrene-block-isobutylene-block-styrene) or "SIBS." This material has been shown to elicit minimal foreign body reaction, inflammation, or capsule formation when implanted in the eye [118]. Similar to the XEN, the dimensions of the MicroShunt are based on the Hagen-Poiseuille equation in an attempt to prevent clinically significant hypotony [116]. In a three-year prospective, non-randomised trial the MicroShunt reduced IOP to the low teens in patients with glaucoma refractory to medical therapy for up to 3 years with only transient adverse events in the first 3 months after surgery [117]. In this study, mean medication IOP was reduced from $23.8 \pm 5.3$ mmHg to $10.7 \pm 3.5$ mmHg at 3 years with a reduction in the mean number of medications from 2.4 ± 0.9 to 0.7 ± 1.1 [117]. The most common complications were transient hypotony (13%) and transient choroidal effusions (8.7%), all of which resolved spontaneously [117]. A prospective, randomized controlled trial comparing the MicroShunt to trabeculectomy is underway.

## Conclusion

Glaucoma remains a common and important cause of visual impairment. The development and advancement of new diagnostic and therapeutic technologies, including novel drugs and drug delivery systems together with new surgical options, will ensure continued improvements in glaucoma detection and treatment.

## References

1. Quigley HA, Broman AT. The number of people with glaucoma worldwide in 2010 and 2020. Br J Ophthalmol. 2006;90:262–7.
2. Keel S, Xie J, Foreman J, et al. Prevalence of glaucoma in the Australian National Eye Health Survey. Br J Ophthalmol. 2018.
3. Tham YC, Li X, Wong TY, Quigley HA, Aung T, Cheng CY. Global prevalence of glaucoma and projections of glaucoma burden through 2040: a systematic review and meta-analysis. Ophthalmology. 2014;121:2081–90.
4. Mwanza JC, Budenz DL, Godfrey DG, et al. Diagnostic performance of optical coherence tomography ganglion cell—inner plexiform layer thickness measurements in early glaucoma. Ophthalmology. 2014;121:849–54.
5. Kuang TM, Zhang C, Zangwill LM, Weinreb RN, Medeiros FA. Estimating lead time gained by optical coherence tomography in detecting glaucoma before development of visual field defects. Ophthalmology. 2015;122:2002–9.
6. Hwang YH, Kim MK, Kim DW. Segmentation errors in macular ganglion cell analysis as determined by optical coherence tomography. Ophthalmology. 2016;123:950–8.
7. Liu Y, Simavli H, Que CJ, et al. Patient characteristics associated with artifacts in spectralis optical coherence tomography imaging of the retinal nerve fiber layer in glaucoma. Am J Ophthalmol. 2015;159:565–76.e2.
8. Sung KR, Wollstein G, Kim NR, et al. Macular assessment using optical coherence tomography for glaucoma diagnosis. Br J Ophthalmol. 2012;96:1452–5.
9. Shieh E, Lee R, Que C, et al. Diagnostic performance of a novel three-dimensional neuroretinal rim parameter for glaucoma using high-density volume scans. Am J Ophthalmol. 2016;169:168–78.
10. Kim SY, Park HY, Park CK. The effects of peripapillary atrophy on the diagnostic ability of Stratus and Cirrus OCT in the analysis of optic nerve head parameters and disc size. Invest Ophthalmol Vis Sci. 2012;53:4475–84.
11. Povazay B, Hofer B, Hermann B, et al. Minimum distance mapping using three-dimensional optical coherence tomography for glaucoma diagnosis. J Biomed Opt. 2007;12:041204.
12. Tsikata E, Lee R, Shieh E, et al. Comprehensive three-dimensional analysis of the neuroretinal rim in glaucoma using high-density spectral-domain optical coherence tomography volume scans. Invest Ophthalmol Vis Sci. 2016;57:5498–508.

13. Mansouri K, Medeiros FA, Tatham AJ, Marchase N, Weinreb RN. Evaluation of retinal and choroidal thickness by swept-source optical coherence tomography: repeatability and assessment of artifacts. Am J Ophthalmol. 2014;157:1022–32.
14. Lee SY, Kwon HJ, Bae HW, et al. Frequency, type and cause of artifacts in swept-source and cirrus HD optical coherence tomography in cases of glaucoma and suspected glaucoma. Curr Eye Res. 2016;41:957–64.
15. Yang Z, Tatham AJ, Weinreb RN, Medeiros FA, Liu T, Zangwill LM. Diagnostic ability of macular ganglion cell inner plexiform layer measurements in glaucoma using swept source and spectral domain optical coherence tomography. PLoS One. 2015;10:e0125957.
16. Hood DC, De Cuir N, Blumberg DM, et al. A single wide-field OCT protocol can provide compelling information for the diagnosis of early glaucoma. Transl Vis Sci Technol. 2016;5:4.
17. Lee KM, Lee EJ, Kim TW, Kim H. Comparison of the abilities of SD-OCT and SS-OCT in evaluating the thickness of the macular inner retinal layer for glaucoma diagnosis. PLoS One. 2016;11:e0147964.
18. Lee WJ, Na KI, Kim YK, Jeoung JW, Park KH. Diagnostic ability of wide-field retinal nerve fiber layer maps using swept-source optical coherence tomography for detection of preperimetric and early perimetric glaucoma. J Glaucoma. 2017;26:577–85.
19. Kim YW, Kim DW, Jeoung JW, Kim DM, Park KH. Peripheral lamina cribrosa depth in primary open-angle glaucoma: a swept-source optical coherence tomography study of lamina cribrosa. Eye (Lond). 2015;29:1368–74.
20. Quigley HA, Addicks EM, Green W, Maumenee AE. Optic nerve damage in human glaucoma: Ii. the site of injury and susceptibility to damage. Arch Ophthalmol. 1981;99:635–49.
21. Burgoyne CF, Downs JC, Bellezza AJ, Suh JK, Hart RT. The optic nerve head as a biomechanical structure: a new paradigm for understanding the role of IOP-related stress and strain in the pathophysiology of glaucomatous optic nerve head damage. Prog Retin Eye Res. 2005;24:39–73.
22. Wan KH, Leung CKS. Optical coherence tomography angiography in glaucoma: a minireview. F1000Res. 2017;6:1686.
23. Abegao Pinto L, Willekens K, Van Keer K, et al. Ocular blood flow in glaucoma—the Leuven Eye Study. Acta Ophthalmol. 2016;94:592–8.
24. Lee EJ, Lee KM, Lee SH, Kim T-W. OCT angiography of the peripapillary retina in primary open-angle glaucoma. Invest Ophthalmol Vis Sci. 2016;57:6265–70.
25. Jia Y, Wei E, Wang X, et al. Optical coherence tomography angiography of optic disc perfusion in glaucoma. Ophthalmology. 2014;121:1322–32.
26. Liu L, Jia Y, Takusagawa HL, et al. Optical coherence tomography angiography of the peripapillary retina in glaucoma. JAMA Ophthalmol. 2015;133:1045–52.
27. Yarmohammadi A, Zangwill LM, Diniz-Filho A, et al. Optical coherence tomography angiography vessel density in healthy, glaucoma suspect, and glaucoma eyes. Invest Ophthalmol Vis Sci. 2016;57:OCT451–OCT9.
28. Shin JW, Sung KR, Lee JY, Kwon J, Seong M. Optical coherence tomography angiography vessel density mapping at various retinal layers in healthy and normal tension glaucoma eyes. Graefes Arch Clin Exp Ophthalmol. 2017;255:1193–202.
29. Geyman LS, Garg RA, Suwan Y, et al. Peripapillary perfused capillary density in primary open-angle glaucoma across disease stage: an optical coherence tomography angiography study. Br J Ophthalmol. 2017;101:1261–8.
30. Cennamo G, Montorio D, Velotti N, Sparnelli F, Reibaldi M, Cennamo G. Optical coherence tomography angiography in pre-perimetric open-angle glaucoma. Graefes Arch Clin Exp Ophthalmol. 2017;255:1787–93.
31. Yarmohammadi A, Zangwill LM, Diniz-Filho A, et al. Relationship between optical coherence tomography angiography vessel density and severity of visual field loss in glaucoma. Ophthalmology. 2016;123:2498–508.

32. Yarmohammadi A, Zangwill LM, Diniz-Filho A, et al. Peripapillary and macular vessel density in patients with glaucoma and single-hemifield visual field defect. Ophthalmology. 2017;124:709–19.
33. Mansoori T, Sivaswamy J, Gamalapati JS, Balakrishna N. Radial peripapillary capillary density measurement using optical coherence tomography angiography in early glaucoma. J Glaucoma. 2017;26:438–43.
34. Mammo Z, Heisler M, Balaratnasingam C, et al. Quantitative optical coherence tomography angiography of radial peripapillary capillaries in glaucoma, glaucoma suspect, and normal eyes. Am J Ophthalmol. 2016;170:41–9.
35. Wang X, Jiang C, Ko T, et al. Correlation between optic disc perfusion and glaucomatous severity in patients with open-angle glaucoma: an optical coherence tomography angiography study. Graefes Arch Clin Exp Ophthalmol. 2015;253:1557–64.
36. Zeboulon P, Leveque PM, Brasnu E, et al. Effect of surgical intraocular pressure lowering on peripapillary and macular vessel density in glaucoma patients: an optical coherence tomography angiography study. J Glaucoma. 2017;26:466–72.
37. Holló G. Influence of large intraocular pressure reduction on peripapillary OCT vessel density in ocular hypertensive and glaucoma eyes. J Glaucoma. 2017;26:e7–e10.
38. Wang X, Jiang C, Kong X, Yu X, Sun X. Peripapillary retinal vessel density in eyes with acute primary angle closure: an optical coherence tomography angiography study. Graefes Arch Clin Exp Ophthalmol. 2017;255:1013–8.
39. Miller DT, Kocaoglu OP, Wang Q, Lee S. Adaptive optics and the eye (super resolution OCT). Eye (Lond). 2011;25:321–30.
40. Roorda A. Adaptive optics for studying visual function: a comprehensive review. J Vis. 2011;11:6.
41. Sommer A, Katz J, Quigley HA, et al. Clinically detectable nerve fiber atrophy precedes the onset of glaucomatous field loss. Arch Ophthalmol. 1991;109:77–83.
42. Kocaoglu OP, Cense B, Jonnal RS, et al. Imaging retinal nerve fiber bundles using optical coherence tomography with adaptive optics. Vision Res. 2011;51:1835–44.
43. Takayama K, Ooto S, Hangai M, et al. High-resolution imaging of retinal nerve fiber bundles in glaucoma using adaptive optics scanning laser ophthalmoscopy. Am J Ophthalmol. 2013;155:870–81.e3.
44. Chen MF, Chui TY, Alhadeff P, et al. Adaptive optics imaging of healthy and abnormal regions of retinal nerve fiber bundles of patients with glaucoma. Invest Ophthalmol Vis Sci. 2015;56:674–81.
45. Hood DC, Chen MF, Lee D, et al. Confocal adaptive optics imaging of peripapillary nerve fiber bundles: implications for glaucomatous damage seen on circumpapillary OCT scans. Transl Vis Sci Technol. 2015;4:12.
46. Hood DC, Lee D, Jarukasetphon R, et al. Progression of local glaucomatous damage near fixation as seen with adaptive optics imaging. Transl Vis Sci Technol. 2017;6:6.
47. Rossi EA, Granger CE, Sharma R, et al. Imaging individual neurons in the retinal ganglion cell layer of the living eye. Proc Natl Acad Sci U S A. 2017;114:586–91.
48. Hood DC, Raza AS, de Moraes CG, Liebmann JM, Ritch R. Glaucomatous damage of the macula. Prog Retin Eye Res. 2013;32:1–21.
49. Curcio CA, Allen KA. Topography of ganglion cells in human retina. J Comp Neurol. 1990;300:5–25.
50. Hood DC, Slobodnick A, Raza AS, de Moraes CG, Teng CC, Ritch R. Early glaucoma involves both deep local, and shallow widespread, retinal nerve fiber damage of the macular region. Invest Ophthalmol Vis Sci. 2014;55:632–49.
51. De Moraes CG, Hood DC, Thenappan A, et al. 24-2 visual fields miss central defects shown on 10-2 tests in glaucoma suspects, ocular hypertensives, and early glaucoma. Ophthalmology. 2017;124:1449–56.

52. Chong LX, McKendrick AM, Ganeshrao SB, Turpin A. Customized, automated stimulus location choice for assessment of visual field defects. Invest Ophthalmol Vis Sci. 2014;55:3265–74.
53. Chong LX, Turpin A, McKendrick AM. Assessing the GOANNA visual field algorithm using artificial scotoma generation on human observers. Transl Vis Sci Technol. 2016;5:1.
54. Rubinstein NJ, McKendrick AM, Turpin A. Incorporating spatial models in visual field test procedures. Transl Vis Sci Technol. 2016;5:7.
55. Bogunović H, Kwon YH, Rashid A, et al. Relationships of retinal structure and Humphrey 24-2 visual field thresholds in patients with glaucoma. Invest Ophthalmol Vis Sci. 2015;56:259–71.
56. Ganeshrao SB, McKendrick AM, Denniss J, Turpin AJO, Science V. A perimetric test procedure that uses structural information. Optom Vis Sci. 2015;92:70–82.
57. Chauhan BC, Garway-Heath DF, Goni FJ, et al. Practical recommendations for measuring rates of visual field change in glaucoma. Br J Ophthalmol. 2008;92:569–73.
58. Wu Z, Saunders LJ, Daga FB, Diniz-Filho A, Medeiros FA. Frequency of testing to detect visual field progression derived using a longitudinal cohort of glaucoma patients. Ophthalmology. 2017;124:786–92.
59. Rao HL, Raveendran S, James V, et al. Comparing the performance of compass perimetry with humphrey field analyzer in eyes with glaucoma. J Glaucoma. 2017;26:292–7.
60. Fogagnolo P, Modarelli A, Oddone F, et al. Comparison of Compass and Humphrey perimeters in detecting glaucomatous defects. Eur J Ophthalmol. 2016;26:598–606.
61. Matsuura M, Murata H, Fujino Y, Hirasawa K, Yanagisawa M, Asaoka R. Evaluating the usefulness of MP-3 microperimetry in glaucoma patients. Am J Ophthalmol. 2018;187:1–9.
62. Zvornicanin E, Zvornicanin J, Hadziefendic B. The use of smart phones in ophthalmology. Acta Inform Med. 2014;22:206–9.
63. Anderson AJ, Bedggood PA, George Kong YX, Martin KR, Vingrys AJ. Can home monitoring allow earlier detection of rapid visual field progression in glaucoma? Ophthalmology. 2017;124:1735–42.
64. Kong YX, He M, Crowston JG, Vingrys AJ. A comparison of perimetric results from a tablet perimeter and humphrey field analyzer in glaucoma patients. Transl Vis Sci Technol. 2016;5:2.
65. Kerr NM, Patel HY, Chew SS, Ali NQ, Eady EK, Danesh-Meyer HV. Patient satisfaction with topical ocular hypotensives. Clin Experiment Ophthalmol. 2013;41:27–35.
66. Robin AL, Novack GD, Covert DW, Crockett RS, Marcic TS. Adherence in glaucoma: objective measurements of once-daily and adjunctive medication use. Am J Ophthalmol. 2007;144:533–40.
67. Hennessy AL, Katz J, Covert D, et al. A video study of drop instillation in both glaucoma and retina patients with visual impairment. Am J Ophthalmol. 2011;152:982–8.
68. Garway-Heath DF, Crabb DP, Bunce C, et al. Latanoprost for open-angle glaucoma (UKGTS): a randomised, multicentre, placebo-controlled trial. Lancet. 2015;385:1295–304.
69. Wang SK, Chang RT. An emerging treatment option for glaucoma: Rho kinase inhibitors. Clin Ophthalmol. 2014;8:883–90.
70. Rao VP, Epstein DL. Rho GTPase/Rho kinase inhibition as a novel target for the treatment of glaucoma. BioDrugs. 2007;21:167–77.
71. Tokushige H, Waki M, Takayama Y, Tanihara H. Effects of Y-39983, a selective Rho-associated protein kinase inhibitor, on blood flow in optic nerve head in rabbits and axonal regeneration of retinal ganglion cells in rats. Curr Eye Res. 2011;36:964–70.
72. Kitaoka Y, Kitaoka Y, Kumai T, et al. Involvement of RhoA and possible neuroprotective effect of fasudil, a Rho kinase inhibitor, in NMDA-induced neurotoxicity in the rat retina. Brain Res. 2004;1018:111–8.
73. Honjo M, Tanihara H, Kameda T, Kawaji T, Yoshimura N, Araie M. Potential role of Rho-associated protein kinase inhibitor Y-27632 in glaucoma filtration surgery. Invest Ophthalmol Vis Sci. 2007;48:5549–57.

74. Tanihara H, Inoue T, Yamamoto T, et al. Phase 1 clinical trials of a selective Rho kinase inhibitor, K-115. JAMA Ophthalmol. 2013;131:1288–95.
75. Tanihara H, Inoue T, Yamamoto T, et al. Phase 2 randomized clinical study of a Rho kinase inhibitor, K-115, in primary open-angle glaucoma and ocular hypertension. Am J Ophthalmol. 2013;156:731–6.
76. Okumura N, Okazaki Y, Inoue R, et al. Rho-associated kinase inhibitor eye drop (Ripasudil) transiently alters the morphology of corneal endothelial cells. Invest Ophthalmol Vis Sci. 2015;56:7560–7.
77. Tanihara H, Inoue T, Yamamoto T, et al. One-year clinical evaluation of 0.4% ripasudil (K-115) in patients with open-angle glaucoma and ocular hypertension. Acta Ophthalmol. 2016;94:e26–34.
78. Tanihara H, Inoue T, Yamamoto T, et al. Additive intraocular pressure-lowering effects of the rho kinase inhibitor Ripasudil (K-115) combined with timolol or latanoprost: a report of 2 randomized clinical trials. JAMA Ophthalmol. 2015;133:755–61.
79. Levy B, Ramirez N, Novack GD, Kopczynski C. Ocular hypotensive safety and systemic absorption of AR-13324 ophthalmic solution in normal volunteers. Am J Ophthalmol. 2015;159:980–5.e1.
80. Wang RF, Williamson JE, Kopczynski C, Serle JB. Effect of 0.04% AR-13324, a ROCK, and norepinephrine transporter inhibitor, on aqueous humor dynamics in normotensive monkey eyes. J Glaucoma. 2015;24:51–4.
81. Serle JB, Katz LJ, McLaurin E, et al. Two phase 3 clinical trials comparing the safety and efficacy of netarsudil to timolol in patients with elevated intraocular pressure: rho kinase elevated IOP treatment trial 1 and 2 (ROCKET-1 and ROCKET-2). Am J Ophthalmol. 2018;186:116–27.
82. Bacharach J, Dubiner HB, Levy B, Kopczynski CC, Novack GD, Group A-CS. Double-masked, randomized, dose-response study of AR-13324 versus latanoprost in patients with elevated intraocular pressure. Ophthalmology. 2015;122:302–7.
83. Lewis RA, Levy B, Ramirez N, et al. Fixed-dose combination of AR-13324 and latanoprost: a double-masked, 28-day, randomised, controlled study in patients with open-angle glaucoma or ocular hypertension. Br J Ophthalmol. 2016;100:339–44.
84. Krauss AH, Impagnatiello F, Toris CB, et al. Ocular hypotensive activity of BOL-303259-X, a nitric oxide donating prostaglandin F2α agonist, in preclinical models. Exp Eye Res. 2011;93:250–5.
85. Nathanson JA, McKee M. Alterations of ocular nitric oxide synthase in human glaucoma. Invest Ophthalmol Vis Sci. 1995;36:1774–84.
86. Weinreb RN, Ong T, Scassellati Sforzolini B, Vittitow JL, Singh K, Kaufman PL. A randomised, controlled comparison of latanoprostene bunod and latanoprost 0.005% in the treatment of ocular hypertension and open angle glaucoma: the VOYAGER study. Br J Ophthalmol. 2015;99:738–45.
87. Medeiros FA, Martin KR, Peace J, Scassellati Sforzolini B, Vittitow JL, Weinreb RN. Comparison of Latanoprostene Bunod 0.024% and Timolol Maleate 0.5% in open-angle glaucoma or ocular hypertension: the LUNAR study. Am J Ophthalmol. 2016;168:250–9.
88. Weinreb RN, Scassellati Sforzolini B, Vittitow J, Liebmann J. Latanoprostene Bunod 0.024% versus Timolol Maleate 0.5% in subjects with open-angle glaucoma or ocular hypertension: the APOLLO study. Ophthalmology. 2016;123:965–73.
89. Perera SA, Ting DS, Nongpiur ME, et al. Feasibility study of sustained-release travoprost punctum plug for intraocular pressure reduction in an Asian population. Clin Ophthalmol. 2016;10:757–64.
90. Brandt JD, Sall K, DuBiner H, et al. Six-month intraocular pressure reduction with a topical bimatoprost ocular insert: results of a phase II randomized controlled study. Ophthalmology. 2016;123:1685–94.
91. Brandt JD, DuBiner HB, Benza R, et al. Long-term safety and efficacy of a sustained-release bimatoprost ocular ring. Ophthalmology. 2017;124:1565–6.

92. Franca JR, Foureaux G, Fuscaldi LL, et al. Bimatoprost-loaded ocular inserts as sustained release drug delivery systems for glaucoma treatment: in vitro and in vivo evaluation. PLoS One. 2014;9:e95461.
93. Lewis R, Christie W, Day D. Bimatoprost sustained-release implants for glaucoma therapy: interim results from a 24-month phase 1/2 clinical trial. In: Paper session presented at The AAO Annual Meeting, Las Vegas, NV; 2015.
94. Lewis RA, Christie WC, Day DG, et al. Bimatoprost sustained-release implants for glaucoma therapy: 6-month results from a phase I/II clinical trial. Am J Ophthalmol. 2017;175:137–47.
95. Glaukos. Glaukos Corporation's iDose™ Travoprost achieves sustained IOP reduction and favorable safety profile in 12-month interim cohort; 2018.
96. Spaeth GL, Idowu O, Seligsohn A, et al. The effects of iridotomy size and position on symptoms following laser peripheral iridotomy. Am J Ophthalmol. 2006;141:427–8.
97. Vera V, Naqi A, Belovay GW, Varma DK, Ahmed II. Dysphotopsia after temporal versus superior laser peripheral iridotomy: a prospective randomized paired eye trial. Am J Ophthalmol. 2014;157:929–35.
98. Srinivasan K, Zebardast N, Krishnamurthy P, et al. Comparison of new visual disturbances after superior versus nasal/temporal laser peripheral iridotomy: a prospective randomized trial. Ophthalmology. 2018;125:345–51.
99. Gunning FP, Greve EL. Lens extraction for uncontrolled angle-closure glaucoma: long-term follow-up. J Cataract Refract Surg. 1998;24:1347–56.
100. Azuara-Blanco A, Burr J, Ramsay C, et al. Effectiveness of early lens extraction for the treatment of primary angle-closure glaucoma (EAGLE): a randomised controlled trial. Lancet. 2016;388:1389–97.
101. Kerr NM, Kumar HK, Crowston JG, Walland MJ. Glaucoma laser and surgical procedure rates in Australia. Br J Ophthalmol. 2016;100:1686–91.
102. Gedde SJ, Schiffman JC, Feuer WJ, et al. Treatment outcomes in the Tube Versus Trabeculectomy (TVT) study after five years of follow-up. Am J Ophthalmol. 2012;153:789–803.e2.
103. Gedde SJ, Feuer WJ, Shi W, et al. Treatment outcomes in the primary tube versus trabeculectomy study after 1 year of follow-up. Ophthalmology. 2018;125:650–63.
104. Glaukos. Glaukos announces FDA approval for the iStent inject® Trabecular Micro-Bypass System; 2018.
105. Ivantis. Ivantis Announces FDA approval for its innovative Hydrus® Microstent Device for Minimally Invasive Glaucoma Surgery (MIGS); 2018.
106. Ivantis. New Data from the HORIZON Trial of the Hydrus® Microstent shows significantly lower IOP and medication use at 24 months in a US Patient Cohort; 2018.
107. Ivantis. Ivantis announces results of landmark prospective, randomized comparative MIGS clinical trial; 2018.
108. FDA. Alcon Research, LTD. Recalls CyPass® Micro-stent Systems due to risk of endothelial cell loss; 2018.
109. Vold S, Ahmed IIK, Craven ER, et al. Two-year COMPASS trial results: supraciliary microstenting with phacoemulsification in patients with open-angle glaucoma and cataracts. Ophthalmology. 2016;123:2103–12.
110. ASCRS. Preliminary ASCRS CyPass Withdrawal Consensus Statement; 2018.
111. Alcon. Alcon announces voluntary global market withdrawal of CyPass Micro-Stent for surgical glaucoma; 2018.
112. Schlenker MB, Gulamhusein H, Conrad-Hengerer I, et al. Efficacy, safety, and risk factors for failure of standalone Ab interno gelatin microstent implantation versus standalone trabeculectomy. Ophthalmology. 2017;124:1579–88.
113. Gedde SJ, Herndon LW, Brandt JD, et al. Postoperative complications in the Tube Versus Trabeculectomy (TVT) study during five years of follow-up. Am J Ophthalmol. 2012;153:804–14.e1.

114. Lewis RA. Ab interno approach to the subconjunctival space using a collagen glaucoma stent. J Cataract Refract Surg. 2014;40:1301–6.
115. Allergan. Allergan Receives FDA Clearance for the XEN® Gel Stent, a New Surgical Treatment for Refractory Glaucoma; 2016.
116. Acosta AC, Espana EM, Yamamoto H, et al. A newly designed glaucoma drainage implant made of poly (styrene-b-isobutylene-b-styrene): biocompatibility and function in normal rabbit eyes. Arch Ophthalmol. 2006;124:1742–9.
117. Batlle JF, Fantes F, Riss I, et al. Three-year follow-up of a novel aqueous humor microshunt. J Glaucoma. 2016;25:e58–65.
118. Arrieta EA, Aly M, Parrish R, et al. Clinicopathologic correlations of poly-(styrene-b-isobutylene-b-styrene) glaucoma drainage devices of different internal diameters in rabbits. Ophthalmic Surg Lasers Imaging Retina. 2011;42:338–45.

# Chapter 5
# Recent Advances in Uveitis

Xia Ni Wu, Lazha Ahmed Talat Sharief, Roy Schwartz,
Þóra Elísabet Jónsdóttir, Anastasia Tasiopoulou,
Ahmed Al-Janabi, Noura Al Qassimi, Amgad Mahmoud,
Sue Lightman, and Oren Tomkins-Netzer

## Introduction

The uveitides are a collection of more than 30 diseases manifesting as intraocular inflammation. Their prevalence is approximately 60–130 per 10,000 people, though they remain a common cause of blindness, accounting for up to 15% of cases [1, 2]. Because uveitis primarily affects young people of working age, it can result in significant, long-lasting morbidity. Early diagnosis and prompt treatment can prevent ocular complications and vision loss in many cases. With the continued advancement of diagnostic techniques and targeted drugs, early identification and rapid inflammatory control is increasingly possible.

## The Standardization of Uveitis Nomenclature

The diagnosis of uveitis relies mainly on the combination of clinical presentation and ancillary tests, including laboratory tests and imaging studies [3]. Most symptoms and signs have low specificity and can appear across different etiologies.

X. N. Wu · L. A. T. Sharief · R. Schwartz · Þ. E. Jónsdóttir · A. Tasiopoulou · A. Al-Janabi
N. Al Qassimi · A. Mahmoud · S. Lightman
Institute of Ophthalmology, University College London, Moorfields Eye Hospital,
London, UK

O. Tomkins-Netzer (✉)
Institute of Ophthalmology, University College London, Moorfields Eye Hospital,
London, UK

Technion, Institute of Technology, Bnai Zion Medical Center, Haifa, Israel
e-mail: o.tomkins-netzer@ucl.ac.uk

© Springer Nature Switzerland AG 2020                                      121
A. Grzybowski (ed.), *Current Concepts in Ophthalmology*,
https://doi.org/10.1007/978-3-030-25389-9_5

This complicates our ability to report on specific diseases or even reach an agreement between treating physicians. To try and address this issue, the Standardization of Uveitis Nomenclature (SUN) Working Group proposed diagnostic criteria and unified nomenclature in describing uveitis [4]. The project categorized uveitis according to anatomical location (anterior, intermediate, posterior, and panuveitis), temporal course (acute, recurrent, and chronic) and disease activity (cells and flare grading). The SUN group then attempted to develop classification criteria for the diagnosis of the leading 25 uveitis entities [5]. They reviewed the clinical and laboratory findings of 5766 cases collected from multinational clinics and examined the diagnostic agreement between uveitis experts. It was concluded that agreement between uveitis experts on the diagnosis of a specific disease entity was moderate in most cases but increased to 99% once a consensus was reached between the experts. Expanding the use of validated and standardized classification criteria will improve the diagnosis and reporting of uveitis.

## Imaging in Uveitis

Imaging modalities continue to evolve, bringing with them new diagnostic abilities and improving patient treatment and follow-up. Conventional fundus photography and fluorescein angiography (FA) are limited by their narrow fields of view. Ultra-wide-field (UWF) imaging provides a 200-degree view of the fundus that can demonstrate pathologies in the retinal periphery and assist in their localization relative to the posterior pole. This enhanced representation of retinal pathology aids in the clinical management and treatment of posterior uveitis (Fig. 5.1a, b) [6]. Aggarwal et al. compared findings in traditional and UWF FA in 33 eyes with posterior uveitis related to tuberculosis (TB) and showed that UWF revealed additional areas of non-perfusion, neovascularization, active vasculitis, and peripheral choroiditis, which influenced treatment decisions in 45.5% of eyes [7]. Similarly, Mesquida et al reviewed 38 eyes with active vasculitis associated with Behçet disease [8]. UWF imaging revealed additional information that resulted in a change of management in 80% of patients and improved disease monitoring in 55%. Conversely, UWF may reveal peripheral vasculitis in an otherwise asymptomatic eye and patient, the clinical significance of which currently remains unknown.

Optical coherence tomography angiography (OCTA) is a novel and noninvasive technique for demonstrating the microvascular blood flow. It produces depth-resolved evaluation of the reflectance data, providing three-dimensional volume information and can be used to isolate vascular structures from the retinal neural network [9]. A valuable use of this imaging modality is in the diagnosis of choroidal neovascularization (CNV), which is a known complication of posterior uveitis. Although FA remains the gold standard for the detection of CNV, it may be limited when differentiating between active inflammatory lesions and inactive lesions with an active CNV. Studies on patients with punctate inner choroidopathy and multifocal choroiditis demonstrate that OCTA is able to depict the vascular elements and

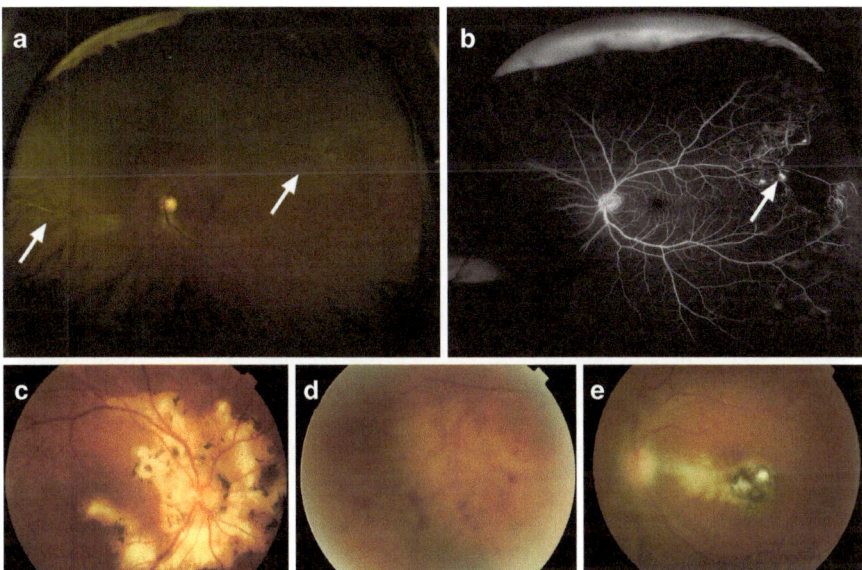

**Fig. 5.1** Infectious Uveitis. (**a**) Ultra-wide-field color images of a patient with occlusive vasculitis related to tuberculosis demonstrating peripheral ghost vessels (arrows) and small retinal hemorrhages. (**b**) Fluorescein angiography showing an area of retinal ischemia in the temporal periphery with neovascularization along the border (arrow). (**c**) Serpiginous-like choroiditis extending from the optic disc. (**d**) Acute retinal necrosis with extensive areas of retinal necrosis, retinitis and retinal hemorrhages. (**e**) Reactivation of ocular toxoplasmosis along the nasal border of an old chorioretinal scar

help differentiate between active inflammation and CNV, both of which leak on FA [10]. This informs subsequent management decisions for immunosuppression and/or anti-angiogenic treatments. Further, the noninvasive nature of OCTA allows its utilisation in patients where conventional FA would be contraindicated such as allergy.

Swept-source optical coherence tomography (SS-OCT) uses a short cavity swept laser with a tunable wavelength of operation instead of the diode laser used in spectral-domain OCT, giving it improved image penetration using a wavelength of 1050 nm and high axial resolution [11]. This method allows better visualization of the choroid together with the retina, aiding in the diagnosis and management of choroidal conditions. Dastiridou et al., analyzed SS-OCT images of 386 eyes with birdshot chorioretinopathy (BSCR) and 59 control eyes and found higher choroidal reflectivity and lower choroidal thickness in inactive BSCR patients compared with active patients and controls, suggesting these as biomarkers for disease activity [12]. Another example of a useful biomarker was demonstrated in Vogt-Koyanagi-Harada syndrome (VKH). A new SS-OCT parameter, "RPE undulation index" which quantitatively describes choroidal deformations, was positively related to both choroidal and retinal thickness, indicating it may be used as a marker of VKH severity [13].

The diagnosis and management of uveitis is heavily reliant on imaging. The rapid development of imaging modalities is expected to further enhance our ability to diagnose and manage uveitis patients. Combinations of the above modalities, including wide-field and swept-source OCTA are promising developments in this regard.

## Advances in the Management of Non-infectious Uveitis

Uveitis may be related to systemic disease in up to 20% of patients and can be the presenting sign in many cases [1]. Ocular findings guide the workup of patients to include tests aimed at identifying related diseases. Presence of systemic disease may influence the management of the ocular inflammation, and inform the need for multidisciplinary input. Diagnostic techniques are continually advancing, establishing more exact disease etiologies and relationships to systemic diseases.

## Anterior Uveitis and Spondyloarthritis

Anterior uveitis (AU) is the most common form of uveitis, accounting for up to a third of cases [1], and up to 60% are also HLA-B27 positive [14]. HLA-B27-associated acute AU (AAU) is the most common form of AU, and is strongly related to underlying systemic disease such as spondyloarthritis (SpA), [15, 16] with many patients having undiagnosed axial SpA. In a study on axial magnetic resonance imaging (MRI) of young AAU patients with chronic back pain, up to a quarter were found to have axial SpA [17]. Studies examining screening algorithms for the diagnosis of SpA among patients with AAU found that 40–50% had undiagnosed SpA [14, 18], with patients who were HLA-B27 positive more likely to be subsequently diagnosed [14]. While treatment of AU is primarily based on topical corticosteroids, systemic disease requires the involvement of rheumatologists and potentially systemic immunosuppression. This can include anti-tumor necrosis factor α (TNFα) agents, which may affect the likelihood of AU reactivation and disease control. Infliximab and adalimumab have been shown to reduce the risk of uveitis flares and the need for ocular treatment [19–25]. Conversely, etanercept is well-known to have little effect on ocular inflammation, and may actually induce intraocular inflammation and result in an increased prevalence of flares [22, 23]. Using screening algorithms to identify previously undiagnosed SpA patients would allow early treatment and disease control, while the choice of drugs can have a direct impact on uveitis control.

## Sarcoidosis

Sarcoidosis is a multisystemic chronic inflammatory disorder of unknown etiology characterized by noncaseating granulomas. Between 30 and 60% of patients develop ocular signs, which can be the presenting complaint in up to 30% of patients [26].

The International Workshop on Ocular Sarcoidosis (IWOS) recently presented the revised guidelines for the diagnosis of ocular sarcoidosis [27]. Patients are considered to have definite ocular sarcoidosis with a positive biospy and compatible uveitis, and presumed or probable disease if they had a combination of ocular signs and positive laboratory findings but no suggestive biopsy (Fig. 5.2a, Table 5.1). Presumed disease requires the presence of bi-hilar lymphadenopathy and two additional intraocular signs; probable disease is defined by three intraocular signs and two other positive investigations. Other tests under consideration for inclusion in future consensus guidelines include serum levels of soluble interleukin (IL)-2 receptor and Krebs von den Lungen (KL)-6. Of note, elevated IL-2 receptor levels were reported to have 98% sensitivity and 94% specificity in ocular sarcoidosis [28].

The use of angiotensin converting enzyme (ACE) levels to diagnose ocular sarcoidosis is of particular interest. ACE can be elevated in many granulomatous pulmonary diseases such as tuberculosis, sarcoidosis and histoplasmosis [29], and its value in the diagnosis of these diseases is controversial. When results of elevated ACE levels were combined with abnormal levels of serum lysozyme from patients with ocular sarcoidosis they had a sensitivity of 61%, which suggests a limited role in diagnosis [30]. In a recent study that examined the value of elevated ACE levels in predicting ocular sarcoidosis from a general non-infectious uveitis population [31], ACE had a sensitivity of 78% and a specificity of 90% for ocular sarcoidosis among adults, with a negative predictive value of 97%. In children the test performed less well and had a sensitivity of 60% and a specificity of 78.5%, but still with a negative predictive value of 96.9%. These results suggest the greatest advantage of testing ACE levels would be in ruling out sarcoidosis in suspected cases, when the levels are within the normal range. It should also be noted that the normal range of ACE levels can vary between laboratories but is generally accepted to be up to 53 μL [31]. Normal ACE levels from children can be even higher and caution should be exercised in their interpretation [32].

Following diagnosis, the treatment of sarcoidosis frequently requires the use of long-term immunosuppression. Similar to other forms of uveitis, treatment is based

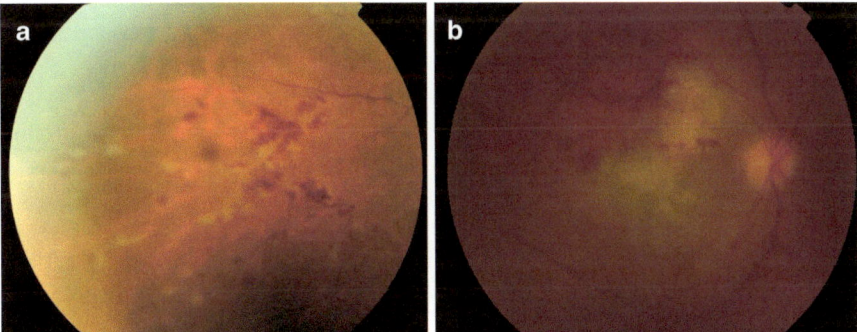

**Fig. 5.2** Non-infectious Uveitis. (**a**) A patient with ocular sarcoidosis demonstrating choroidal granulomas and retinal vasculitis with hemorrhages. (**b**) A case of Behçet disease manifesting as retinitis with occlusive vasculitis

**Table 5.1** IWOS revised diagnostic criteria for ocular sarcoidosis

| **Clinical signs** |
| --- |
| 1. Mutton-fat KPs (large and small) and/or iris nodules at pupillary margin (Koeppe) or in stroma (Busacca) |
| 2. Trabecular meshwork nodules and/or tent-shaped PAS |
| 3. Snowballs/string of pearls vitreous opacities |
| 4. Multiple chorioretinal peripheral lesions (active and atrophic) |
| 5. Nodular and/or segmental periphlebitis (± candle wax drippings) and/or macroaneurysm in an inflamed eye |
| 6. Optic disc nodule(s)/granuloma(s) and/or solitary choroidal nodule |
| 7. Bilaterality |
| **Systemic investigations** |
| 1. Bilateral hilar lymphadenopathy on chest X-ray and/or chest CT scan |
| 2. Negative tuberculin test or interferon-gamma releasing assays |
| 3. Serum angiotensin converting enzyme elevated |
| 4. Serum lysozyme elevated |
| 5. Bronchoalveolar lavage fluid CD4/CD8 ratio elevated (> 3.5) |
| 6. PET positive (abnormal accumulation of gallium-67 scintigraphy or 18F-fluorodeoxyglucose) |
| 7. Lymphopenia (< 1000 cells/uL) |
| 8. Parenchymal lung changes consistent with sarcoidosis as determined by pulmonologists or radiologists |

*KP* keratic precipitate; *PAS* peripheral anterior synechiae; *CT* computed tomography; *PET* positron emission tomography

on a drug escalation approach beginning with systemic corticosteroids [33, 34], followed by 2nd-line immunosuppressive agents and biologics as needed. Sarcoidosis appears to have a relatively good response to corticosteroids, and while these patients are seen to need more corticosteroids than other causes of uveitis, they are less likely to need 2nd-line treatment [35, 36]. The majority of patients respond to treatment and visual acuity is maintained [37], with macular edema and cataract the main causes of vision loss.

# Behçet's Disease

Behçet's disease (BD) is a chronic inflammatory disorder of unknown etiology that predominates along the ancient 'Silk Route' from southern Europe, Turkey to Japan [38, 39]. The disease manifests as an immune-mediated systemic vasculitis involving small, medium, and large arteries and veins (Fig. 5.2b) [40]. Ocular involvement occurs in up to 50% of patients and ranges from a chronic panuveitis to vasculitis, resulting in vision loss in many cases [41, 42]. While the disease is classically characterized by the triad of recurrent oral and genital aphthous ulcers, ocular inflammation and skin lesions [43], many patients do not present with the full set of signs and diagnosis is based on matching diagnostic criteria. HLA-B51 has some association with the disease (sensitivity 51%, specificity 71%) but is not part of the diagnostic criteria and should mainly be used to support the diagnosis [15, 44]. Several diagnostic criteria have been proposed; the International Criteria for BD (ICBD) is currently the most commonly used [45]. These criteria comprise of a scoring system of seven items including ocular findings, genital ulcers, oral ulcers, skin lesions, neurological manifestations, vascular manifestations and a positive pathergy test [45]. The minimum score for a patient to be classified as having BD is 4. The criteria demonstrate a high sensitivity (94.8%), but a lower specificity (90.5%). Interestingly, a UK cohort study which used the newer ICBD 2014 classification in a predominantly UK population showed even lower specificity and suggested reversion to older classification systems for UK populations [46].

Behçet's disease is a potentially blinding condition, secondary to macular ischaemia, dense vitritis, and macular edema [42, 47]. Treatment must be started immediately and maintained long-term to prevent disease progression, second eye involvement, ocular complications and vision loss. Treatment is based on the use of systemic immunosuppression, and while corticosteroids are used as the 1st-line agent, studies demonstrate that BD is particularly responsive to treatment with anti-TNFα agents [48–51]. The recent licensing of adalimumab for the treatment of refractory uveitis recognized this particular affinity and adalimumab is available in some countries for most BD-related uveitis patients immediately following treatment failure with corticosteroids, without the need of first attempting a 2nd-line agent. Other studies suggest that refractory BD-related uveitis is also highly responsive to interferon α2a [52–54], which can be considered for such cases. Treatment results in visual acuity stabilization, extended disease remission and prolonged time to relapse.

## Systemic Treatment for Non-infectious Uveitis

Choice of treatment for non-infectious uveitis is influenced by the disease laterality, systemic involvement, course and natural history, and tolerability to the drugs. In many cases, long-term treatment is required to maintain disease control and issues of extended exposure and systemic side effects influence treatment choice. Oral corticosteroids are crucial for acute management while the slower acting immunosuppressive agents are important as 2nd-line treatment and as steroid-sparing agents [55]. Conventional immunosuppressants include antimetabolites (methotrexate, mycophenolate mofetil, azathioprine), calcineurin inhibitors (cyclosporine, tacrolimus), and alkylating agents (cyclophosphamide, chlorambucil). Newer biologic agents used in uveitis are the anti-TNFα inhibitors infliximab and adalimumab.

Corticosteroids are the cornerstone of uveitis management and are delivered either locally or systemically. They work quickly and effectively for most inflammatory conditions, are widely studied and generally well tolerated [55]. The aim of treatment is to achieve complete control of the disease with resolution of all intraocular inflammation, while maintaining a long-term steroid dose of ≤7.5 mg prednisolone per day, which significantly reduces the risk of systemic side effects [56]. Use of 2nd-line immunosuppressive agents and biologics is advocated as steroid-sparing treatment when inflammatory control is not achieved, maintained at low corticosteroid doses, or when the side effects are intolerable. Second-line immunosuppressive agents achieve disease control in up to 50% of cases and while none are licensed for treating uveitis, methotrexate and mycophenolate mofetil are commonly used [2, 57]. Treatment requires continual monitoring of blood counts as well as hepatic function, and side effects can restrict the use of these drugs.

The increasing understanding of the inflammatory cascade and in particular, evidence supporting Th-17 cells as mediators of uveitis, has led to the identification of cytokines that influence these cells and the development of specific biologic drugs. Current candidate molecules for treatment include pro-inflammatory cytokines such as TNFα, IL-6, IL-17 as well as vascular endothelial growth factor (VEGF) [58]. Most of the information on clinical use of biologics in uveitis focuses on anti-TNFα drugs. Infliximab is a chimeric monoclonal antibody to TNFα and adalimumab is a fully human monoclonal antibody. Both drugs appear to be effective for treating uveitis and in particular, uveitis related to juvenile idiopathic arthritis (JIA), BD, and HLA-B27-associated uveitis [20, 59]. In 2016 the results of two randomized, placebo-controlled trials resulted in the U.S. Food and Drug Administration approving adalimumab for the treatment of non-infectious, intermediate, posterior or panuveitis. The VISUAL I & II studies demonstrated that treatment with adalimumab resulted in an almost 50% reduction in relapse rates following a rapid tapering of systemic corticosteroids [60, 61]. Patients with either active uveitis (VISUAL I) and inactive uveitis (VISUAL II) had reduced rates of treatment failure and vision loss, compared to patients given placebo. A follow-up study (VISUAL III) demonstrated that 60% of patients with active uveitis at baseline were able to achieve quiescence by week 78, with 66% of them steroid-free [62]. 74% of patients who were inactive at baseline also maintained quiescence at week 78. Adalimumab was further demonstrated to be an effective adjunctive treatment to methotrexate for the management of patients with JIA-related uveitis. Those receiving adalimumab had a 27% treatment failure rate compared to 60% among placebo-treated patients [63]. Several studies have attempted to compare the effect of treating uveitis between infliximab and adalimumab and did not find a significant difference [64–66]. Adalimumab is currently indicated as a 3rd-line agent for refractory uveitis that failed corticosteroids and at least one other immunosuppressive agent, although it is licensed as 2nd-line for BD in some countries.

Studies on tocilizumab, an IL-6 receptor antagonist, suggest that repeat infusions can result in effective control of intraocular inflammation over 6–12 months [67–70]. Currently, treatment with tocilizumab is not licensed for uveitis and is considered only in cases that failed anti-TNFα agents. Sarilumab, another IL-6 receptor antibody, demonstrated less efficacy at controlling intraocular inflammation, though it demonstrated a more pronounced effect on macular edema [71]. Secukinumab, an anti IL-17A antibody, has demonstrated mixed results. Three randomized controlled studies failed to demonstrate a significant effect for subcutaneous drug administration [72], while a trial examining intravenous infusions *resulted in* showed improved inflammatory control and remission rates [73].

## Use of Local Treatment for Non-infectious Uveitis

Local treatment for uveitis includes the use of topical drops as well as periocular and intraocular injections. Intraocular steroids are used as monotherapy or as an adjunctive to systemic immunosuppression [74, 75]. Intravitreal injections of triamcinolone acetate (2–4 mg) are routinely used for controlling posterior uveitis, vitritis, and macular edema [76]. The injections are effective in controlling the intraocular inflammation, reducing macular edema, and improving vision, with few systemic side effects. A single injection can last up to three months and can be repeated as needed. However ocular side effects are common, predominantly raised intraocular pressure and cataract progression [76, 77]. The bioerodible dexamethasone implant Ozurdex (Allergan, Irvine, CA) is licensed for use in non-infectious non-anterior uveitis to control intraocular inflammation, reduce vitreous haze and macular edema, and improve vision [78].

Long-term corticosteroid implants are also used for controlling uveitis and there are currently two commercially available intravitreal fluocinolone acetonide implants (0.59 mg), a surgically inserted implant (Retisert; Bausch & Lomb, Bridgewater, NJ) and an injectable insert (Iluvien; Alimera Sciences, Aldershot, UK). These implants continually release a steady dose of steroids into the vitreous up to 2.5 years. The Multicenter Uveitis Steroid Treatment (MUST) trial and follow-up study (MUST-FS) was a prospective, randomized, multicenter study designed to compare conventional systemic therapy with oral corticosteroids and immunosuppression against the surgically inserted fluocinolone acetonide implant [79]. The study randomized 255 patients (479 eyes with uveitis) to either treatment arm and by 2 years found there was no difference with regards to visual acuity, though the implant was superior in inflammatory control [80]. Patients who completed the study were followed up to 7 years with the results remaining steady for an additional 30 months and only lost at the 7 years timepoint, when the group receiving systemic treatment achieved an average visual benefit of 7.1 letters [79]. It is thought that inflammatory relapses once the steroid implant wears out results in chorioretinal scarring and visual penalty. Ocular side effects were greater in the implant group, with 45% of eyes requiring glaucoma surgery and 90% requiring cataract surgery. However, visual function improved following cataract surgery and remained comparable [81], with many patients remaining disease free for many years, without the need for additional systemic treatment. The injectable fluocinolone acetate insert is currently under investigation as a treatment for non-infectious uveitis and preliminary results form a prospective, randomized, multicenter study comparing it to sham injections suggest that by 12 months the risk of disease recurrence was significantly reduced (38% vs. 98%), though the risk of cataract development was higher (33% vs. 12%) [82].

To identify the preferred local treatment approach to uveitic macular edema, the Periocular and Intravitreal Corticosteroids for Uveitis Macular Edema (POINT) trial compared the relative efficacy of periocular triamcinolone, intravitreal triamcinolone and the intravitreal dexamethasone implant [83]. The study randomized 192 patients (235 eyes with uveitic macular edema) to one of the three treatment arms and followed them for 6 months. The primary endpoint was the change in central subfield thickness (CST) at 8 weeks. The study found that while all treatment arms resulted in improved CST, for those receiving intravitreal triamcinolone injections or the dexamethasone implant the change was greater than for those receiving periocular triamcinolone (39%, 46% and 23%, respectively). Both intravitreal treatment arms were superior in resolving macular edema and improving visual acuity, though there was no difference between them.

Other options for local treatment include the use of intravitreal methotrexate injections (400 µg/0.1 mL), which may be effective for up to 4 months in refractory cases [84, 85], or intravitreal biologic agents such as sirolimus. A study examining the effect of an intravitreal injection of 440 µg of sirolimus demonstrated a significant improvement in intraocular inflammation and vitreous haze, while maintaining visual acuity and allowing up to 77% of patients to taper their systemic immunosuppression [86]. The follow-up study did not reach primary outcomes and was therefore not approved by the FDA. Other small cohort studies suggest that while visual acuity may improve, in some eyes the treatment induced inflammation [87, 88]. The current available data is not sufficiently robust to conclude about the role of intravitreal anti-TNFα agents for the treatment of noninfectious uveitis.

Anti-vascular endothelial growth factor agents are routinely used for the treatment of macular edema secondary to diabetic retinopathy and retinal vein occlusions [89, 90]. While its role in these diseases is well established, the evidence in ocular inflammation is less clear and relies mainly on small case series. A recent study of uncommon causes of macular edema compared monthly injections of ranibizumab to sham treatment and included 21 patients with uveitis-related macular edema. At two months, the treated group had a greater gain in visual acuity and CST, however by 12 months the effect on CST was lost [91]. A second study comparing repeated monthly injections of bevacizumab to intravitreal triamcinolone for the treatment of refractory CME in eyes with inactive uveitis found that by 24 months, both treatments resulted in improvement in CST and visual acuity [92]. The study suggests bevacizumab may have a role in the management of refractory CME in quiescent eyes. The Macular Edema Ranibizumab vs. Intravitreal Anti-inflammatory Therapy (MERIT) trial is currently recruiting and will attempt to compare the efficacy of ranibizumab and intravitreal steroids in treating uveitic macular edema.

## Advances in the Management of Infectious Uveitis

When considering infectious causes of uveitis, damage to ocular structures is caused by both the pathogen and the immune system. In many instances, ophthalmologists are required to begin treatment before a firm diagnosis is reached and therapy is routinely initiated with a combination of anti-microbial and immunosuppressive drugs. Once a definitive diagnosis is reached, the unnecessary treatments are stopped. While anti-microbial treatment is guided by pathogen sensitivity, the unique structure of the eye, in particular the function of the blood-ocular and blood retinal barriers, further complicates the choice of treatment.

Identifying possible infectious pathogens is primarily based on serum serology and cultures obtained from ocular biopsies. Polymerase chain reaction (PCR) is a method used to identify genetic material and is used in the diagnosis of infectious uveitis. It is both sensitive (85–90.2%) and highly specific (67–93.9%) and can be used to test for the DNA or RNA of a pathogen [93–95]. It can be applied to small volume samples, such as are obtained from the anterior chamber or vitreous biopsies, is suitable for diagnosing ocular infectious diseases and is comparable to the results of cultures [95–97]. The method can be applied to the diagnosis of infectious endophthalmitis, ocular toxoplasmosis and herpetic-related uveitis [98–100]. In cases of anterior uveitis with sectoral iris atrophy, distinguishing the causative agent particularly between herpes simplex virus, varicella zoster virus and cytomegalovirus, influences the choice, dose, and length of antiviral treatments [101].

## Acute Retinal Necrosis

Acute retinal necrosis (ARN) is a retinal infection occurring in either immunocompetent or immunocompromised patients caused by viruses from the herpesviridae family, particularly herpes simplex virus and varicella zoster virus. The infection results in extensive retinal necrosis, typically beginning in the retinal periphery and progressing towards the posterior pole (Fig. 5.1d). Patient visual outcome is generally poor and early, aggressive treatment is warranted to prevent vision loss and retinal complications, such as retinal detachment [102]. Treatment includes the use of systemic antivirals, particularly intravenous (IV) aciclovir with systemic corticosterois and adjunctive intravitreal injections of antiviral drugs. Alternatively, intravenous aciclovir can be substituted with oral valaciclovir, a prodrug of aciclovir, which has good bioavailability and results in comparable intravitreal concentrations of the active drug. Pharmacokinetic modeling predicted equivalent vitreal concentrations between valaciclovir 1.5/2.0 g three times a day and IV aciclovir 700 mg every 8 h. Intravitreal drug levels exceeded the 50% inhibitory concentration for varicella zoster virus [103]. Using oral drugs allows patients to be managed in an outpatient setting, though strict monitoring is still required. While severe vision loss still occurs in up to 50% of eyes [104, 105], a study comparing both treatment approaches found no difference in final visual acuity [106]. Vision loss is most commonly related to the development of retinal detachment that occurs in up to 60% of eyes [98, 106, 107]. The concurrent use of intravitreal injections, either foscarnet 2.4 mg/0.1 mL or ganciclovir 2–5 mg/0.05–0.1 mL, may have a greater therapeutic effect and several case series suggest that rates of retinal detachment and vision loss may be reduced [108, 109]. The value of early prophylactic barrier laser remains unclear with conflicting results from retrospective case series. The American Academy of Ophthalmology recently concluded that initial oral or IV antiviral treatment with adjunctive intravitreal foscarnet is an effective therapeutic approach, and that the role of prophylactic laser retinopexy remains unclear [98].

## Tuberculosis-Related Uveitis

Tuberculosis (TB) is a worldwide problem caused by *Mycobacterium tuberculosis*, and results in extensive morbidity and mortality [110]. The majority of people exposed to tuberculosis remain asymptomatic and the disease is described as latent TB. Diagnosis relies on positive testing, such as the Mantoux test or interferon gamma release assays, amongst other investigations [111]. Ocular involvement classically presents as choroidal granulomas, chronic panuveitis, and/or occlusive retinal vasculitis (Fig. 5.1a, b). The mechanism of ocular disease in latent TB remains unclear. Serpiginous choroiditis accounts for up to half the cases associated with TB [112, 113], particularly in endemic regions (Fig. 5.1c). While anti-TB treatment is clearly indicated in patients with signs of active pulmonary or extrapulmonary TB infection, treatment of those with latent TB is inconsistent, particularly if the ocular phenotype is atypical. While the ocular inflammation is managed with local and systemic immunosuppressive drugs, several studies have suggested that systemic anti-TB treatment may reduce uveitis recurrence rates [114–118]. If the ophthalmologist suspects the uveitis to be related to latent TB and decides to initiate immunosuppressive treatment, a full six month anti-TB course is advocated and therapy should be given in coordination with infectious disease specialists. In particular, patients should be treated for latent TB prior to commencing anti-TNFα immunosuppression given the increased risk of infection.

## Toxoplasmosis

*Toxoplasma gondii*, an intracellular protozoan parasite, is a common pathogen infecting approximately 30% of the global population [119]. The life cycle of the parasite is linked to that of cats, and in regions where cats are common up to 90% of the population are seropositive (e.g. Brazil, Paris) [120]. Ocular infection is common and primary infection may be either congenital or following ingestion of contaminated food or drink. Most primary infections are asymptomatic and cases that are brought to clinical attention are typically reactivations along the border of an old chorio-retinal scar (Fig. 5.1e). Active infection can appear as a chorioretinitis with vitritis and occasionally AU. While diagnosis is based on clinical presentation and positive serum serology for *Toxoplasma gondii*, identifying the retinal lesions in the presence of severe inflammation and dense vitritis may be difficult and a high level of suspicion is needed [121]. Although toxoplasmosis in an immunocompetent patient is a self-limiting disease, treatment is considered when active inflammation is located near structures that are important for visual function (optic disc, macula and main retinal blood vessels) or when symptoms affect visual function. Treatment is based on a combination of anti-parasitic agents and anti-inflammatory drugs [122], and while the classic triad of pyrimethamine, sulfadiazine and folinic acid is commonly used, other treatment protocols are also suggested. Alternative treatment approaches include the use of oral or intravitreal clindamycin or oral trimethoprim and sulfamethoxazole [123, 124]. The latter is given twice a day and is considerably easier for patients to follow. Several studies examined the efficacy of these different treatment options though none demonstrated a clear advantage [123]. In a recent statement, the American Academy of Ophthalmology concluded there was no clinical evidence to support an advantage to using any particular treatment and choice of protocol should be based on clinical experience [125]. The use of prophylactic treatment following reactivation continues to be debated and several studies demonstrated that antibiotic treatment for up to a year could reduce the risk of reactivation by as much as 90% [126–129]. The risk of reactivation may continue to be reduced after stopping treatment for up to three years [130], though there is no clear recommendation for continuing prophylactic treatment [125, 127]. Long-term prophylactic treatment should be considered in patients with increased risk of reactivation, immunocompromised patients, or those with multiple previous recurrences [125, 131].

The last decade has seen an exponential increase in diagnostic and treatment tools available to the ophthalmologist, with the ensuing advancement in research, knowledge, and management. Precise imaging methods, utilizing wide-angle imaging and combined techniques, will help identify active inflammation even in the retinal periphery and will distinguish it from other retinal lesions, such as neovascularization. The increasing use of biologic agents and intravitreal drugs will also result in better control of intraocular inflammation and less systemic side effects related to systemic corticosteroids. Longer acting agents, with less ocular and systemic side effects will help manage the disease in these otherwise healthy patients and promote their continued independence and productivity.

# References

1. Tomkins-Netzer O, Talat L, Bar A, et al. Long-term clinical outcome and causes of vision loss in patients with uveitis. Ophthalmology. 2014;121(12):2387–92.
2. Jabs DA. Immunosuppression for the Uveitides. Ophthalmology. 2018;125(2):193–202.
3. Jabs DA, Busingye J. Approach to the diagnosis of the uveitides. Am J Ophthalmol. 2013;156(2):228–36.
4. Jabs DA, Nussenblatt RB, Rosenbaum JT. Standardization of uveitis nomenclature for reporting clinical data. Results of the First International Workshop. Am J Ophthalmol. 2005;140(3):509–16.
5. Jabs DA, Dick A, Doucette JT, et al. Interobserver agreement among uveitis experts on uveitic diagnoses: the standardization of uveitis nomenclature experience. Am J Ophthalmol. 2018;186:19–24.
6. Campbell JP, Leder HA, Sepah YJ, et al. Wide-field retinal imaging in the management of noninfectious posterior uveitis. Am J Ophthalmol. 2012;154(5):908–11 e2.
7. Aggarwal K, Mulkutkar S, Mahajan S, et al. Role of ultra-wide field imaging in the management of tubercular posterior uveitis. Ocul Immunol Inflamm. 2016;24(6):631–6.
8. Mesquida M, Llorenc V, Fontenla JR, et al. Use of ultra-wide-field retinal imaging in the management of active Behcet retinal vasculitis. Retina. 2014;34(10):2121–7.
9. Spaide RF, Fujimoto JG, Waheed NK. Optical coherence tomography angiography. Retina. 2015;35(11):2161–2.
10. Levison AL, Baynes KM, Lowder CY, et al. Choroidal neovascularisation on optical coherence tomography angiography in punctate inner choroidopathy and multifocal choroiditis. Br J Ophthalmol. 2017;101(5):616–22.
11. Lavinsky F, Lavinsky D. Novel perspectives on swept-source optical coherence tomography. Int J Retina Vitreous. 2016;2:25.
12. Dastiridou AI, Bousquet E, Kuehlewein L, et al. Choroidal imaging with swept-source optical coherence tomography in patients with birdshot chorioretinopathy: choroidal reflectivity and thickness. Ophthalmology. 2017;124(8):1186–95.
13. Hosoda Y, Uji A, Hangai M, et al. Relationship between retinal lesions and inward choroidal bulging in Vogt-Koyanagi-Harada disease. Am J Ophthalmol. 2014;157(5):1056–63.
14. Juanola X, Loza Santamaria E, Cordero-Coma M, Group SW. Description and prevalence of spondyloarthritis in patients with anterior uveitis: the SENTINEL Interdisciplinary Collaborative Project. Ophthalmology. 2016;123(8):1632–6.
15. Bodis G, Toth V, Schwarting A. Role of human leukocyte antigens (HLA) in autoimmune diseases. Rheumatol Ther. 2018;5(1):5–20.
16. Wakefield D, Yates W, Amjadi S, McCluskey P. HLA-B27 anterior uveitis: immunology and immunopathology. Ocul Immunol Inflamm. 2016;24(4):450–9.
17. Sykes MP, Hamilton L, Jones C, Gaffney K. Prevalence of axial spondyloarthritis in patients with acute anterior uveitis: a cross-sectional study utilising MRI. RMD Open. 2018;4(1):e000553.
18. Haroon M, O'Rourke M, Ramasamy P, et al. A novel evidence-based detection of undiagnosed spondyloarthritis in patients presenting with acute anterior uveitis: the DUET (Dublin Uveitis Evaluation Tool). Ann Rheum Dis. 2015;74(11):1990–5.
19. Kim M, Won JY, Choi SY, et al. Anti-TNFalpha treatment for HLA-B27-positive ankylosing spondylitis-related uveitis. Am J Ophthalmol. 2016;170:32–40.
20. Levy-Clarke G, Jabs DA, Read RW, et al. Expert panel recommendations for the use of anti-tumor necrosis factor biologic agents in patients with ocular inflammatory disorders. Ophthalmology. 2014;121(3):785–96 e3.
21. Guignard S, Gossec L, Salliot C, et al. Efficacy of tumour necrosis factor blockers in reducing uveitis flares in patients with spondylarthropathy: a retrospective study. Ann Rheum Dis. 2006;65(12):1631–4.

22. Wendling D, Prati C. Paradoxical effects of anti-TNF-alpha agents in inflammatory diseases. Expert Rev Clin Immunol. 2014;10(1):159–69.
23. Fabiani C, Vitale A, Lopalco G, et al. Different roles of TNF inhibitors in acute anterior uveitis associated with ankylosing spondylitis: state of the art. Clin Rheumatol. 2016;35(11):2631–8.
24. Braun J, Davis J, Dougados M, et al. First update of the international ASAS consensus statement for the use of anti-TNF agents in patients with ankylosing spondylitis. Ann Rheum Dis. 2006;65(3):316–20.
25. Rudwaleit M, Rodevand E, Holck P, et al. Adalimumab effectively reduces the rate of anterior uveitis flares in patients with active ankylosing spondylitis: results of a prospective open-label study. Ann Rheum Dis. 2009;68(5):696–701.
26. Ma S, Rogers SL, Hall AJ, et al. Sarcoidosis related uveitis: clinical presentations, disease course and rates of systemic disease progression after uveitis diagnosis. Am J Ophthalmol. 2019;198:30–6.
27. Mochizuki M, Smith JR, Takase H for the International Workshop on Ocular Sarcoidosis Study Group, et al. Revised criteria of International Workshop on Ocular Sarcoidosis (IWOS) for the diagnosis of ocular sarcoidosis. Br J Ophthalmol. 2019;103:1418–22.
28. Gundlach E, Hoffmann MM, Prasse A, et al. Interleukin-2 receptor and angiotensin-converting enzyme as markers for ocular sarcoidosis. PLoS One. 2016;11(1):e0147258.
29. Sahin O, Ziaei A, Karaismailoglu E, et al. The serum angiotensin converting enzyme and lysozyme levels in patients with ocular involvement of autoimmune and infectious diseases. BMC Ophthalmol. 2016;16:19.
30. Acharya NR, Browne EN, Rao N, et al. Distinguishing features of ocular sarcoidosis in an international cohort of uveitis patients. Ophthalmology. 2018;125(1):119–26.
31. Niederer RL, Al-Janabi A, Lightman SL, et al. Serum angiotensin-converting enzyme has a high negative predictive value in the investigation for systemic sarcoidosis. Am J Ophthalmol. 2018;194:82–7.
32. Rodriguez GE, Shin BC, Abernathy RS, et al. Serum angiotensin-converting enzyme activity in normal children and in those with sarcoidosis. J Pediatr. 1981;99(1):68–72.
33. Matsou A, Tsaousis KT. Management of chronic ocular sarcoidosis: challenges and solutions. Clin Ophthalmol. 2018;12:519–32.
34. Rothova A. Ocular involvement in sarcoidosis. Br J Ophthalmol. 2000;84(1):110–6.
35. Niederer RL, Sharief L, Bar A, et al. Predictors of long-term visual outcome in intermediate uveitis. Ophthalmology. 2017;124(3):393–8.
36. Lee SY, Lee HG, Kim DS, et al. Ocular sarcoidosis in a Korean population. J Korean Med Sci. 2009;24(3):413–9.
37. Miserocchi E, Modorati G, Di Matteo F, et al. Visual outcome in ocular sarcoidosis: retrospective evaluation of risk factors. Eur J Ophthalmol. 2011;21(6):802–10.
38. Kaneko F, Togashi A, Saito S, et al. Behcet's disease (Adamantiades-Behcet's disease). Clin Dev Immunol. 2011;2011:681956.
39. Zouboulis CC. Epidemiology of Adamantiades-Behcet's disease. Ann Med Interne (Paris). 1999;150(6):488–98.
40. Hatemi G, Yazici Y, Yazici H. Behcet's syndrome. Rheum Dis Clin North Am. 2013;39(2):245–61.
41. Fabiani C, Alio JL. Local (topical and intraocular) therapy for ocular Adamantiades-Behcet's disease. Curr Opin Ophthalmol. 2015;26(6):546–52.
42. Figus M, Posarelli C, Albert TG, et al. A clinical picture of the visual outcome in Adamantiades-Behcet's disease. Biomed Res Int. 2015;2015:120519.
43. Arayssi T, Hamdan A. New insights into the pathogenesis and therapy of Behcet's disease. Curr Opin Pharmacol. 2004;4(2):183–8.
44. Zamecki KJ, Jabs DA. HLA typing in uveitis: use and misuse. Am J Ophthalmol. 2010;149(2):189–93 e2.
45. International Team for the Revision of the International Criteria for Behcet's D. The International Criteria for Behcet's Disease (ICBD): a collaborative study of 27 countries on the sensitivity and specificity of the new criteria. J Eur Acad Dermatol Venereol. 2014;28(3):338–47.

46. Blake T, Pickup L, Carruthers D, et al. Birmingham Behcet's service: classification of disease and application of the 2014 International Criteria for Behcet's disease (ICBD) to a UK cohort. BMC Musculoskelet Disord. 2017;18(1):101.
47. Amer R, Alsughayyar W, Almeida D. Pattern and causes of visual loss in Behcet's uveitis: short-term and long-term outcomes. Graefes Arch Clin Exp Ophthalmol. 2017;255(7):1423–32.
48. Cunningham ET Jr, Tugal-Tutkun I, Khairallah M, et al. Behcet uveitis. Ocul Immunol Inflamm. 2017;25(1):2–6.
49. Keino H, Okada AA, Watanabe T, et al. Efficacy of infliximab for early remission induction in refractory uveoretinitis associated with Behcet disease: a 2-year follow-up study. Ocul Immunol Inflamm. 2017;25(1):46–51.
50. Martin-Varillas JL, Calvo-Rio V, Beltran E, et al. Successful optimization of adalimumab therapy in refractory uveitis due to Behcet's disease. Ophthalmology. 2018;125(9):1444–51.
51. Fabiani C, Vitale A, Emmi G, et al. Efficacy and safety of adalimumab in Behcet's disease-related uveitis: a multicenter retrospective observational study. Clin Rheumatol. 2017;36(1):183–9.
52. Lightman S, Taylor SR, Bunce C, et al. Pegylated interferon-alpha-2b reduces corticosteroid requirement in patients with Behcet's disease with upregulation of circulating regulatory T cells and reduction of Th17. Ann Rheum Dis. 2015;74(6):1138–44.
53. Diwo E, Gueudry J, Saadoun D, et al. Long-term efficacy of interferon in severe uveitis associated with Behcet disease. Ocul Immunol Inflamm. 2017;25(1):76–84.
54. Hasanreisoglu M, Cubuk MO, Ozdek S, et al. Interferon alpha-2a therapy in patients with refractory Behcet uveitis. Ocul Immunol Inflamm. 2017;25(1):71–5.
55. Tomkins-Netzer O, Talat L, Ismetova F, et al. Immunomodulatory therapy in uveitis. Dev Ophthalmol. 2016;55:265–75.
56. Suhler EB, Thorne JE, Mittal M, et al. Corticosteroid-related adverse events systematically increase with corticosteroid dose in noninfectious intermediate, posterior, or panuveitis: post hoc analyses from the VISUAL-1 and VISUAL-2 trials. Ophthalmology. 2017;124(12):1799–807.
57. Rathinam SR, Babu M, Thundikandy R, et al. A randomized clinical trial comparing methotrexate and mycophenolate mofetil for noninfectious uveitis. Ophthalmology. 2014;121(10):1863–70.
58. Weinstein JE, Pepple KL. Cytokines in uveitis. Curr Opin Ophthalmol. 2018;29(3):267–74.
59. Taylor SR, Singh J, Menezo V, et al. Behcet disease: visual prognosis and factors influencing the development of visual loss. Am J Ophthalmol. 2011;152:1059–66.
60. Jaffe GJ, Dick AD, Brezin AP, et al. Adalimumab in patients with active noninfectious uveitis. N Engl J Med. 2016;375(10):932–43.
61. Nguyen QD, Merrill PT, Jaffe GJ, et al. Adalimumab for prevention of uveitic flare in patients with inactive non-infectious uveitis controlled by corticosteroids (VISUAL II): a multicentre, double-masked, randomised, placebo-controlled phase 3 trial. Lancet. 2016;388(10050):1183–92.
62. Suhler EB, Adan A, Brezin AP, et al. Safety and efficacy of adalimumab in patients with noninfectious uveitis in an ongoing open-label study: VISUAL III. Ophthalmology. 2018;125(7):1075–87.
63. Ramanan AV, Dick AD, Jones AP, et al. Adalimumab plus methotrexate for uveitis in juvenile idiopathic arthritis. N Engl J Med. 2017;376(17):1637–46.
64. Vallet H, Seve P, Biard L, et al. Infliximab versus adalimumab in the treatment of refractory inflammatory uveitis: a Multicenter Study from the French Uveitis Network. Arthritis Rheumatol. 2016;68(6):1522–30.
65. Deitch I, Amer R, Tomkins-Netzer O, et al. The effect of anti-tumor necrosis factor alpha agents on the outcome in pediatric uveitis of diverse etiologies. Graefes Arch Clin Exp Ophthalmol. 2018;256(4):801–8.

66. Fabiani C, Vitale A, Rigante D, et al. Comparative efficacy between adalimumab and inflix-imab in the treatment of non-infectious intermediate uveitis, posterior uveitis, and panuveitis: a retrospective observational study of 107 patients. Clin Rheumatol. 2019;38:407–15.
67. Sepah YJ, Sadiq MA, Chu DS, et al. Primary (month-6) outcomes of the STOP-uveitis study: evaluating the safety, tolerability, and efficacy of tocilizumab in patients with noninfectious uveitis. Am J Ophthalmol. 2017;183:71–80.
68. Tappeiner C, Mesquida M, Adan A, et al. Evidence for tocilizumab as a treatment option in refractory uveitis associated with juvenile idiopathic arthritis. J Rheumatol. 2016;43(12):2183–8.
69. Atienza-Mateo B, Calvo-Rio V, Beltran E, et al. Anti-interleukin 6 receptor tocilizumab in refractory uveitis associated with Behcet's disease: multicentre retrospective study. Rheumatology (Oxford). 2018;57(5):856–64.
70. Calvo-Rio V, de la Hera D, Beltran-Catalan E, et al. Tocilizumab in uveitis refractory to other biologic drugs: a study of 3 cases and a literature review. Clin Exp Rheumatol. 2014;32(4 Suppl 84):S54–7.
71. Heissigerova J, Callanan D, de Smet MD, et al. Efficacy and safety of sarilumab for noninfectious uveitis of posterior segment: outcomes from the phase 2 SATURN trial. Ophthalmology. 2019;126:428–37.
72. Dick AD, Tugal-Tutkun I, Foster S, et al. Secukinumab in the treatment of noninfectious uveitis: results of three randomized, controlled clinical trials. Ophthalmology. 2013;120(4):777–87.
73. Letko E, Yeh S, Foster CS, et al. Efficacy and safety of intravenous secukinumab in non-infectious uveitis requiring steroid-sparing immunosuppressive therapy. Ophthalmology. 2015;122(5):939–48.
74. Sharief LAT, Lightman S, Tomkins-Netzer O. Using local therapy to control noninfectious uveitis. Ophthalmology. 2018;125(3):329–31.
75. Tomkins-Netzer O, Lightman S, Drye L, et al. Outcome of treatment of uveitic macular edema: the multicenter uveitis steroid treatment trial 2-year results. Ophthalmology. 2015;122(11):2351–9.
76. Kok H, Lau C, Maycock N, et al. Outcome of intravitreal triamcinolone in uveitis. Ophthalmology. 2005;112(11):1916 e1–7.
77. Sallam A, Taylor SR, Habot-Wilner Z, et al. Repeat intravitreal triamcinolone acetonide injections in uveitic macular oedema. Acta Ophthalmol. 2012;90:e323–5.
78. Lowder C, Belfort R Jr, Lightman S, et al. Dexamethasone intravitreal implant for noninfectious intermediate or posterior uveitis. Arch Ophthalmol. 2011;129(5):545–53.
79. Writing Committee for the Multicenter Uveitis Steroid Treatment T, Follow-up Study Research G, Kempen JH, et al. Association between long-lasting intravitreous fluocinolone acetonide implant vs systemic anti-inflammatory therapy and visual acuity at 7 years among patients with intermediate, posterior, or panuveitis. JAMA. 2017;317(19):1993–2005.
80. Kempen JH, Altaweel MM, Holbrook JT, et al. Randomized comparison of systemic anti-inflammatory therapy versus fluocinolone acetonide implant for intermediate, posterior, and panuveitis: the multicenter uveitis steroid treatment trial. Ophthalmology. 2011;118(10):1916–26.
81. Sen HN, Abreu FM, Louis TA, et al. Cataract surgery outcomes in uveitis: the multicenter uveitis steroid treatment trial. Ophthalmology. 2016;123(1):183–90.
82. Jaffe GJ, Foster S, Pavesio C, et al. Effect of an injectable fluocinolone acetonide insert on recurrence rates in noninfectious uveitis affecting the posterior segment: 12-month results. Ophthalmology. 2019;126:601–10.
83. Multicenter Uveitis Steroid Treatment Trial Research Group, Thorne JE, et al. Periocular triamcinolone vs. intravitreal triamcinolone vs. intravitreal dexamethasone implant for the treatment of uveitic macular edema: the periocular vs. intravitreal corticosteroids for uveitic macular edema (POINT) trial. Ophthalmology. 2019;126:283–95.

84. Taylor A, Sheng KC, Herrero LJ, et al. Methotrexate treatment causes early onset of disease in a mouse model of Ross River virus-induced inflammatory disease through increased monocyte production. PLoS One. 2013;8(8):e71146.
85. Julian K, Langner-Wegscheider BJ, Haas A, et al. Intravitreal methotrexate in the management of presumed tuberculous serpiginous-like choroiditis. Retina. 2013;33(9):1943–8.
86. Nguyen QD, Merrill PT, Clark WL, et al. Intravitreal sirolimus for noninfectious uveitis: a phase III Sirolimus Study Assessing Double-masKed Uveitis TReAtment (SAKURA). Ophthalmology. 2016;123(11):2413–23.
87. Shanmuganathan VA, Casely EM, Raj D, et al. The efficacy of sirolimus in the treatment of patients with refractory uveitis. Br J Ophthalmol. 2005;89(6):666–9.
88. Nguyen QD, Sadiq MA, Soliman MK, et al. The effect of different dosing schedules of intravitreal Sirolimus, a mammalian target of rapamycin (mTOR) inhibitor, in the treatment of non-infectious uveitis (An American Ophthalmological Society Thesis). Trans Am Ophthalmol Soc. 2016;114:T3.
89. Wells JA, Glassman AR, Ayala AR, et al. Aflibercept, Bevacizumab, or Ranibizumab for diabetic macular edema: two-year results from a comparative effectiveness randomized clinical trial. Ophthalmology. 2016;123(6):1351–9.
90. Ho M, Liu DT, Lam DS, Jonas JB. Retinal vein occlusions, from basics to the latest treatment. Retina. 2016;36(3):432–48.
91. Staurenghi G, Lai TYY, Mitchell P, et al. Efficacy and safety of Ranibizumab 0.5 mg for the treatment of macular edema resulting from uncommon causes: twelve-month findings from PROMETHEUS. Ophthalmology. 2018;125(6):850–62.
92. Lasave AF, Zeballos DG, El-Haig WM, et al. Short-term results of a single intravitreal bevacizumab (avastin) injection versus a single intravitreal triamcinolone acetonide (kenacort) injection for the management of refractory noninfectious uveitic cystoid macular edema. Ocular immunology and inflammation. 2009;17:423–30.
93. Kharel Sitaula R, Janani MK, Madhavan HN, et al. Outcome of polymerase chain reaction (PCR) analysis in 100 suspected cases of infectious uveitis. J Ophthalmic Inflamm Infect. 2018;8(1):2.
94. Majumder PD, Sudharshan S, Biswas J. Laboratory support in the diagnosis of uveitis. Indian J Ophthalmol. 2013;61(6):269–76.
95. Sandhu HS, Hajrasouliha A, Kaplan HJ, et al. Diagnostic utility of quantitative polymerase chain reaction versus culture in endophthalmitis and uveitis. Ocul Immunol Inflamm. 2019;27:578–82.
96. Thompson PP, Kowalski RP. A 13-year retrospective review of polymerase chain reaction testing for infectious agents from ocular samples. Ophthalmology. 2011;118(7):1449–53.
97. Bispo PJM, Davoudi S, Sahm ML, et al. Rapid detection and identification of uveitis pathogens by qualitative multiplex real-time PCR. Invest Ophthalmol Vis Sci. 2018; 59(1):582–9.
98. Schoenberger SD, Kim SJ, Thorne JE, et al. Diagnosis and treatment of acute retinal necrosis: a report by the American Academy of Ophthalmology. Ophthalmology. 2017;124(3):382–92.
99. Hong BK, Lee CS, Van Gelder RN, Garg SJ. Emerging techniques for pathogen discovery in endophthalmitis. Curr Opin Ophthalmol. 2015;26(3):221–5.
100. Sugita S, Shimizu N, Watanabe K, et al. Use of multiplex PCR and real-time PCR to detect human herpes virus genome in ocular fluids of patients with uveitis. Br J Ophthalmol. 2008;92(7):928–32.
101. Neumann R, Barequet D, Rosenblatt A, et al. Herpetic anterior uveitis—analysis of presumed and pcr proven cases. Ocul Immunol Inflamm. 2019;27:211–8.
102. Butler NJ, Moradi A, Salek SS, et al. Acute retinal necrosis: presenting characteristics and clinical outcomes in a cohort of polymerase chain reaction-positive patients. Am J Ophthalmol. 2017;179:179–89.
103. Liu T, Jain A, Fung M, et al. Valacyclovir as initial treatment for acute retinal necrosis: a pharmacokinetic modeling and simulation study. Curr Eye Res. 2017;42(7):1035–8.

104. Sims JL, Yeoh J, Stawell RJ. Acute retinal necrosis: a case series with clinical features and treatment outcomes. Clin Exp Ophthalmol. 2009;37(5):473–7.
105. Lau CH, Missotten T, Salzmann J, et al. Acute retinal necrosis features, management, and outcomes. Ophthalmology. 2007;114(4):756–62.
106. Baltinas J, Lightman S, Tomkins-Netzer O. Comparing treatment of acute retinal necrosis with either oral valacyclovir or intravenous acyclovir. Am J Ophthalmol. 2018;188:173–80.
107. Tibbetts MD, Shah CP, Young LH, et al. Treatment of acute retinal necrosis. Ophthalmology. 2010;117(4):818–24.
108. Yeh S, Suhler EB, Smith JR, et al. Combination systemic and intravitreal antiviral therapy in the management of acute retinal necrosis syndrome. Ophthalmic Surg Lasers Imaging Retina. 2014;45(5):399–407.
109. Wong R, Pavesio CE, Laidlaw DA, et al. Acute retinal necrosis: the effects of intravitreal foscarnet and virus type on outcome. Ophthalmology. 2010;117(3):556–60.
110. WHO Global Tuberculosis Report. 2015. World Health Organization; 2015.
111. Dyrhol-Riise AM, Gran G, Wentzel-Larsen T, et al. Diagnosis and follow-up of treatment of latent tuberculosis; the utility of the QuantiFERON-TB Gold In-tube assay in outpatients from a tuberculosis low-endemic country. BMC Infect Dis. 2010;10:57.
112. Nazari Khanamiri H, Rao NA. Serpiginous choroiditis and infectious multifocal serpiginoid choroiditis. Surv Ophthalmol. 2013;58(3):203–32.
113. Agrawal R, Gunasekeran DV, Agarwal A, et al. The Collaborative Ocular Tuberculosis Study (COTS)-1: a multinational description of the spectrum of choroidal involvement in 245 patients with tubercular uveitis. Ocul Immunol Inflamm. 2019;29:1–11.
114. La Distia Nora R, van Velthoven ME, Ten Dam-van Loon NH, et al. Clinical manifestations of patients with intraocular inflammation and positive QuantiFERON-TB gold in-tube test in a country nonendemic for tuberculosis. Am J Ophthalmol. 2014;157(4):754–61.
115. Bansal R, Gupta A, Gupta V, et al. Role of anti-tubercular therapy in uveitis with latent/manifest tuberculosis. Am J Ophthalmol. 2008;146(5):772–9.
116. Ang M, Hedayatfar A, Wong W, et al. Duration of anti-tubercular therapy in uveitis associated with latent tuberculosis: a case-control study. Br J Ophthalmol. 2012;96(3):332–6.
117. Sanghvi C, Bell C, Woodhead M, et al. Presumed tuberculous uveitis: diagnosis, management, and outcome. Eye (Lond). 2011;25(4):475–80.
118. Tomkins-Netzer O, Leong BCS, Zhang X, et al. Effect of antituberculous therapy on uveitis associated with latent tuberculosis. Am J Ophthalmol. 2018;190:164–70.
119. Liu Q, Wang ZD, Huang SY, et al. Diagnosis of toxoplasmosis and typing of *Toxoplasma gondii*. Parasit Vectors. 2015;8:292.
120. Villard O, Cimon B, L'Ollivier C, et al. Serological diagnosis of *Toxoplasma gondii* infection: recommendations from the French National Reference Center for Toxoplasmosis. Diagn Microbiol Infect Dis. 2016;84(1):22–33.
121. Bosch-Driessen LE, Berendschot TT, Ongkosuwito JV, et al. Ocular toxoplasmosis: clinical features and prognosis of 154 patients. Ophthalmology. 2002;109(5):869–78.
122. Jasper S, Vedula SS, John SS, et al. Corticosteroids as adjuvant therapy for ocular toxoplasmosis. Cochrane Database Syst Rev. 2017;(1):CD007417.
123. Zhang Y, Lin X, Lu F. Current treatment of ocular toxoplasmosis in immunocompetent patients: a network meta-analysis. Acta Trop. 2018;185:52–62.
124. Bosch-Driessen LH, Verbraak FD, Suttorp-Schulten MS, et al. A prospective, randomized trial of pyrimethamine and azithromycin vs pyrimethamine and sulfadiazine for the treatment of ocular toxoplasmosis. Am J Ophthalmol. 2002;134(1):34–40.
125. Kim SJ, Scott IU, Brown GC, et al. Interventions for toxoplasma retinochoroiditis: a report by the American Academy of Ophthalmology. Ophthalmology. 2013;120(2):371–8.
126. Silveira C, Belfort R Jr, Muccioli C, et al. The effect of long-term intermittent trimethoprim/sulfamethoxazole treatment on recurrences of toxoplasmic retinochoroiditis. Am J Ophthalmol. 2002;134(1):41–6.
127. Pradhan E, Bhandari S, Gilbert RE, et al. Antibiotics versus no treatment for toxoplasma retinochoroiditis. Cochrane Database Syst Rev. 2016;(5):CD002218.

128. Borkowski PK, Brydak-Godowska J, Basiak W, et al. The impact of short-term, intensive antifolate treatment (with pyrimethamine and sulfadoxine) and antibiotics followed by long-term, secondary antifolate prophylaxis on the rate of toxoplasmic retinochoroiditis recurrence. PLoS Negl Trop Dis. 2016;10(8):e0004892.

129. Felix JP, Lira RP, Zacchia RS, et al. Trimethoprim-sulfamethoxazole versus placebo to reduce the risk of recurrences of *Toxoplasma gondii* retinochoroiditis: randomized controlled clinical trial. Am J Ophthalmol. 2014;157(4):762–6 e1.

130. Fernandes Felix JP, Cavalcanti Lira RP, Cosimo AB, et al. Trimethoprim-sulfamethoxazole versus placebo in reducing the risk of toxoplasmic retinochoroiditis recurrences: a three-year follow-up. Am J Ophthalmol. 2016;170:176–82.

131. Reich M, Mackensen F. Ocular toxoplasmosis: background and evidence for an antibiotic prophylaxis. Curr Opin Ophthalmol. 2015;26(6):498–505.

# Chapter 6
# Recent Developments in Maculopathy

Francesco Bandello, Marco Battista, Maria Brambati, Vincenzo Starace, Alessandro Arrigo, and Maurizio Battaglia Parodi

## Introduction

The diagnosis and treatment of maculopathies underwent almost a complete revolution over the last years, thank to the introduction of multimodal imaging and intravitreal treatments. Furthermore, research activity is currently introducing more advanced therapeutic and diagnostic techniques.

The aim of this chapter is to provide an overview on the recent developments both in diagnostic and therapeutic fields of maculopathies.

## *Advances in Retinal Imaging Techniques*

Retinal imaging benefited from a great progress in last decades and years. Nowadays, the recent imaging techniques along with the improvement of old diagnostic methods allow a more and more detailed assessment of anatomy of macular region (Fig. 6.1), a better diagnosis of macular pathologies and improved evaluation of the response to treatment.

### Fluorescein Angiography

Fluorescein Angiography (FA) has been in use in ophthalmologic practice since 1961, when two medical students from Indiana University described and demonstrated the technique [1]. FA requires the intravenous injection of fluorescein dye,

F. Bandello · M. Battista · M. Brambati · V. Starace · A. Arrigo (✉) · M. Battaglia Parodi
Department of Ophthalmology, Vita-Salute San Raffaele University, Ospedale San Raffaele, Milan, Italy

© Springer Nature Switzerland AG 2020
A. Grzybowski (ed.), *Current Concepts in Ophthalmology*,
https://doi.org/10.1007/978-3-030-25389-9_6

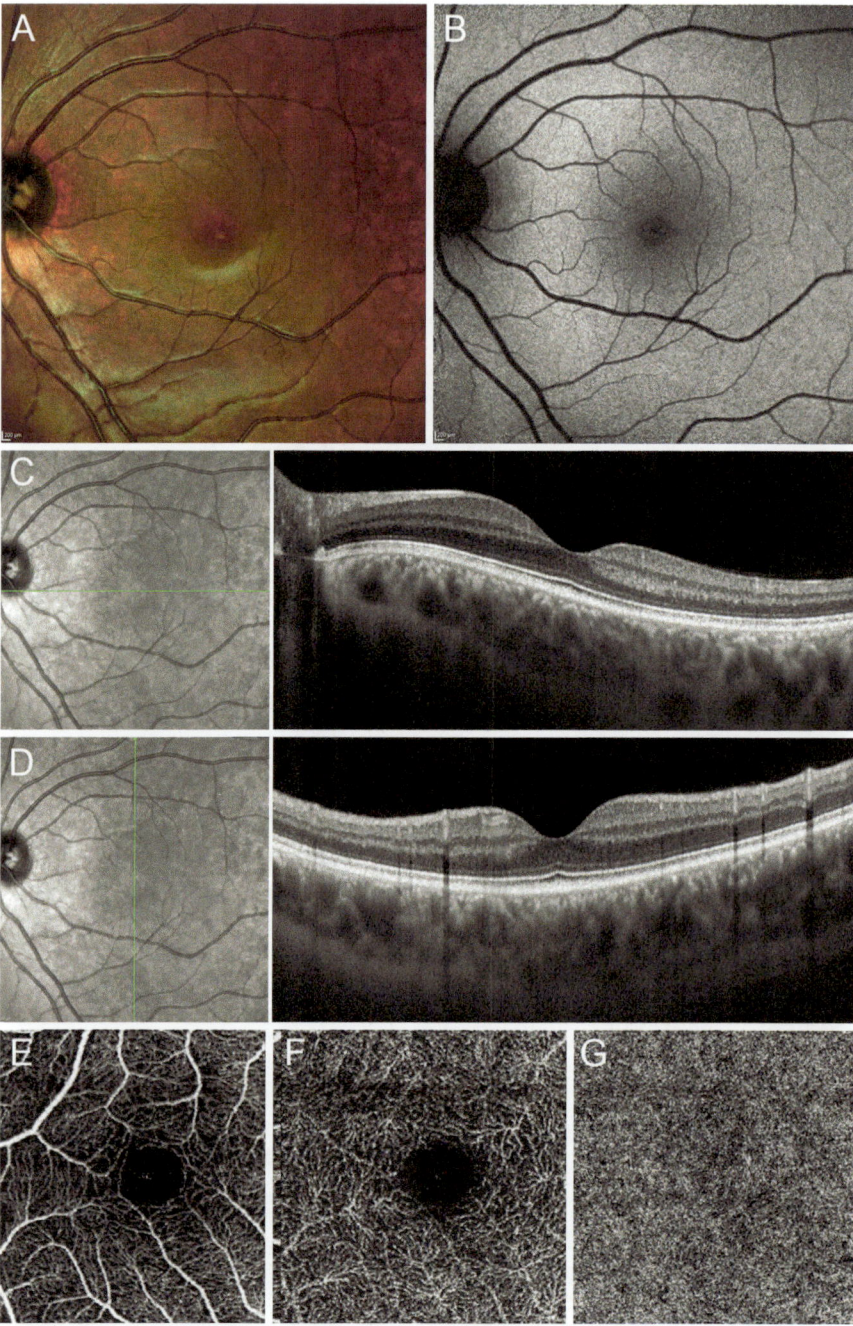

**Fig. 6.1** Multimodal imaging in a healthy subject. Multicolor (**a**) and fundus autofluorescence (**b**) images show the integrity of posterior pole structure, with the physiologic distribution of autofluorescence signal coming from the retinal pigment epithelium cells. Horizontal (**c**) and vertical (**d**) structural OCT scans show the normal reflectivity properties of retinal and choroidal layers. OCTA is able to accurately reconstruct retinal vascular network, namely superficial (**e**), deep (**f**) and choriocapillary (**g**) plexa

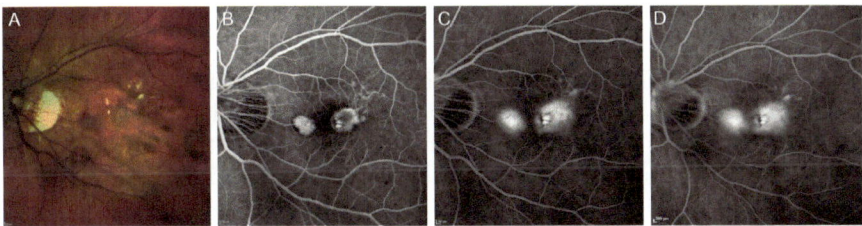

**Fig. 6.2** Fluorescein angiography in a case of myopic choroidal neovascularization. Multicolor (**a**) image shows the characteristic features of a myopic fundus, including retinal thinning and peripapillary atrophy. Moreover, an altered foveal reflex is also detected. FA examination clearly shows the presence of two classic CNV, being detectable already in early phase (**b**), with progressive leakage phenomena in intermediate (**c**) and late (**d**) phases

which rapidly reaches eye circulation. White light passes through a blue excitation filter, and the blue light is absorbed by fluorescein molecules, which in turn emit light in the yellow-green spectrum. A barrier filter allows capturing only light emitted from the excited fluorescein, and the images are recorded. First FA images were recorded on photographic film; nowadays images are recorded digitally, thus allowing easier data analysis, storing and sharing, which can be easily stored and shared. Newer angiography devices support also movie capturing, making the interpretation of the vascular filling details, more identifiable.

FA has been an indispensable tool for diagnosis of macular diseases (Fig. 6.2), but at present its use is diminishing. More recent imaging modalities provide more comprehensive evaluation of the macular anatomy and function. Furthermore, FA has some limitations: it requires an invasive dye injection with a limited transit window and it has limited resolution. Still, angiography contribution remains still valid to the assessment of vascular integrity: in contrast to OCT-A, fluorescein angiography is a dynamic examination which show vessel filling and leakage [2].

The indications of Fluorescein Angiography, Indocyanine Green Angiography and Optical Coherence tomography Angiography are reported in Table 6.1.

**Indocyanine Green Angiography**

Indocyanine Green Angiography (ICGA) was originally described by Yannuzzi in 1992 [3]. Indocyanine green is a water-soluble dye which is almost completely bound to serum proteins (98%), thus its diffusion through choriocapillaris is limited. The retention of the dye in the choroidal circulation makes indocyanine green angiography ideal for imaging of choroidal circulation. As well as FA, ICGA is invasive and requires intravenous injection of the dye.

Nowadays, ICGA is recommended only for a small group of chorioretinal disorders, including some forms of neovascularization in age-related macular degeneration (Fig. 6.3) (occult choroidal neovascularization and choroidal neovascularization with subretinal hemorrhage), other neovascular maculopathies, chronic central serous chorioretinopathy, choroidal hemangiomas, and posterior uveitis [4].

## Optical Coherence Tomography

Optical Coherence Tomography (OCT) is a non-invasive imaging modality which allows to acquire retinal cross-section in vivo. Since its original introduction in 1991 [5], OCT has revolutionized the retinal imaging and the evaluation of the macular pathologies. Diagnosis of maculopathy, previously based on fundus biomicroscopic examination, retinography or FA, in most of cases now relies upon OCT detailed contribution. OCT can quantitatively measure retinal thickness and evaluate qualitative anatomic changes, such as intraretinal or subretinal fluid.

**Table 6.1** Indications of fluorescein angiography, indocyanine green angiography and optical coherence tomography angiography in macular diseases

| | Fluorescein angiography | Indocyanine green angiography | Optical coherence tomography angiography |
|---|---|---|---|
| Indications | • Neovascular age related macular degeneration<br>• Diabetic retinopathy<br>• Retinal vein occlusion<br>• Retinal artery occlusion<br>• Genetical macular dystrophy<br>• Central serous chorioretinopathy<br>• Uveitic macular edema | • Occult choroidal neovascularization<br>• Choroidal neovascularization with subretinal hemorrhage<br>• Central serous chorioretinopathy | • Neovascular age related macular degeneration<br>• Diabetic retinopathy<br>• Retinal vein occlusion<br>• Retinal artery occlusion<br>• Genetical macular dystrophy<br>• Central serous chorioretinopathy<br>• Uveitic macular edema |

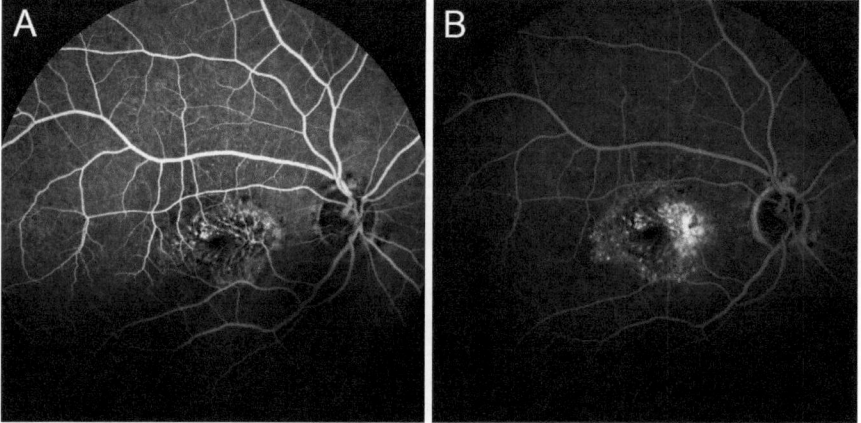

**Fig. 6.3** Multimodal imaging of a choroidal neovascularization secondary to age-related macular degeneration. Early (**a**) and late (**b**) FA phases show the presence of a CNV with the typical pinpoints alterations. ICGA is able to better detect the entire neovascular network, respectively in early (**c**) and late (**d**) phases. Structural OCT (**e**) confirms the presence of a subretinal mixed reflectivity lesion, together with the presence of subretinal fluid and intraretinal cysts

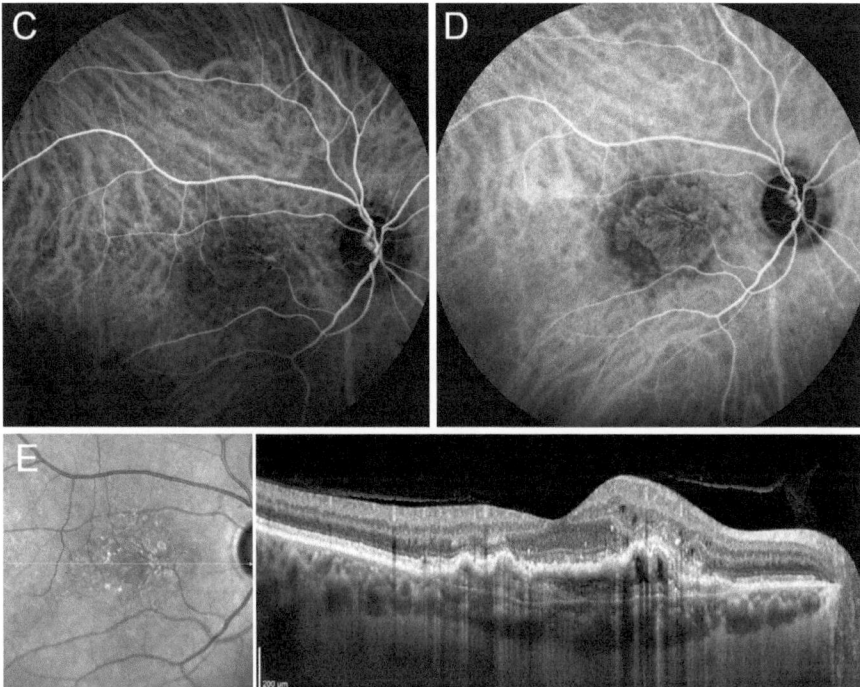

**Fig. 6.3** (continued)

First OCT devices used time-domain technology (TD-OCT), allowing approximately 400 A-scans per second and with a resolution of 10–15 microns. The clinical utility of TD-OCT was inadequate until the implementation of spectral domain technology (SD-OCT), which instead allowed 20,000–80,000 A-scans per second. SD-OCT (introduced in 2002) significantly improved the image resolution (2–8 microns) and reduced motion artifacts [6]. The swept-source OCT (SS-OCT) is a more recent technology allowing high spatial resolution and better tissue penetration. SS-OCT has a scan rate of 100,000 scans per second, and some prototype models could reach up to 400,000 scans per second (Table 6.2) [7]. The increased number of acquisitions improves the area of the retina evaluated and the visualization of retinal structures. SS-OCT allows the simultaneous detailed evaluation of the vitreous and the choroid, enabling to better visualize the choroidal structures, as well as the sub-RPE pathology [8]. However, improvement of OCT technology is still ongoing. Adaptive Optics OCT (AO-OCT) devices dynamically adjust their optical characteristics to compensate for monochromatic aberrations occurring naturally in the eye. Overcoming current AO-OCT limitations (narrow depth focus, restricted field of view) that nowadays do not allow its widespread use, its improved resolution could achieve a better understanding of normal and pathologic retinal function. Furthermore,

**Table 6.2** Comparison between different commercially available optical coherence tomography devices

|  | Time domain | Spectral domain | Swept source |
|---|---|---|---|
| Commercialization | 1996 | 2006 | 2012 |
| Acquisition (A-scans per second) | 400 | 20,000–80,000 | 100,000–400,000 |
| Resolution | 10–15 µm | 2–8 µm | 2–8 µm |
| Characteristics | A moving reference mirror is required, limiting the acquisition rate of the technology Mostly inadequate for current clinical use | Higher sensitivity than TD-OCT High scanning speed and axial resolution and good visualization of retinal layers It has limited penetration with noticeable signal drop-off with depth | Higher sensitivity than TD-OCT, with very high scanning speeds, and minimal signal drop-off with depth It has high spatial resolution and better tissue penetration (from vitreous to choroid) |

it could improve the quality of images from eyes with more aberrations, achieving better performance of the automated segmentation algorithms. Polarization-Sensitive OCT (PS-OCT) is an innovative technology that detects polarization changes in circularly polarized light; polarization of retinal structure (such as the RPE) may improve the detection of macular disease and give the opportunity for earlier intervention [9].

**Optical Coherence Tomography Angiography**

Optical coherence tomography angiography (OCTA) is a recent imaging technique based on OCT, which allows the study of blood vessels in the eye. OCTA uses the variation in OCT signal caused by moving particles (such as red blood cells) in order to infer blood flow. To discriminate the moving particles from static tissue, OCTA devices perform repeated scans at the same location, and the changes of the OCT signal in consecutive scans are employed to visualize the microvasculature [10].

OCTA has many applications in retinal and choroidal vascular imaging, with special focus on the macular disorders.

In age related macular degeneration (AMD), OCTA allows the detection of choroidal neovascularization (CNV), and a more detailed visualization of its structure than dye-based angiography examinations.

In diabetic retinopathy OCTA can show microaneurysms, appearing as focally dilated saccular or fusiform capillaries in the superficial and deep retinal capillary plexa. It is important to remark that not all microaneurysms seen on fluorescein angiography can be detect by OCTA, and vice-versa. OCTA can also visualize the retinal areas of non-perfusion in all the ischemic retinopathies.

OCTA is useful to confirm the clinical diagnosis of retinal vein occlusion or retinal artery occlusion, as it can identify the areas of capillary nonperfusion and retinal ischaemia, and moreover it can detect the presence of collateral vessels, capillary telangiectasia and microaneurysms.

OCTA in also used in genetical macular dystrophy in order to evaluate the damages in retinal plexa and choriocapillaris, and also to detect the presence of CNV.

OCTA could be useful in improving the knowledge of uveitic macular edema, even if there are few studies so far [11].

OCTA has several advantages over dye-based techniques: it is not invasive and fast, it does not have to respect a narrow time window, it has a better vascular definition. OCTA has also some limitations, notably the frequent presence of image artifacts, which are similar and derived from artifacts that occur in OCT. Even if OCTA is a new imaging technique without definitive clinical indications, it is already a fundamental tool in the diagnosis and management of macular pathologies. The comparison between Fluorescein Angiography and OCTA techniques is provided in Table 6.3.

## Fundus Autofluorescence

Fundus autofluorescence (FAF) imaging is a rapid and noninvasive technique. It is used mainly to evaluate retinal pigment epithelial function, as the predominant source of autofluorescence in the macula is lipofuscin granules.

Blue autofluorescence is the intrinsic fluorescence emitted by lipofuscin granules when stimulated by blue light. With retinal aging, lipofuscin granules accumulate in the RPE cells. Normal macula shows a reduced autofluorescence in its center due to the blockage of luteal pigments (lutein and zeaxanthin), while the rest of the macula shows a diffuse autofluorescence signal. Other structure such as the blood vessels and the optic disc appear black because they do not have autofluorescent material [12]. In contrast to blue autofluorescence, green-light autofluorescence imaging is less affected by macular pigments, and it could probably allow a more precise evaluation of small central changes [13].

FAF is extremely useful to uninvasively evaluate all types of maculopathies (Table 6.4) (Fig. 6.4). Both augmentation or reduction of autofluorescence can be pathological. For example, in Best vitelliform dystrophy the autofluorescence signal is increased because of the accumulation of waste material (Fig. 6.5), while in geographic atrophy the signal is decreased because of the loss of RPE cells (Fig. 6.6).

Near-infrared autofluorescence imaging (NIR-AF) in another autofluorescence technique, which evaluates melanin and its distribution throughout the RPE and choroid. NIR-AF can be performed to detect melanin in different macular pathologies (AMD, inherited macular dystrophies, diabetic macular edema, central serous chorioretinopathy). This technique can extend our ways of studying the foveal involvement in macular diseases, since the higher concentration of melanin is present at the level of the fovea. Even if NIR-AF is easily performed with commercially available instruments, it has some limitations, and further research is needed to better understand and to standardize NIR-AF imaging [14].

**Table 6.3** Comparison between fluorescein angiography and OCTA techniques

| Techniques | Microaneurysms | IRMA | DME | Ischemic areas | Neovascularization | Neovascularization growth | Secondary vascular branching | Peripheral vascular arcades | Anastomotic loops |
|---|---|---|---|---|---|---|---|---|---|
| Fluorescein angiography | Yes | Yes | Yes | Yes | Yes | No | No | No | No |
| OCTA | Yes | Yes | Yes | Yes | Yes | Yes | Yes | Yes | Yes |

**Table 6.4** Fundus autofluorescence indications

- Age related macular degeneration
  - Drusen
  - Neovascular age related macular degeneration
  - Geographic atrophy
- Hereditary macular dystrophy
  - Best macular dystrophy
  - Stargardt macular dystrophy
  - Rod-cone dystrophies
  - Pattern dystrophies
- Areas of retinal atrophy
- Retinal areas of pigment accumulation
- White dot syndromes
- Optic disk drusen

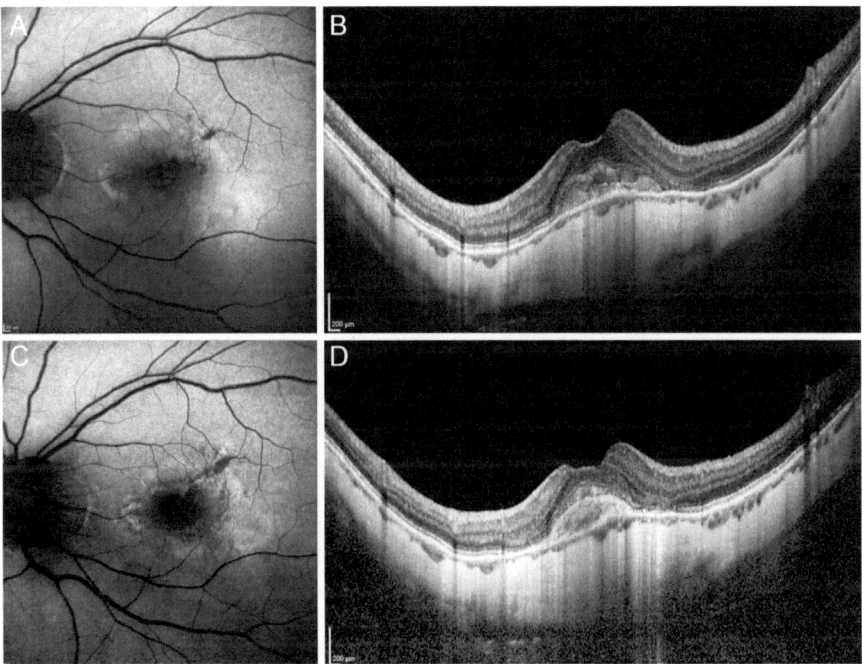

**Fig. 6.4** Fundus autofluorescence in a myopic CNV. At baseline, fundus autofluorescence shows the presence of macular autofluorescence changes, with an increase of hypoautofluorescent signal (**a**); structural OCT clearly detects the presence of a subretinal hyperreflective lesion, together with the presence of subretinal fluid (**b**). After anti-VEGF injections, fundus autofluorescence shows an increase of hypoautofluorescent signal, interpretable as increased atrophy (**c**), confirmed also by structural OCT (**d**)

## New Perspectives: Artificial Intelligence and Telemedicine

In this section the main features of multimodal imaging have been discussed, showing the very useful role of these methodologies in clinical practice (Fig. 6.7).

Artificial intelligence has a great potential to improve medical activity and health care quality. Several studies have demonstrated that artificial intelligence software

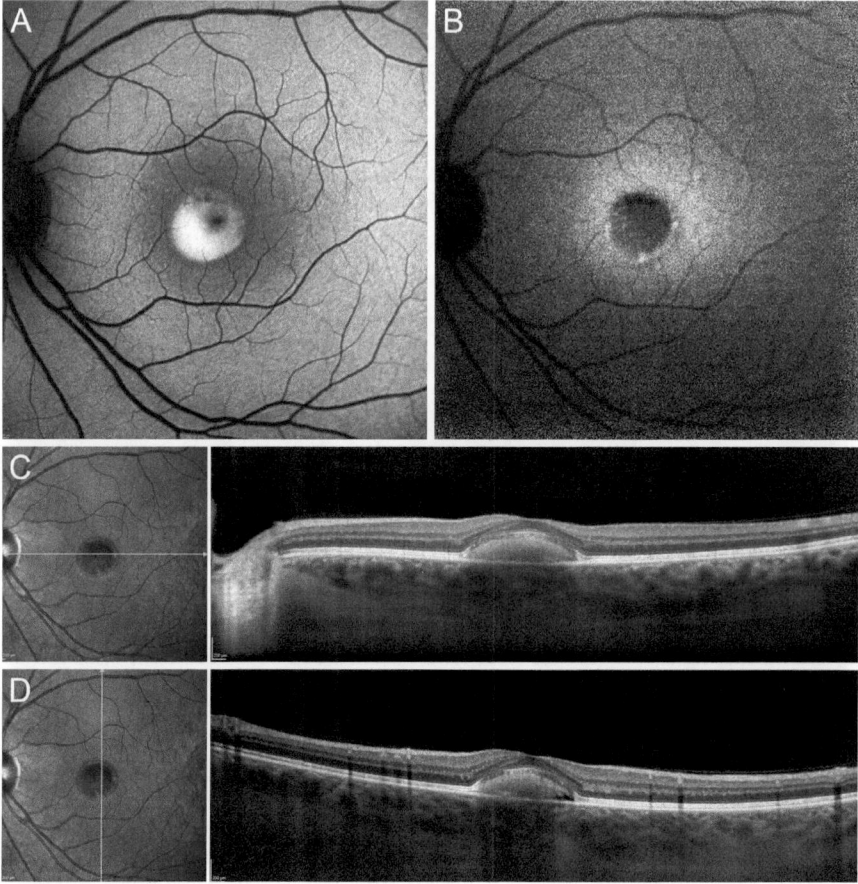

**Fig. 6.5** Multimodal imaging in a case of Best disease. The vitelliform material appears hyperautofluorescent (**a**) and it masks the signal provided by melanin in NIR-AF (**b**). Structural OCT (**c**, **d**) clearly shows the vitelliform acculumation, with rarefaction of outer retinal layers and normally reflective inner layers

can identify retinal diseases with the same or better accuracy than human specialists, even if their role in medical decision-making is still controversial. Nowadays, the most encouraging results are obtained for age related macular degeneration and diabetic retinopathy [15].

Another important implementation in maculopathy care could be portable devices. For example, a portable and self-measuring OCT system may reduce the cost of managing chronic maculopathy by providing easily accessible and continuous retinal monitoring [16].

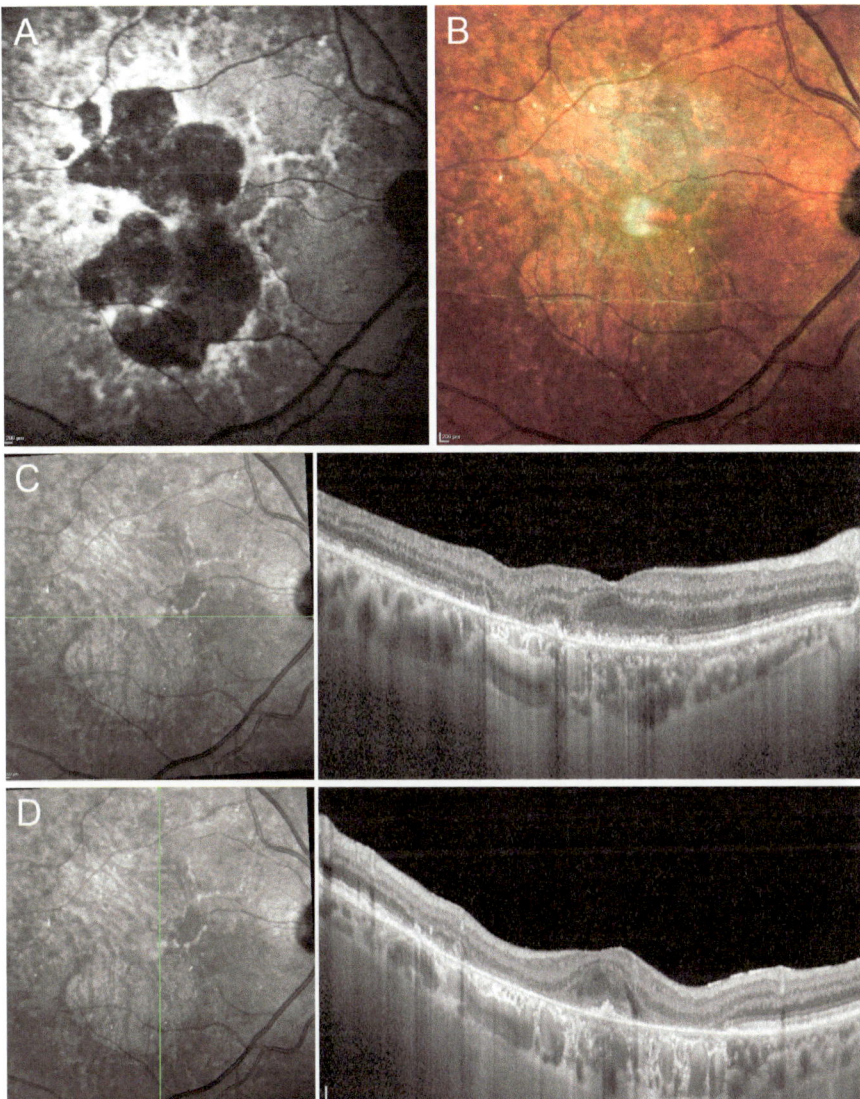

**Fig. 6.6** Multimodal imaging in a case of geographic atrophy. FAF image (**a**) clearly shows the hypoautofluorescent region, affected by the atrophic process. The hyperautofluorescent perilesional signal is typical of GA. The posterior pole atrophy is also confirmed by multicolor image (**b**), showing a marked depigmentation. Structural OCT (**c**, **d**) clearly shows the atrophy of the outer retinal layers, with window effect artifact interesting the choroid, the latter caused by the lack of light absorption caused by the atrophy of the retinal pigment epithelium

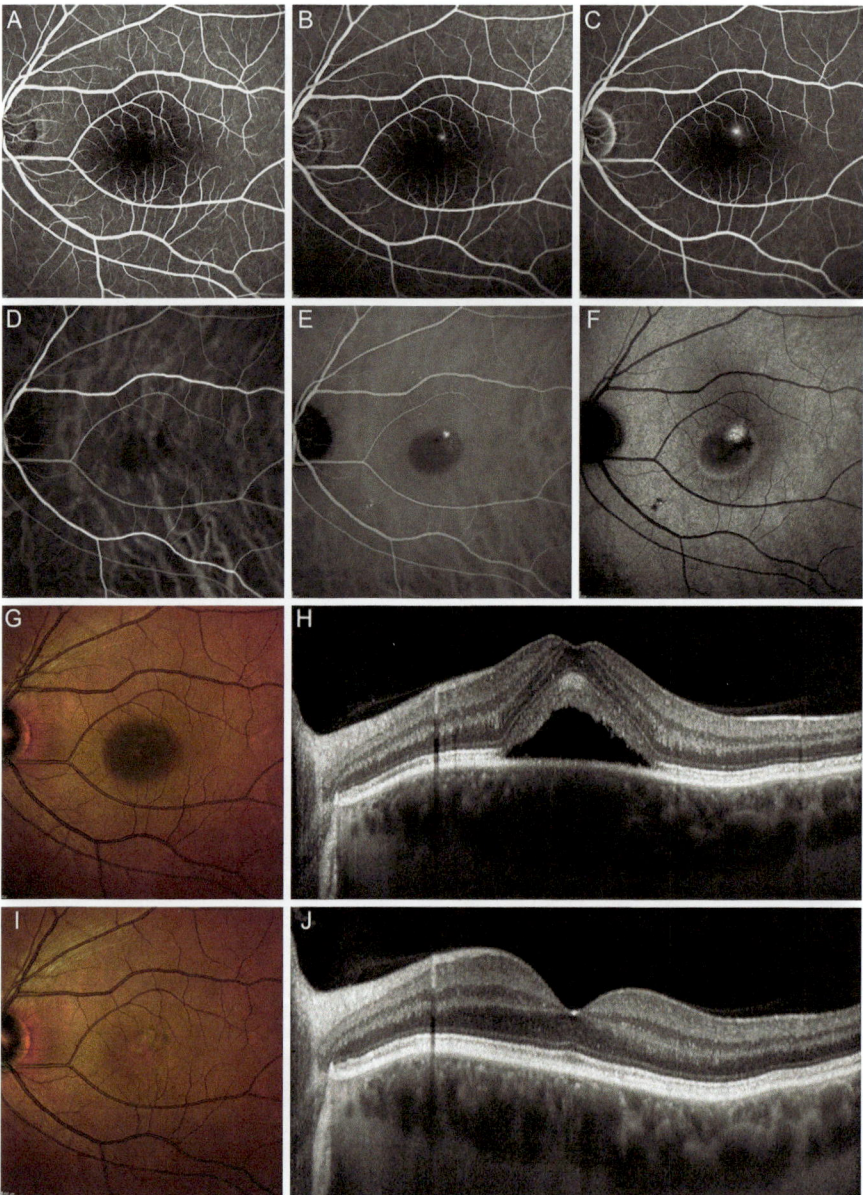

**Fig. 6.7** Multimodal imaging in a case of central serous chorioretinopathy. FA shows the presence of a fugal hyperfluorescent point, increasing in dimension from early (**a**) to intermediate and late phases (**b, c**). ICGA confirms the presence of the fugal point in all three phases (**d–f**); moreover, it shows a masking effect secondary to the presence of massive fluid. This latter is accurately detected by multicolor image (**g**) and structural OCT (**h**), accurately documenting the loss of physiologic foveal profile. After the treatment with eplerenone, both multicolor image (**i**) and structural OCT (**j**) document the restoration of macular features

## *Advances in Intravitreal Treatments*

Choroidal neovascularization (CNV) due to neovascular AMD (nAMD) is the cause of AMD-related severe vision loss among people aged 55 years or older in western countries. Anti-vascular endothelial growth factor (anti-VEGF) agents, delivered intravitreally, arrest the angiogenic process and stop the growth of abnormal blood vessels in the eye (Fig. 6.8). The aim of this therapy is to prevent disease evolution, vision loss and, in some cases, improve vision [17].

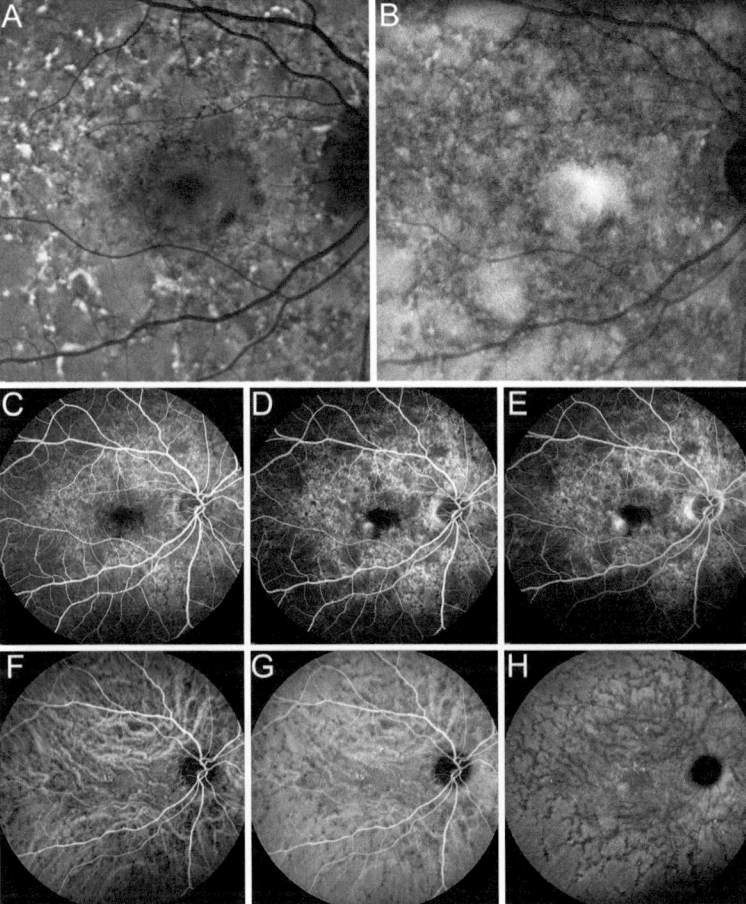

**Fig. 6.8** Multimodal imaging in a case of Stargardt disease complicated by the onset of a choroidal neovascularization. Blue (**a**) and near-infrared (**b**) autofluorescence images are very useful to document the distribution and extension of atrophic alterations, hypo- and hyperautofluorescent flecks. Early, intermediate and late phases of FA (**c–e**) and ICGA (**f–h**) exams detect the presence of a CNV, associated with sparse diffuse alterations extended also over the vascular arcades. Structural OCT shows an hyperreflective lesion associated with subretinal fluid (**i**), with complete recovery of exudation with stabilization of lesion size after anti-VEGF intravitreal treatment (**j**)

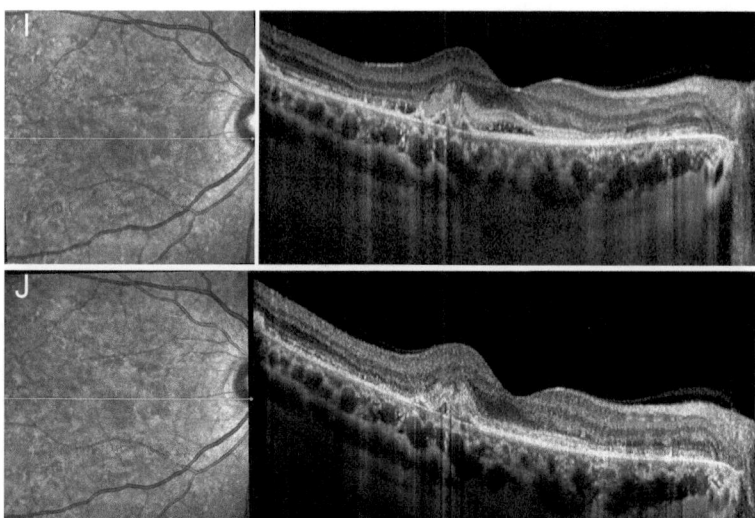

**Fig. 6.8** (continued)

Currently the two main drugs used to treat nAMD are Ranibizumab and Aflibercept. Bevacizumab, (Avastin; Genentech/Roche), does not have approval from the US Food and Drug Administration (FDA) and the National Institute for Health and Care Excellence for the treatment of AMD. Clinical trials have demonstrated similar efficacy of Bevacizumab and Ranibizumab. However, questions remain regarding serious systemic and ocular side effects of Bevacizumab. Whereas ranibizumab is provided in single-dose vials, bevacizumab requires compounding, which may increase the risk of ocular infections [18, 19].

Ranibizumab was the first treatment for neovascular AMD that offered a realistic hope for vision improvement.

The registration studies (ANCHOR and MARINA trials) analyzed the use of Ranibizumab versus photodynamic therapy in classic membranes and versus placebo in occult neovascularization. These trials established vision improvement in Ranibizumab groups and vision loss in the comparator groups. FDA approved Ranibizumab for the treatment of AMD in 2007 [20, 21].

Aflibercept, formerly known as VEGF-Trap, is another anti-VEGF drug that was approved for the treatment of nAMD by the FDA in 2011, after the results of VIEW 1 and 2 trials [22, 23]. These studies demonstrated that aflibercept is an effective therapy for nAMD and it can be administered every 2 months [22].

Angiogenesis can be inhibited with different treatments, which have been studied with excellent outcomes in the clinical trials but with less successful results using real-world data. The targets of these new therapies are: better efficacy, longer duration of action and simultaneous effects on VEGF blockade and prevention of atrophy and scarring. Between these new drugs, Brolucizumab and Abicipar pegol showed positive outcomes in phase 2 trials and now are being studied in phase 3 trials [24].

Brolucizumab (RTH258) is a humanized single-chain antibody fragment that inhibits all isoforms of VEGF-A. It was developed by ESBATech (discovery to phase 2a), Alcon Laboratories (phase 2b) and Novartis (phase 3).This drug has a small molecular weight (26 kDa) in comparison to Aflibercept and Ranibizumab (respectively 115 kDa and 48 kDa). This enables Brolucizumab to penetrate tissues and to be removed more rapidly from systemic circulation compared to larger molecules. Two different trials (HAWK and HARRIER) were designed to compare the efficacy and safety of Brolucizumab versus Aflibercept in subjects with nAMD. These studies showed important results in term of visual acuity and duration of action. Moreover, Brolucizumab seemed to be superior to Aflibercept in reducing intraretinal and subretinal fluid by OCT at different time-points [25, 26].

Abicipar pegol (Allergan) is a recombinant protein of the designed ankyrin repeat protein (DARPin) family. DARPins are small, single-domain antibody mimetic proteins that can selectively bind to a target protein with high affinity and specificity. In comparison to Ranibizumab, Abicipar showed a higher affinity for VEGF-A and a longer half-life. SEQUOIA and CEDAR are two clinical trials designed to evaluate the safety and efficacy of Abicipar versus Ranibizumab in nAMD. After 52 weeks both studies achieved non-inferiority in vision compared to Ranibizumab. However, patients treated with Abicipar presented more ocular adverse events following the treatment, most notably in the form of intraocular inflammation as uveitis, vitritis and vasculitis. Most of these episodes were classified as mild or moderate and over 80% of them were treated and responded to topical corticosteroid [27].

Another interesting molecule with anti-angiogenic effects is Squalamine (OHR-102). This drug is delivered to the eye in the form of an eye drop. IMPACT study was performed on this new drug, comparing squalamine eye drops plus Ranibizumab versus Ranibizumab monotherapy. This study showed positive outcomes in term of visual acuity and, at present, a phase 3 study is ongoing to evaluate the efficacy and safety of squalamine eye drops [24].

Diabetic macular edema (DME) is a severe complication of diabetic retinopathy and is characterized by breakdown of the blood-retina barrier and increased vascular permeability.

Currently therapeutic strategies for DME includes focal/grid laser photocoagulation, intravitreal anti-VEGF or corticosteroid treatment [28].

Fluocinolone acetonide intravitreal implant 0.19 mg (Iluvien) is a nonbiodegradable, injectable corticosteroid implant. It has been approved in 2013 as a treatment option of DME in patients with pseudophakia who have been previously treated with corticosteroids and didn't have a clinically significant rise in intraocular pressure. Iluvien lasts 36 months and contains 0.19 mg of fluocinolone acetonide which is released at an average rate of 0.2 µg/day [29].

The Fluocinolone Acetonide in Diabetic Macular Edema (FAME) registration studies consisted of two identical, double masked, sham-controlled, multicenter, phase 3 studies— trial A and trial B—and included 956 patients with DME. Patients were randomized to receive Iluvien or placebo. Participants who received Iluvien showed a significantly improvement in best-corrected visual acuity (BCVA) than sham injection. The Iluvien implant also significantly reduced foveal thickness at 24 months. These effects last 36 months. Consistent with corticosteroid class-specific adverse events, the most significant concerns in the use of Iluvien are ocular hypertension and cataract. Raised IOP was treated with medical therapy in most patients, with only <5% requiring incisional IOP-lowering surgery. These results have been also supported by real-world studies [30].

## Advances in Other Non-surgical Treatments

New perspectives for the treatment of maculopathies regard gene therapy and new technological devices, namely artificial retinal microchips.

Many hopes dwell in gene therapy. The eye has been at the perfect candidate for translational gene therapy because of its small, enclosed structure, immune privilege, and easy accessibility. The availability of animal models and the opportunity to take in vivo imaging techniques allows for noninvasive and sensible monitoring of the effects of gene delivery. Two strategies have been adopted in gene therapy: gene augmentation or gene disrupting/silencing [31]. The former consists in an insertion of a mutant gene in the host cell through a vector. The latter employs editing tools, as RNA interference or nucleases [32, 33], for gene suppression and many studies on animal model are searching for possible applications in human ocular disease. Gene augmentation may be use for AR and XL diseases and is the most experimented strategy worldwide. The gene of interest could be delivered as DNA, or alternatively as mRNA or mRNA analog. Viral vectors represent the preferred choice to transfer nucleic acids in cells. Adenovirus and Lentivirus have the best qualities for this task. Adeno-associated virus is the more used vector in ophthalmology due to its efficiency, persistence and poor immunogenicity [34]. Adeno-associated virus (AAV) belongs to capside virus with no envelope and has small dimension (19–21 nm). AAV has low risk of mutagenesis because it remains in episomal form in the nucleus [35]. AAV is the chosen vector for RPE65 trials [36, 37]. The limiting factor in AAV use is the packaging capacity of 4.8 kb [38]. Moreover, regulatory elements are necessary for the procedure and so the capacity is further reduced to 3 kb [39]. For this reason, large genes as ABCA4 and MY07A (7 kb) could not be inserted in AAV carriers [40]. The use of dual AAV carrier has been developed to overcome the issue [41]. The genetic material is packed as two distinct fragments and delivered to the cell and then recombining through homologous recombination or trans-splicing methodic [42]. The AAV serotypes more studied and used in ocular gene therapy are AAV2, AAV5 and AAV8. Different capsid proteins confer diverse target tropism and transduction efficiency [43–45]. The AAV2 is able to efficiently transduce RPE cells, photoreceptors cells and retinal ganglion cells [43]. Recent studies suggest that the antibody response triggered by a first injection could limit the transduction in the other eye [46].

Lentiviral vectors derive form variant of human immunodeficiency virus type 1 [47]. The cargo capacity is larger than AAV viruses: 8–10 kb [48]. After transduction the gene inserted are reverse transcribed into the host genome and then expressed

[49]. Insertional mutagenesis is a risk since the integration. In preclinical studies lentivirus seemed effective in targeting RPE cell, but not photoreceptors [50].

Subretinal and intravitreal injection are the strategies to deliver the virus carriers in the eye. The first method targets RPE cells, photoreceptors and Muller cells. In almost all human clinical trials has been used to deliver RPE65 [51]. Observed complications for subretinal injection are macular hole, retinal tears, inability to detach the retina whit multiple injection attempts, cataract, long recovery time because of large volume injected [36, 52, 53]. Intravitreal injection targets retinal ganglion cells and the virus molecules are directly injected in the hyaloid [54]. Immunologic and inflammatory responses, transient elevation in intraocular pressure are the main complications [55–57].

Nanoparticles (NPs) can also be used for gene therapy alternatively to viral carrier [58]. NPs, usually lipid-based, were developed to be internalized by the cell and to be capable of transferring the carried genetic material to the nucleus, escaping from the endosome. Lipid NPs are stable, biocompatible, no inflammatory-induce molecules [59]. Large plasmid DNA up to 20 kb could be transferred by NPs [60]. Two preclinical studies efficaciously treated a Rs1h deficient X-linked retinoschisis in a mouse model through NPs injections [61, 62]. NPs disadvantages compared to viral carriers are lower gene expression and lack of specificity to the different types of retinal cells [59].

Viral vectors with subretinal/intravitreal injection, and in particular AAV, and gene augmentation strategy have been used for the most completed and ongoing human trials. Voretigene neparvovec-rzyl (trade name of Luxturna) was approved in December 2017 as the first gene therapy for inherited retinal degenerations by Food and Drug Administration. It consists in AAV2 viral vectors carrying human RPE65 DNA driven by a CMV enhancer targeting RPE cells through subretinal injection [63, 64].

Retinitis pigmentosa and Leber's Congenital Amaurosis (LCA) would benefit from Voretigene therapy. Mutations in RPE65 account for approximately 2% of autosomal recessive RP and 16% of LCA [65]. Results from the first 2 years of this clinical trial showed that RPE65 gene replacement therapy was not associated with serious adverse events, and improvement in at least one measure of visual function was observed in 9/12 subjects, with the trend for improvement being observed in the younger patients [66]. In the 3, 4, 5 years after treatment no safety issues were observed and progression of photoreceptors degeneration was slower in early age patients [67].

Gene therapy must be completed before the onset of cell death caused by the disease. Retinal degeneration progression was seen in a human LCA study with gene therapy, despite a visual acuity improvement [58]. Perfect timing is therefore crucial.

The first multicentre nonrandomised open-label clinical trial in choroideremia patients reported encouraging results using an AAV2 [68]. After 2 years, the median visual acuity increased by 4.5 letters in the treated eyes versus 1.5 letters loss in the untreated eyes [69, 70]. Association with OCTA information may contribute to a more precise localization of gene therapy in the attempt to maximize the functional improvement [71].

Gene therapy approach is an exciting researching field in IRD and an actual clinical option after Voretigene launch in RPE65 mediated diseases. Cargo capacity remains a limiting factor and new researches are needed to find new vectors or modify the current ones. We hope that new data and technological improvement will lead to perfectionated the results in treated patients and extend gene therapy effectiveness to other IRD.

Gene therapy approach may help maintain visual acuity in the early onset of the disease, while electric stimulation through electrodes attempt to a partial restoration of the vision using the remaining retinal network [72]. After photoreceptors degeneration the inner retinal cells may continue to survive and be operative for many years despite neural remodeling [73].

Two different strategies of implants have been performed: implantation of electrode arrays epiretinally in connection with retinal ganglion cells or implantation of the microchip in the subretinal space, substituting photoreceptors [74–76]. External image and data processing are necessary for the first approach to bypass retinal image analysis, while the subretinal implants try to restore the normal connections. RP has been targeted for this kind of approach from the beginning, due to primarily photoreceptor degeneration. Microchip is constituted by photodiodes, which convert light energy in electric energy. The electric response can be driven and translated by still vital bipolar cells. Electrical stimulation pattern maintains its retinotopic orientation because the normal retinal network is employed. This is experimentally confirmed when patient read letters and combine them to words or have is acuity assessed by presenting Landolt C-rings [77, 78]. Instead direct stimulation of ganglion cells needs a learning/processing of the signal [79]. The subretinal space is a privileged space and immunological reactions or scarring processes are low into it. The epiretinal implant could lead to epiretinal membrane formation or neural atrophy (Table 6.5) [80].

However, the electric signal must be amplified by the microchip before conveying to bipolar cells, because the normal signal energy is not sufficient to stimulate a diseased retina [81]. So, an induction coil located under the skin beneath the ear was developed to confer relay power to the chip and is connected to the orbital part with a subperiosteal cable [82]. The surgical procedure with subretinal approach is complex and requires an high precision to fix the implant in an exact position. For this reason, the scheduled time for a subretinal surgery implant is 5–8 h vs 1.5–4 h for epiretinal implant surgery [83]. The subretinal microphotodiode-array has so far been implanted in 64 patients (September 2017; data provided by Retina Implant

**Table 6.5** Pros and cons in the choice of epiretinal and subretinal implantation

|  | Pros | Cons |
|---|---|---|
| Epiretinal implantation strategy | Easier and faster surgical procedure (1.5–4 h) | Learning training needed, epiretinal membrane or atrophy in situ formation |
| Subretinal implantation strategy | Direct stimulation of bypolar cells, retinotopic orientation of the image, reduced scarring and immunologic responses | Complex and long surgical procedure (5–8 h), signal needed to be amplified |

AG, Reutlingen, Germany). Durability is a great issue: RETINA IMPLANT Alpha AMS has significantly improved the previous results, reaching a half-life of at least 5 years [82]. One thousand six hundred micro-photodiodes and electrodes are located in an area of 2.8 mm × 2.8 mm. Energy and control signals are transferred to the micro-photodiodes via a subretinal, trans-scleral polyimide foil and a subperiosteal silicone cable, which originates from a secondary coil in the retro-auricular space under the skin. The coil received energy from a primary coil, attached magnetically behind the ear. The primary coil, in turn, receives energy and controls from a small hand-held device, provided with controls for the user and engineers.

The implantation surgery begins with the retro-auricular part. Then intraocular surgery follows with the preparation of a scleral flap, temporally closed with a suture. Next step is the three-port complete vitrectomy and the sub-retinal bleb creation to avoid retinal injuries from the guide foil or the implant. The retina is lifted with 41-gauge sub-retinal injection of balancer salt solution. After the bleb, the scleral flap is re-opened and the guide foil is inserted through a choroidal incision into the subretinal bleb and the pushed tangentially to the ocular surface. The guide foil is thus adjusted in the correct position. The implant can easily be advanced between the RPE and the guide foil and then this latter is carefully removed. The scleral flap is closed, and the silicone mesh of the implant secured to the sclera over the flap. Fluid/air exchange is performed, and the eye filled with silicone oil. Explantation was part of the first protocol (2005–2009). According to recent data, 4 of 64 patients underwent re-implantation with RETINA IMPLANT Alpha AMS. All re-implantations have been performed in the exact same locations as the primary surgery and, clearly, surgery is considerably more difficult than explantation. A multicentered trial with RETINA IMPLANT Alpha AMS in 15 blind patients was performed in Germany [82]. Implant-mediated visual perception was seen in 13/15 patients. At second month, 11/13 patients passed the light perception test, while motion detection was possible for two out of 11 patients when the implant was switched ON at the first month. 2/13 patients were able to distinguish Landolt C-rings up to 20/1111 and 20/546 and able to discriminate the orientation of gratings with a spatial frequency of 0.66 and 1 cpd. Implant-mediated visual perception was generally stable over the observation period of 12 months [82].

Microchip implants are a modern and feasible approach to IRD and new technological developments and studies are required to better understand the maximum potential of this surgery [84–86].

## Conclusion

In conclusion, the future perspectives on the diagnosis and treatment of maculopathies will undergo to even more advanced methodologies and will led ophthalmologists to an optimistic era were patients will benefit from more fine and precocious diagnosis, as well as in treatments able to act against the pathological mechanisms of macular diseases, preventing the onset and progression of complications like atrophy.

# References

1. Novotny HR, Alvis DL. A method of photographing fluorescence in circulating blood in the human retina. Circulation. 1961;24:82–6.
2. Marmor MF, Ravin JG. Fluorescein angiography: insight and serendipity a half century ago. Arch Ophthalmol. 2011;129(7):943–8.
3. Yannuzzi LA, Slakter JS, Sorenson JA, Guyer DR, Orlock DA. Digital indocyanine green videoangiography and choroidal neovascularization. Retina. 1992;12(3):191–223.
4. Yannuzzi LA. Indocyanine green angiography: a perspective on use in the clinical setting. Am J Ophthalmol. 2011;151:745–751.e1.
5. Huang D, Swanson EA, Lin CP, et al. Optical coherence tomography. Science. 1991;254:1178–81.
6. Wojtkowski M, Leitgeb R, Kowalczyk A, et al. In vivo human retinal imaging by Fourier Domain optical coherence tomography. J Biomed Opt. 2002;7:457–63.
7. Postaid B, Baumann B, Huang D, et al. Ultrahigh speed 1050 nm swept source/Fourier domain OCT retinal and anterior segment imaging at 100,000 to 400,000 axial scans per second. Opt Express. 2010;18:200029–48.
8. Lavinsky F, Lavinsky D. Novel perspectives on swept-source optical coherence tomography. Int J Retina Vitreous. 2016;2:25. eCollection 2016.
9. Gabriele ML, Wollstein G, Ishikawa H, et al. Optical coherence tomography: history, current status, and laboratory work. Invest Ophthalmol Vis Sci. 2011;52(5):2425–36.
10. Kashani AH, Chen CL, Gahm JK, et al. Optical coherence tomography angiography: a comprehensive review of current methods and clinical applications. Prog Retin Eye Res. 2017;60:66–100.
11. Tan ACS, Tan GS, Denniston AK, et al. An overview of the clinical applications of optical coherence tomography angiography. Eye (Lond). 2018;32(2):262–86.
12. Frampton GK, Kalita N, Payne L, et al. Fundus autofluorescence imaging: systematic review of test accuracy for the diagnosis and monitoring of retinal conditions. Eye (Lond). 2017;31(7):995–1007.
13. Wolf-Schnurrbusch UE, Wittwer VV, Ghanem R, et al. Blue light versus green light autofluorescence: lesion size of areas with geographic atrophy. Invest Ophthalmol Vis Sci. 2011;52:9497–502.
14. Maryse LL, Carroll J, Skala MC. Imaging retinal melanin: a review of current technologies. J Biol Eng. 2018;12:29.
15. Ting DSW, Pasquale LR, Peng L, et al. Artificial intelligence and deep learning in ophthalmology. Br J Ophthalmol. 2019;103(2):167–75.
16. Maloca P, Hasler PW, Barthelmes D, et al. Safety and feasibility of a novel sparse optical coherence tomography device for patient-delivered retina home monitoring. Transl Vis Sci Technol. 2018;7(4):8.
17. Solomon SD, Lindsley K, Vedula SS, Krzystolik MG, Hawkins BS. Anti-vascular endothelial growth factor for neovascular age-related macular degeneration. Cochrane Database Syst Rev. 2014;8(8):CD005139.
18. Gower EW, Stein JD, Shekhawat NS, et al. Geographic and demographic variation in use of ranibizumab versus bevacizumab for neovascular age-related macular degeneration in the United States. Am J Ophthalmol. 2017;184:157–66.
19. CATT Research Group, Martin DF, Maguire MG, et al. Ranibizumab and bevacizumab for neovascular age-related macular degeneration. N Engl J Med. 2011;364(20):1897–908.
20. Rofagha S, Bhisitkul RB, Boyer DS, Sadda SR, Zhang K. Seven-year outcomes in ranibizumab-treated patients in ANCHOR, MARINA, and HORIZON: a multicenter cohort study (SEVEN-UP). Ophthalmology. 2013;120(11):2292–9.
21. Brown DM, Kaiser PK, Michels M, et al. Ranibizumab versus verteporfin for neovascular age-related macular degeneration. N Engl J Med. 2006;355:1432–44.

22. Heier JS, Brown DM, Chong V, et al. Intravitreal aflibercept (VEGF trap-eye) in wet age-related macular degeneration. Ophthalmology. 2012;119:2537–48.
23. Schmidt-Erfurth U, Kaiser PK, Korobelnik JF, et al. Intravitreal aflibercept injection for neovascular age-related macular degeneration: ninety-six-week results of the VIEW studies. Ophthalmology. 2014;121(1):193–201.
24. Schlottmann PG, Alezzandrini AA, Zas M, Rodriguez FJ, Luna JDWL. New treatment modalities for neovascular age-related macular degeneration. Asia Pac J Ophthalmol (Phila). 2017;6:514–9.
25. Dugel PU, Jaffe GJ, Sallstig P, et al. Brolucizumab versus aflibercept in participants with neovascular age-related macular degeneration: a randomized trial. Ophthalmology. 2017;124(9):1296–304.
26. Wykoff CC, Hariprasad SM, Zhou B. Innovation in neovascular age-related macular degeneration: consideration of brolucizumab, abicipar, and the port delivery system. Ophthalmic Surg Lasers Imaging Retina. 2018;49(12):913–7.
27. Khurana R. Safety and efficacy of abicipar in patients with neovascular age-related macular degeneration. Lect Present Am Acad Ophthalmol 2018 Annu Meet Oct 27, Chicago; 2018.
28. Syed YY. Fluocinolone acetonide intravitreal implant 0.19 mg (ILUVIEN): a review in diabetic macular edema. Drugs. 2017;77:575–83.
29. Massa H, Nagar AM, Vergados A, Dadoukis P, Patra S, Panos GD. Intravitreal fluocinolone acetonide implant (ILUVIEN®) for diabetic macular oedema: a literature review. J Int Med Res. 2019;47(1):31–43.
30. Campochiaro PA, Brown DM, Pearson A, et al. Long-term benefit of sustained-delivery fluocinolone acetonide vitreous inserts for diabetic macular edema. Ophthalmology. 2011;118(4):626–635.e2.
31. Arbabi A, Liu A, Ameri H. Gene therapy for inherited retinal degeneration. J Ocul Pharmacol Ther. 2019;35(2):79–97.
32. Millington-Ward S, Chadderton N, O'Reilly M, et al. Suppression and replacement gene therapy for autosomal dominant disease in a murine model of dominant retinitis pigmentosa. Mol Ther. 2011;19:642–9.
33. Gaj T, Gersbach CA, Barbas CF 3rd. ZFN, TALEN, and CRISPR/Cas-based methods for genome engineering. Trends Biotechnol. 2013;31(7):397–405.
34. Daya S, Berns KI. Gene therapy using adeno-associated virus vectors. Clin Microbiol Rev. 2008;21:583–93.
35. Tenenbaum L, Lehtonen E, Monahan PE. Evaluation of risks related to the use of adeno-associated virus-based vectors. Curr Gene Ther. 2003;3:545–65.
36. Bainbridge JW, Smith AJ, Barker SS, et al. Effect of gene therapy on visual function in Leber's congenital amaurosis. N Engl J Med. 2008;358:2231–9.
37. Hauswirth WW, Aleman TS, Kaushal S, et al. Treatment of leber congenital amaurosis due to RPE65 mutations by ocular subretinal injection of adeno-associated virus gene vector: short-term results of a phase I trial. Hum Gene Ther. 2008;19:979–90.
38. Naso MF, Tomkowicz B, Perry WL 3rd, Strohl WR. Adeno-associated virus (AAV) as a vector for gene therapy. BioDrugs. 2017;31:317–34.
39. Bennett J. Taking stock of retinal gene therapy: looking back and moving forward. Mol Ther. 2017;25:1076–94.
40. Cashman SM, Sadowski SL, Morris DJ, Frederick J, Kumar-Singh R. Intercellular trafficking of adenovirus-delivered HSV VP22 from the retinal pigment epithelium to the photoreceptors—implications for gene therapy. Mol Ther. 2002;6:813–23.
41. Trapani I, Colella P, Sommella A, et al. Effective delivery of large genes to the retina by dual AAV vectors. EMBO Mol Med. 2014;6:194–211.
42. Ghosh A, Yue Y, Duan D. Efficient transgene re-constitution with hybrid dual AAV vectors carrying the minimized bridging sequences. Hum Gene Ther. 2011;22:77–83.
43. Allocca M, Mussolino C, Garcia-Hoyos M, et al. Novel adeno-associated virus serotypes efficiently trans- duce murine photoreceptors. J Virol. 2007;81:11372–80.

44. Allocca M, Manfredi A, Iodice C, Di Vicino U, Auricchio A. AAV-mediated gene replacement, either alone or in combination with physical and pharmacological agents, results in partial and transient protection from photoreceptor degeneration associated with betaPDE deficiency. Invest Ophthalmol Vis Sci. 2011;52:5713–9.
45. Martin KR, Klein RL, Quigley HA. Gene delivery to the eye using adeno-associated viral vectors. Methods. 2002;28:267–75.
46. Li Q, Miller R, Han PY, et al. Intraocular route of AAV2 vector administration defines humoral immune response and therapeutic potential. Mol Vis. 2008;14:1760–9.
47. Greenberg KP, Lee ES, Schaffer DV, Flannery G. Gene delivery to the retina using lentiviral vectors. Adv Exp Med Biol. 2006;572:255–66.
48. Balaggan KS, Ali RR. Ocular gene delivery using lentiviral vectors. Gene Ther. 2012;19:145–53.
49. White M, Whittaker R, Gandara C, Stoll EA. A guide to approaching regulatory considerations for lentiviral-mediated gene therapies. Hum Gene Ther Methods. 2017;28:163–76.
50. Harvey AR, Kamphuis W, Eggers R, et al. Intravitreal injection of adeno-associated viral vectors results in the transduction of different types of retinal neurons in neonatal and adult rats: a comparison with lentiviral vectors. Mol Cell Neurosci. 2002;21:141–57.
51. Ameri H. Prospect of retinal gene therapy following commercialization of voretigene neparvovec-rzyl for retinal dystrophy mediated by RPE65 mutation. J Curr Ophthalmol. 2018;30:1–2.
52. Maguire AM, Simonelli F, Pierce EA, et al. Safety and efficacy of gene transfer for Leber's congenital amaurosis. N Engl J Med. 2008;358:2240–8.
53. Bennett J, Wellman J, Marshall KA, et al. Safety and durability of effect of contralateral-eye administration of AAV2 gene therapy in patients with childhood-onset blindness caused by RPE65 mutations: a follow-on phase 1 trial. Lancet. 2016;388:661–72.
54. Dudus L, Anand V, Acland GM, et al. Persistent transgene product in retina, optic nerve and brain after intraocular injection of rAAV. Vis Res. 1999;39:2545–53.
55. Dalkara D, Byrne LC, Klimczak RR, et al. In vivo-directed evolution of a new adeno-associated virus for therapeutic outer retinal gene delivery from the vitreous. Sci Transl Med. 2013;5:189ra176.
56. Mace E, Caplette R, Marre O, et al. Targeting channelrhodopsin-2 to ON-bipolar cells with vitreally administered AAV restores ON and OFF visual responses in blind mice. Mol Ther. 2015;3:7–16.
57. Feuer WJ, Schiffman JC, Davis JL, et al. Gene therapy for Leber hereditary optic neuropathy: initial results. Ophthalmology. 2016;123:558–70.
58. Adijanto J, Naash MI. Nanoparticle-based technologies for retinal gene therapy. Eur J Pharm Biopharm. 2015;95(Pt B):353–67.
59. Wang Y, Rajala A, Cao B, et al. Cell-specific promoters enable lipid-based nanoparticles to deliver genes to specific cells of the retina in vivo. Theranostics. 2016;6:1514–27.
60. Fink TL, Klepcyk PJ, Oette SM, et al. Plasmid size up to 20kbp does not limit effective in vivo lung gene transfer using compacted DNA nanoparticles. Gene Ther. 2006;13:1048–51.
61. Apaolaza PS, Del Pozo-Rodriguez A, Torrecilla J, et al. Solid lipid nanoparticle-based vectors intended for the treatment of X-linked juvenile retinoschisis by gene therapy: in vivo approaches in Rs1h-deficient mouse model. J Control Release. 2015;217:273–83.
62. Apaolaza PS, Del Pozo-Rodriguez A, Solinis MA, et al. Structural recovery of the retina in a retinoschisin-deficient mouse after gene replacement therapy by solid lipid nanoparticles. Biomaterials. 2016;90:40–9.
63. Bennicelli J, Wright JF, Komaromy A, et al. Reversal of blindness in animal models of leber congenital amaurosis using optimized AAV2-mediated gene transfer. Mol Ther. 2008;16:458–65.
64. Jacobson SG, Aleman TS, Cideciyan AV, et al. Identifying photoreceptors in blind eyes caused by RPE65 mutations: prerequisite for human gene therapy success. Proc Natl Acad Sci U S A. 2005;102:6177–82.

65. Morimura H, Fishman GA, Grover SA, Fulton AB, Berson EL, Dryja TP. Mutations in the RPE65 gene in patients with autosomal recessive retinitis pigmentosa or leber congenital amaurosis. Proc Natl Acad Sci U S A. 1998;95(6):3088–93.
66. Weleber RG, Pennesi ME, Wilson DJ, et al. Results at 2 years after gene therapy for RPE65-deficient Leber congenital amaurosis and severe early-childhood-onset retinal dystrophy. Ophthalmology. 2016;123:1606–20.
67. Pennesi ME, Weleber RG, Yang P, et al. Results at 5 years after gene therapy for RPE65-deficient retinal dystrophy. Hum Gene Ther. 2018. [Epub ahead of print].
68. Cideciyan AV, Jacobson SG, Beltran WA, et al. Human retinal gene therapy for Leber congenital amaurosis shows advancing retinal degeneration despite enduring visual improvement. Proc Natl Acad Sci U S A. 2013;110:E517–25.
69. MacLaren RE, Groppe M, Barnard AR, et al. Retinal gene therapy in patients with choroideremia: initial findings from a phase 1/2 clinical trial. Lancet. 2014;383:1129–37.
70. MacLaren RE, Xue K, Barnard A, et al. Gene therapy for choroideremia in a multicenter dose escalation phase I/II clinical trial. Invest Ophthalmol Vis Sci. 2018;59:1195.
71. Battaglia Parodi M, Arrigo A, McLaren RE, et al. Vascular alterations revealed with optical coherence tomography angiography in patients with choroideremia. Retina. 2019;39(6):1200–5.
72. Mitsios A, Dubis AM, Moosajee M. Choroideremia: from genetic and clinical phenotyping to gene therapy and future treatments. Ther Adv Ophthalmol. 2018;10:2515841418817490.
73. Zrenner E, Bartz-Schmidt KU, Benav H, et al. Subretinal electronic chips allow blind patients to read letters and combine them to words. Proc Biol Sci. 2010;278:1489–97.
74. Jones BW, Marc RE. Retinal remodeling during retinal degeneration. Exp Eye Res. 2005;81(2):123–37.
75. Yanai D, Weiland JD, Mahadevappa M, Greenberg RJ, Fine YI, Humayun MS. Visual performance using a retinal prosthesis in three subjects with retinitis pigmentosa. Am J Ophthalmol. 2007;143:820–7.
76. Hornig R, Laube T, Walter P, et al. A method and technical equipment for an acute human trial to evaluate retinal implant technology. J Neural Eng. 2005;2(1):S129–34.
77. Gerding H, Benner FP, Taneri S. Experimental implantation of epiretinal retina implants (EPI-RET) with an IOL-type receiver unit. J Neural Eng. 2007;4:S38–49.
78. Eysel UT, Walter P, Gekeler F, et al. Optical imaging reveals 2-dimensional patterns of cortical activation after local retinal stimulation with sub- and epiretinal visual prostheses. Investig Ophthalmol Vis Sci. 2002;43:ARVO E-Abstract 4486.
79. Eckhorn R, Wilms M, Schanze T, et al. Visual resolution with retinal implants estimated from recordings in cat visual cortex. Vis Res. 2006;46:2675–90.
80. Eckmiller R. Learning retina implants with epiretinal contacts. Ophthalmic Res. 1997;29:281–9.
81. Tran BK, Wolfensberger TJ. Retina-implant interaction after 16 months follow-up in a patient with an Argus II prosthesis. Klin Monatsbl Augenheilkd. 2017;234:538–40.
82. Stelzle M, Stett A, Brunner B, et al. Electrical properties of micro-photodiode arrays for use as artificial retina implant. Biomed Microdevices. 2001;3:133–42.
83. Stingl K, Bach M, Bartz-Schmidt KU, et al. Safety and efficacy of subretinal visual implants in humans: methodological aspects. Clin Exp Optom. 2013;96:4–13.
84. Stingl K, Schippert R, Bartz-Schmidt KU, et al. Interim results of a multicenter trial with the new electronic subretinal implant Alpha AMS in 15 patients blind from inherited retinal degenerations. Front Neurosci. 2017;11:445.
85. Luo YH, da Cruz L. The Argus((R)) II retinal prosthesis system. Prog Retin Eye Res. 2016;50:89–107.
86. Gekeler K, Bartz-Schmidt KU, Sachs H, et al. Implantation, removal and replacement of subretinal electronic implants for restoration of vision in patients with retinitis pigmentosa. Curr Opin Ophthalmol. 2018;29(3):239–47.

# Chapter 7
# Recent Developments in Vitreo-Retinal Surgery

**Sana Idrees, Ajay E. Kuriyan, Stephen G. Schwartz, Jean-Marie Parel, and Harry W. Flynn Jr**

## History of Vitrectomy

"Open sky" vitrectomy technique, termed diapupillary resection, was described by Tsugio Dodo for partial removal of a vitreous hemorrhage from a patient in Japan in 1955 [1, 2]. However, the Western world likely did not hear about this technique until 1968 when David Kasner also described an "open sky" technique for vitreous removal using cellulose sponges and scissors. This technique was initially used to address vitreous loss during cataract surgery (Fig. 7.1) and subsequently used to remove opacified vitreous in the setting of amyloidosis [3].

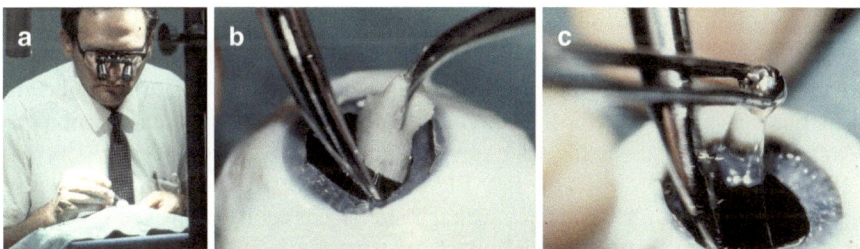

**Fig. 7.1** (**a**) Dr. David Kasner demonstrating open sky technique for vitreous removal using cellulose sponges and scissors on a cadaver eye. (**b**, **c**) High magnification of cadaver eye vitreous removal

S. Idrees · A. E. Kuriyan
Flaum Eye Institute, University of Rochester Medical Center, Rochester, NY, USA

S. G. Schwartz · J.-M. Parel · H. W. Flynn Jr (✉)
Bascom Palmer Eye Institute, University of Miami, Miami, FL, USA
e-mail: HFlynn@med.miami.edu

© Springer Nature Switzerland AG 2020                                                    165
A. Grzybowski (ed.), *Current Concepts in Ophthalmology*,
https://doi.org/10.1007/978-3-030-25389-9_7

**Fig. 7.2** Dr. Robert
Machemer performing pars
plana vitrectomy

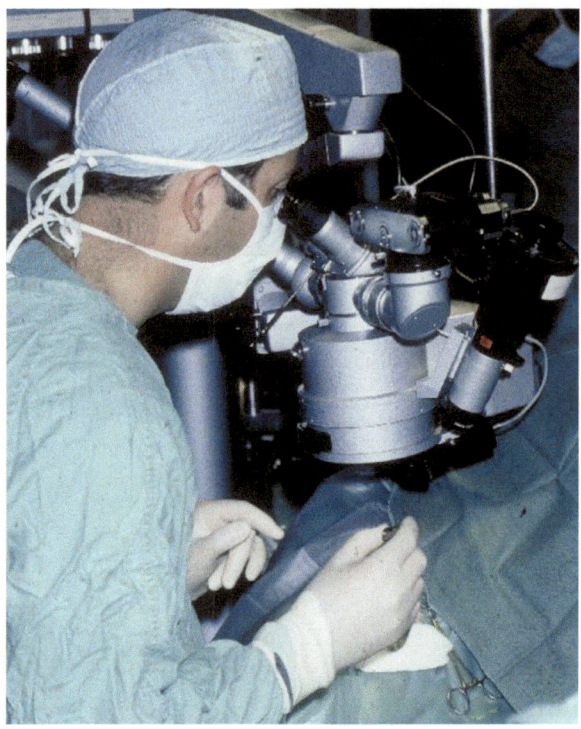

The introduction of modern pars plana vitrectomy (PPV) is generally credited
to Robert Machemer (Fig. 7.2) as he was responsible for developing the first
automated system for vitreous removal with controlled intraocular pressure in
1970 [4]. Machemer and Helmut Buettner initially designed a vitrectomy device
with a drill bit and tiny electric motor encased in a blunt hypodermic needle.
Suction was added to remove the vitreous more effectively, and an infusion tube
was soldered to the outside of the hypodermic needle to prevent globe collapse
[5]. Machemer performed his first PPV on April 20, 1970 on a diabetic patient
with a non-clearing vitreous hemorrhage and visual acuity improved from 2/200
to 20/50 [4]. Subsequently, a collaboration between Jean-Marie Parel (Fig. 7.3a)
and Machemer led to the development of the vitreous infusion suction cutter
(VISC, Fig. 7.3b) and the fiberoptic endoillumination used in early PPV. The
VISC was developed as an instrument which cut vitreous, removed debris from
the eye by suction, while simultaneously infusing Ringer's solution [6, 7]. Early
vitrectomy was performed using a VISC that was 17 gauge and 1.5 mm in diameter inserted through a 2.1 mm scleral incision [6, 8].

   In 1971, Gholam Peyman (Fig. 7.4a) described a technique using a vitrophage
(Fig. 7.4b) to remove and replace the vitreous [9]. In 1974, Conor O'Malley and
Ralph Heintz developed the first three port 20-gauge pars plana vitrectomy system,
separating the components of vitreous cutting, infusion, and illumination [10]. In
1985, Machemer and Dyson Hickingbotham introduced the first 20-gaugetrocar/

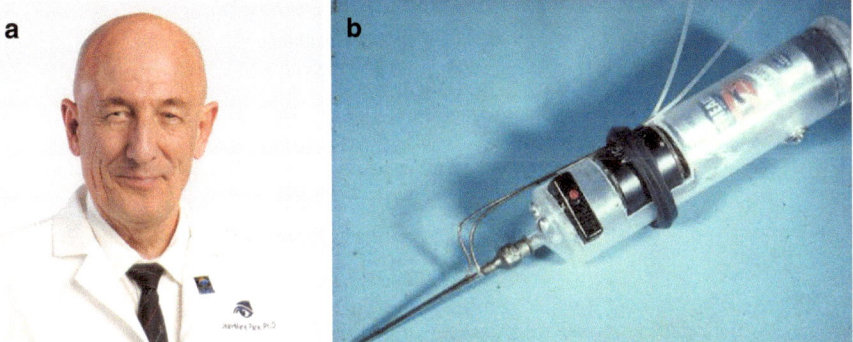

**Fig. 7.3** (**a**) Dr. Gholam Peymann, who developed the vitrophage. (**b**) Photo of the vitrophage

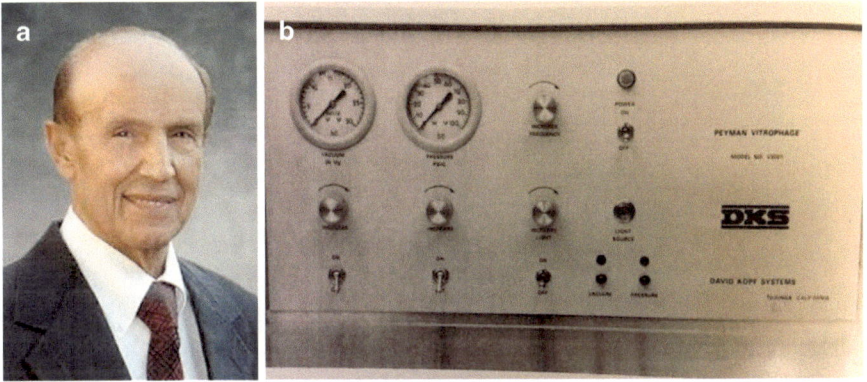

**Fig. 7.4** (**a**) Dr. Jean-Marie Parel, who developed the vitreous infusion suction cutter (VISC) with Dr. Robert Machemer. (**b**) Photo of the VISC

cannula system to allow for easier passage and interchangeability of instruments in an attempt to reduce the risk of iatrogenic retinal tears or retinal detachment [11]. Subsequently, 20-gauge vitrectomy became standard treatment for decades.

In 1990, Eugene de Juan and Hickingbotham developed 25-gauge vitrectomy instrumentation, including a vitreous cutter, microscissors, and vitreous membrane dissector. At that time, use of 25 gauge instruments was limited to select cases requiring high precision due to slow vitreous removal speeds [12]. Peyman described a 23 gauge vitrectomy system in 1990 [13]. In 2002, Gildo Fujii introduced a 25 gauge operating system, the Transconjunctival Sutureless Vitrectomy System, allowing for self-sealing transconjunctival sclerotomies. This method popularized the widespread use of small gauge PPV [14, 15]. In 2005, Claus Eckardt introduced 23 gauge instrumentation as an alternative to 25 gauge PPV [16]. Yusuke Oshima pioneered a 27 gauge vitrectomy system in 2010 [17].

When PPV was first utilized it was generally reserved for the more severe, selected cases, such as non-clearing vitreous hemorrhage and complex retinal

**Table 7.1** Diseases commonly considered amenable to pars plana vitrectomy

1. Retinal or choroidal detachment
    (a) Retinal detachment
        • Rhegmatogenous
        • Traction
        • Combined traction/rhegmatogenous
    (b) Choroidal detachment
        • Serous
        • Hemorrhagic
2. Proliferative vitreoretinopathy
3. Vitreous opacities
    (a) Vitreous hemorrhage
    (b) Other opacities
4. Vitreomacular interface disorders
    (a) Epiretinal membrane
    (b) Macular hole
    (c) Vitreomacular traction
5. Inflammatory disorders
    (a) Endophthalmitis
    (b) Posterior segment uveitis
        • Infectious
        • Noninfectious
6. Complications of anterior segment surgery
    (a) Retained lens material
    (b) Dislocated intraocular lens
7. Trauma
    (a) Intraocular foreign body

detachment [18]. However, evolution of vitreoretinal ancillary equipment and surgical techniques has allowed increases in the utilization of vitrectomy and indications for vitrectomy surgery (Table 7.1). Today, PPV is the most commonly performed surgical procedure by retinal specialists.

## Perioperative Considerations

Vitrectomy can be performed with general or local anesthesia, including regional with or without topical anesthesia [19]. Traditionally, vitrectomy was more often performed with general anesthesia, but recently local anesthesia is also popular [20]. General anesthesia may be used when the procedure is expected to be long or painful. Additionally, patients with claustrophobia, anxiety, or dementia may benefit from surgery with general anesthesia. However, use of general anesthesia decreases turnover time, increases procedural costs, and has increased systemic risks compared to local anesthesia with monitored anesthesia care [21].

Regional block with monitored anesthesia care allows the patient to remain awake during the procedure. Several methods of local anesthesia may been used, including retrobulbar, peribulbar, sub-Tenon's, and topical anesthesia [20]. Retrobulbar anesthesia generally provides excellent anesthesia and akinesia but is associated with small risks of retrobulbar hemorrhage and scleral perforation [22]. Peribulbar anesthesia is associated with fewer risks but is somewhat less effective than retrobulbar anesthesia and may require a longer time to produce adequate effects. Sub-Tenon's anesthesia is administered in the posterior sub-Tenon's space and provides rapid anesthesia and akinesia [22]. Topical anesthesia involves the use of anesthetic drops on the ocular surface. It has been reported effective in select patients for vitreoretinal surgery [23]. However, due to relatively long procedure times for most vitreo-retinal surgery, it has not been widely adopted. In-office PPV with local anesthesia has also been reported, but is not widely practiced [24].

## Vitrectomy Systems

Berkeley Bioengineering in 1974 developed the first three-port, 20G system known as the Ocutome 800 (Fig. 7.5). It had a lightweight pneumatic probe with axial cutting and surgeon foot pedal controlled on-off aspiration. It was followed by the Coopervision Ocutome 8000, which had the first linear aspiration system, integrated light source, and connected fragmenter. These early companies are no longer in existence or are not involved in vitrectomy surgical instruments. Another early vitrectomy system was the MID Labs MicroVit system, which produced the first high-quality disposable pneumatic cutter [25]. The Daisy (Storz) (Fig. 7.6) was introduced in 1986 and had multiple functions including irrigation/aspiration, anterior and posterior vitrectomy, bipolar coagulation, automated scissors, illumination, air exchange and phacoemulsification and fragmentation. The Daisy was followed by the Premiere system. Storz was acquired by Bausch + Lomb in 1997, and the combined organization produced the Millennium Microsurgical System (Fig. 7.7) that year. Also in 1997, Alcon introduced the Accurus (Fig. 7.8).

**Fig. 7.5** Ocutome 800 machine

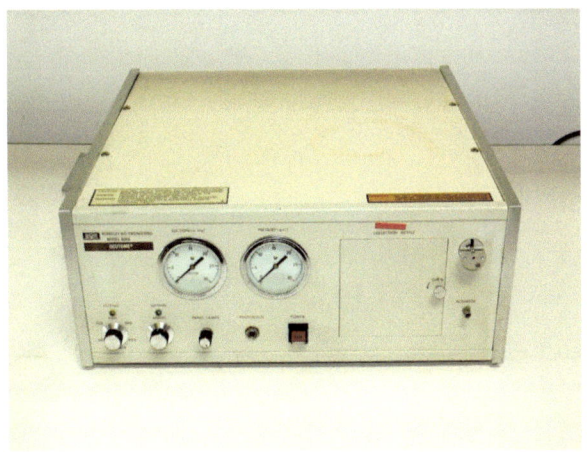

**Fig. 7.6** Storz Daisy machine (Photo courtesy of Bausch + Lomb)

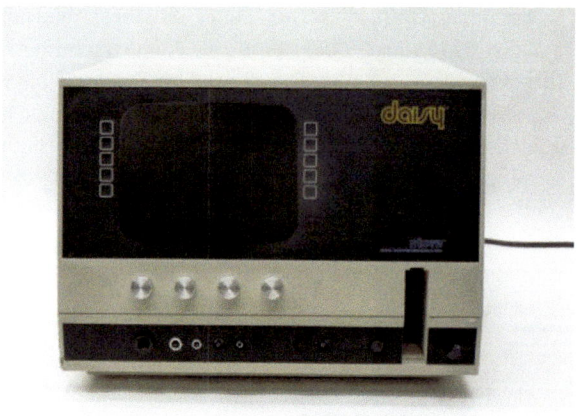

**Fig. 7.7** Bausch + Lomb Millenium Microsurgical System (Photo courtesy of Bausch + Lomb)

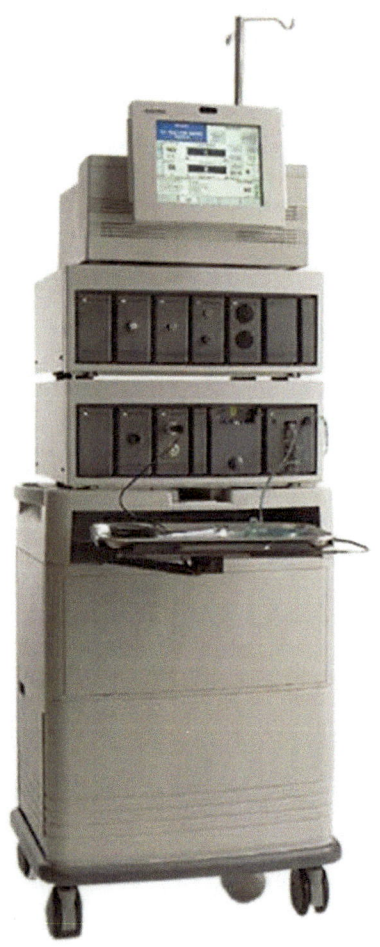

**Fig. 7.8** Alcon Accurus
machine (Photo courtesy
of Alcon)

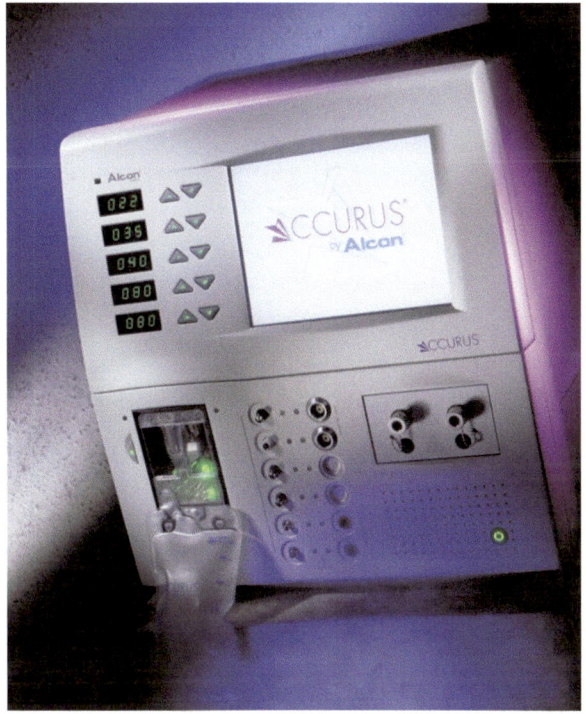

Currently, the most commonly used vitrectomy systems include the Constellation (Alcon, 2008), Enhanced Visual Acuity (EVA, DORC, Zuidland, the Netherlands, 2015), and the Stellaris PC/Stellaris Elite (Bausch + Lomb, Bridgewater, NJ, USA, 2010/2017). The Constellation vitrectomy system (Fig. 7.9) has a dual pneumatic vitreous cutter with increased cut rates up to 10,000 cpm, radiofrequency identification recognition technology to regulate light intensity based upon the probe gauge size, surgeon-controlled duty cycle, integrated laser, and torsional anterior segment phacoemulsification. The Constellation has capacity for 20, 23, 25, and 27 gauge instrumentation. The EVA vitrectomy system (Fig. 7.10) utilizes a two-dimensional vitreous cutter with a cut rate of up to 16,000 cpm, high flow infusion cannula, and instrumentation for 23, 25, and 27 gauge vitrectomy.

The Stellaris PC (Fig. 7.11), has vitreous cutters with cut rates of up to 5000 cpm. It also has a dual light source, color filters for differentiated viewing, and instrumentation for 20, 23, and 25 gauge vitrectomy [26]. The Stellaris Elite Vision Enhancement System (Bausch + Lomb, 2017), offers single port 20, 23, and 25 gauge vitreous cutters with cut rates up to 7500 cpm, and bi-blade 25 and 27 gauge vitrectomy cutters which cut in two directions per cycle with cut rates up to 15,000 cpm. The Stellaris Elite (Fig. 7.12) is also compatible with the ultrasound vitreous cutter, which uses ultrasound energy to liquefy vitreous (instead of cutting it with the traditional guillotine cutter) and remove it using a port that is continuously open. The equivalent cut rate of the hypersonic vitrector (Fig. 7.13) is up to 1.7 million cpm.

**Fig. 7.9** Alcon
Constellation machine
(Photo courtesy of Alcon)

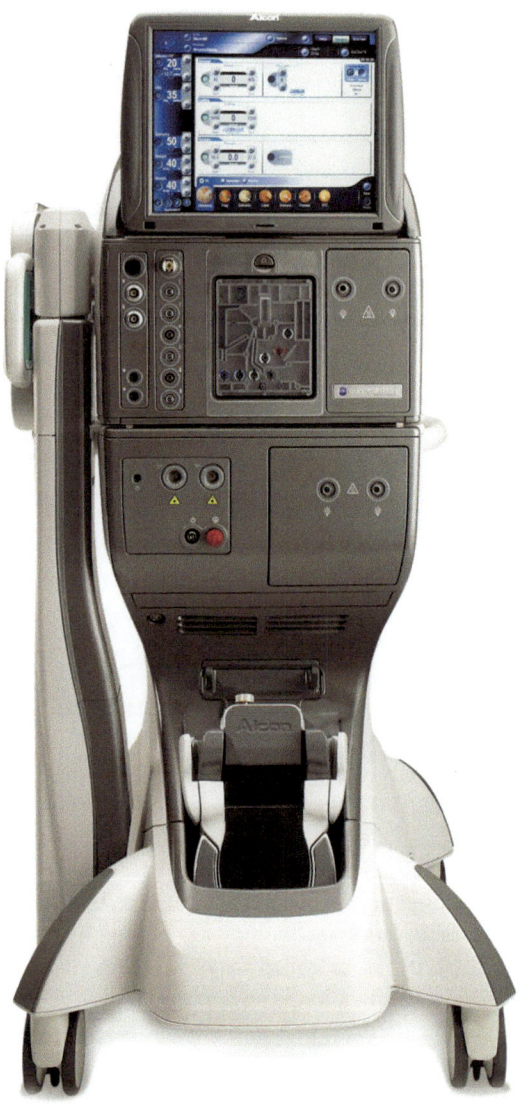

## Cannula-Trocar Systems

After the mid-1970s, PPV was largely performed with 20 gauge instrumentation, requiring conjunctival incisions and sclerotomies measuring approximately 0.9 mm in diameter. With 20G surgery trochars were optional. More recently, the growing use of transconjunctival small-gauge has necessitated the use of cannulated sclerotomies. Fujii first reported a 25 gauge transconjunctival sutureless vitrectomy

**Fig. 7.10** DORC EVA
machine (Photo courtesy
of DORC)

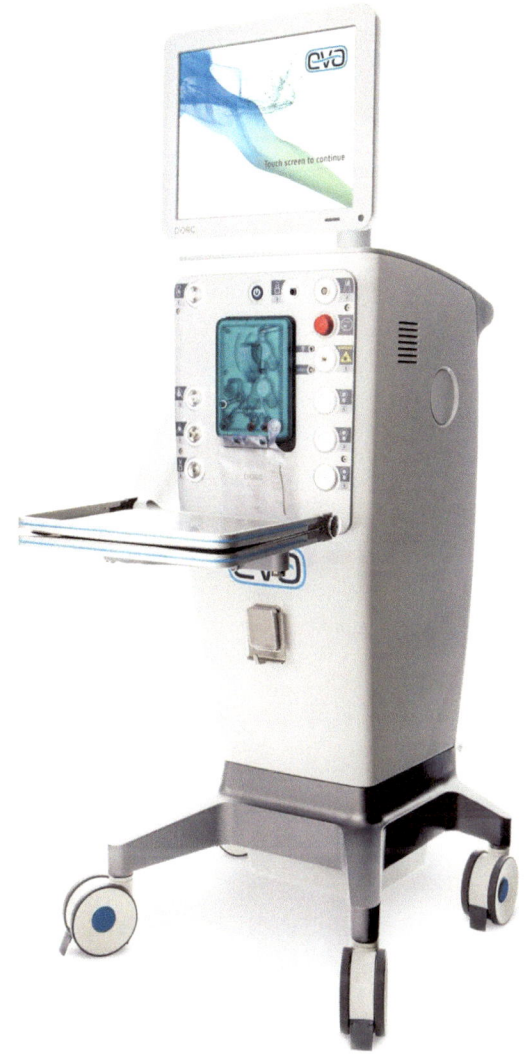

system using microtrocars and cannulas in 2002 [14, 15]. The use of smaller gauge vitrectomy instrumentation has reduced the scleral incision diameter to 0.72 mm for 23 gauge, 0.55 mm for 25 gauge, and 0.40 mm for 27 gauge (Fig. 7.14) [14, 16, 17].

Advantages of cannulas include maintaining the alignment between the conjunctiva and sclera, minimizing wound border trauma and allowing easier and faster interchangeability of instrument and infusion sites [27]. Less traumatic insertion and removal of instruments is thought to contribute to a decreased risk of iatrogenic retinal tears. Additional benefits of the cannula-trocar system include increased

**Fig. 7.11** Bausch + Lomb
Stellaris PC (Photo
courtesy of Bausch +
Lomb)

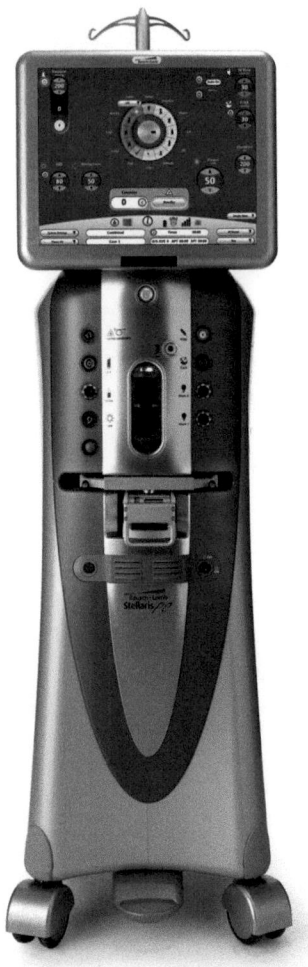

likelihood of self-sealing sclerotomy closure, decreased post-operative discomfort, decreased risk of inflammatory reaction secondary to suture use, and post-operative atrophy and thinning of the sclerotomy site [28]. However, the relatively small internal diameter of the cannula sleeve limits the radius of curvature of smaller gauge intraocular scissors and results in decreased efficiency of intraocular scissors for membrane cutting and dissection compared to intraocular scissors used in 20 gauge vitrectomy [29]. Currently, most vitreoretinal procedures are performed with 23 or 25 gauge transconjunctival cannula-trocar systems, and 20G vitrectomy systems are usually limited to select cases, such as severe posterior segment trauma or intraocular foreign body [30].

**Fig. 7.12**  Bausch + Lomb Stellaris Elite (Photo courtesy of Bausch + Lomb)

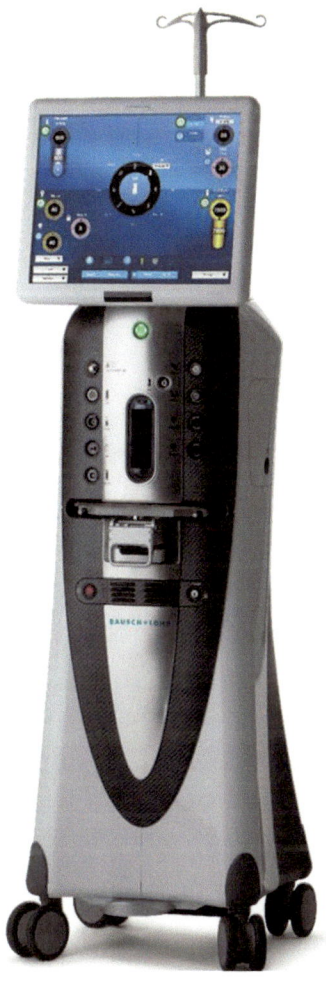

**Fig. 7.13**  Bausch + Lomb hypersonic vitrector (Photo courtesy of Bausch + Lomb)

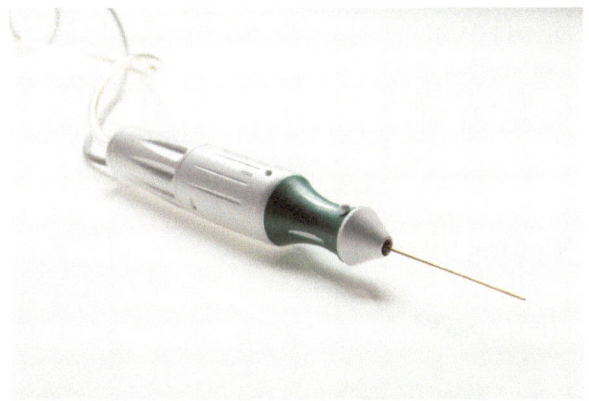

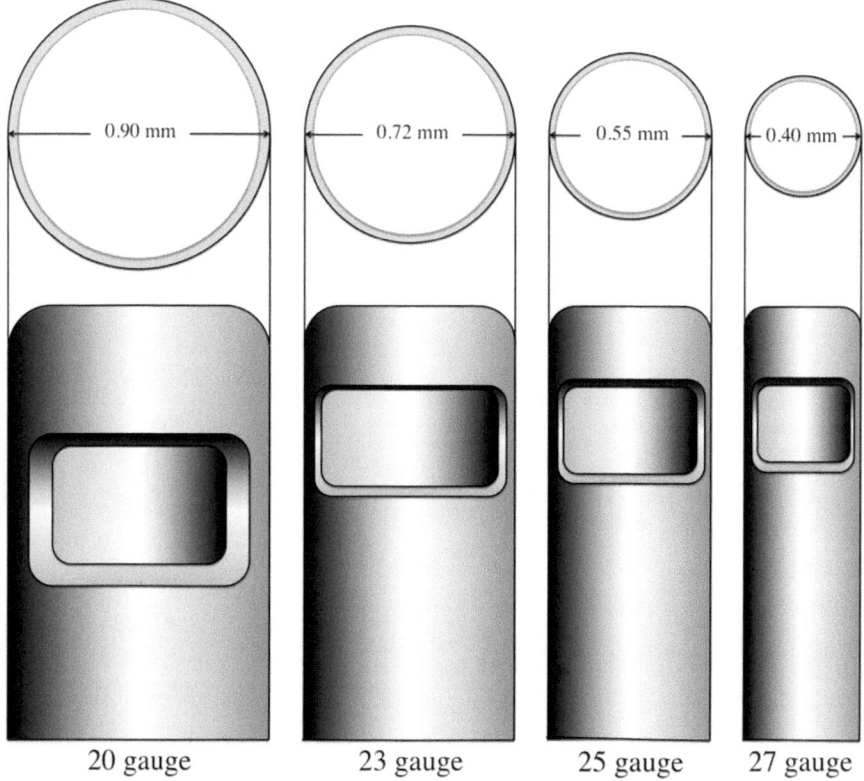

**Fig. 7.14** 20, 23, 25, and 27 gauge vitrectomy probes

Valved cannulas have become popular since they minimize egress of fluid and elimi-nate the need for cannula plugs during instrument exchange. The practical advantages of valved cannulas are more stable intraocular fluidics and improved control of intraocular pressure. Valved cannulas are reported to be comparable to their non-valved counter-parts with regards to functional and anatomical outcomes as well as post-operative com-plications. Valved cannulas can have the disadvantage of increased friction between the instrument and valve and difficult insertion of soft or flexible tip instruments [31, 32]. A valved cannula design can also cause intraocular pressure build-up during air-silicone oil exchange, and venting extensions have been introduced to prevent this.

## Viewing Systems

### *Microscopes*

Enhancements in the optics and illumination of operating microscopes contribute to optimization of the retina surgeon's view. In 1954, Littmann produced the earli-est modern operating microscope with a constant working distance and the ability to change magnification with a revolving Galilean turret, and paraxial illumination [33]. The Galilean turret allowed for different magnifications at a constant working distance, with lenses selected by turning a knob. Paraxial illumination utilized light tubes with bulbs attached to the mounting of the body of the microscope to illuminate the field of view and focus light at the working distance for the microscope, providing better depth perception for surgeons. The ability to move the microscope in the $x$- and $y$-axis and control the movement through a foot pedal were major advancements that improved visualization for vitreous surgery, developed by Parel and Machemer in the 1970s (Fig. 7.15) [34]. An additional advancement was incorporating a beam splitter to provide coaxial viewing for through additional oculars to allow for assistant observation through the microscope (Fig. 7.16) [34]. Over the next several decades, ocular microscopes continued to become more sophisticated with improved light sources and optics to enable improved viewing of the vitreous and retina.

A recent advancement in microscopes for vitreoretinal surgery is the availability of intraoperative real-time optical coherence tomography (OCT) integrated into the surgical microscope. Currently, OCT-integrated microscopes are available from Carl Zeiss Meditec (Fig. 7.17, Jena, Germany) and Leica Microsystems (Bannockburn,

**Fig. 7.15** Early microscope with foot pedal control (Reproduced with permission from Parel, J-M., R. Machemer, and W. Aumayr. "A New Concept for Vitreous Surgery: 5. An Automated Operating Microscope." *American journal of ophthalmology* 77.2 (1974): 161–168)

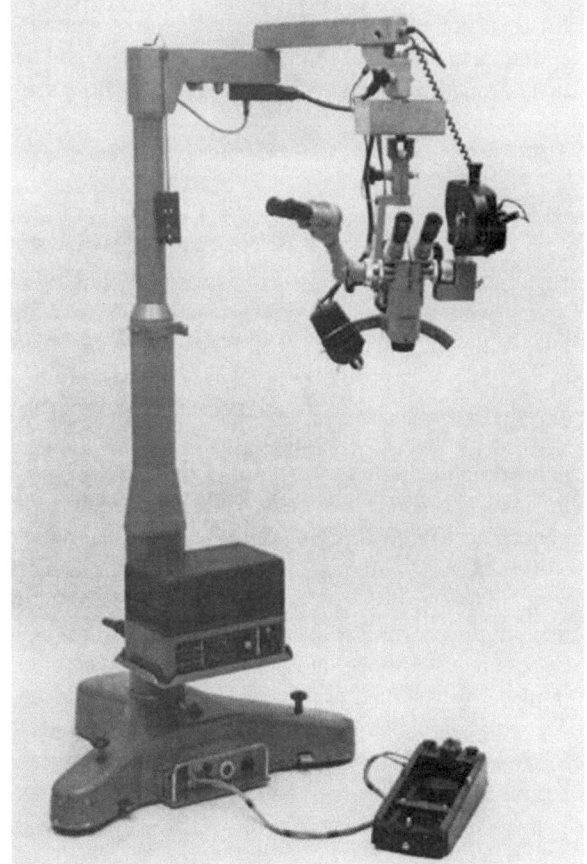

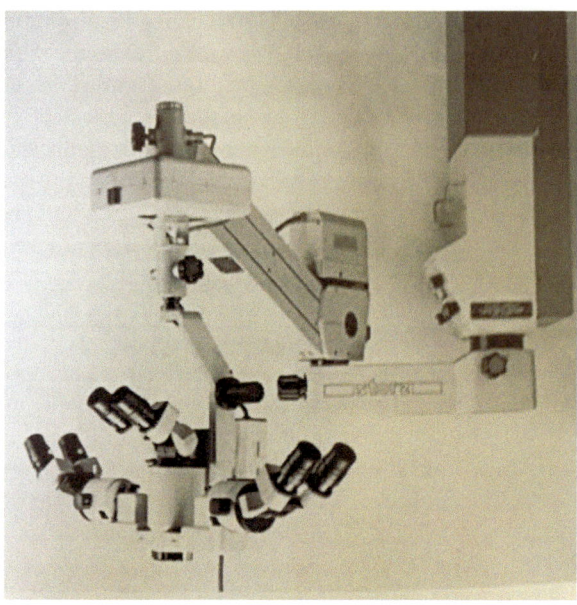

**Fig. 7.16** Early microscope with beam-splitter to allow for assistant viewing

IL, US). Potential uses advantages of intraoperative OCT include confirmation of epiretinal and internal limiting membrane removal and potentially better visualization of membrane peeling in select cases without using retinal dyes [35].

## *Lenses*

Historically, vitreoretinal surgery was performed with planoconcave or biconcave lenses under an operating microscope, which gave a limited field of view, approximately 20–35° (Fig. 7.18) [36]. Prism lenses were used to increase the field of view to 60° [37]. Wide-angle viewing systems that are now available provide increased visualization and access to the peripheral vitreous and retina. Wide-angle viewing systems provide a panoramic view of the retina through the principles of binocular indirect ophthalmoscopy and may require an image inverter mounted on the operating microscope. The two main types of wide-angle viewing systems are contact and noncontact (Table 7.2) [38–42].

Contact lens wide-angle viewing systems provide better image resolution, contrast, and stereopsis than noncontact systems. With direct contact with the cornea, they eliminate corneal aberrations and minimize reflective surfaces [38, 39]. The lenses are either fixed into place using a ring sutured to the sclera or they are held in place by a skilled assistant [39, 43]. The field of view and magnification vary depending upon the lens used.

Noncontact wide-field viewing systems use a lens that is placed above the cornea producing an inverted image, and they use an internal or separate prism system

**Fig. 7.17** Lumera 700 with the Resight 700 intraoperative OCT (Photo courtesy of ZEISS)

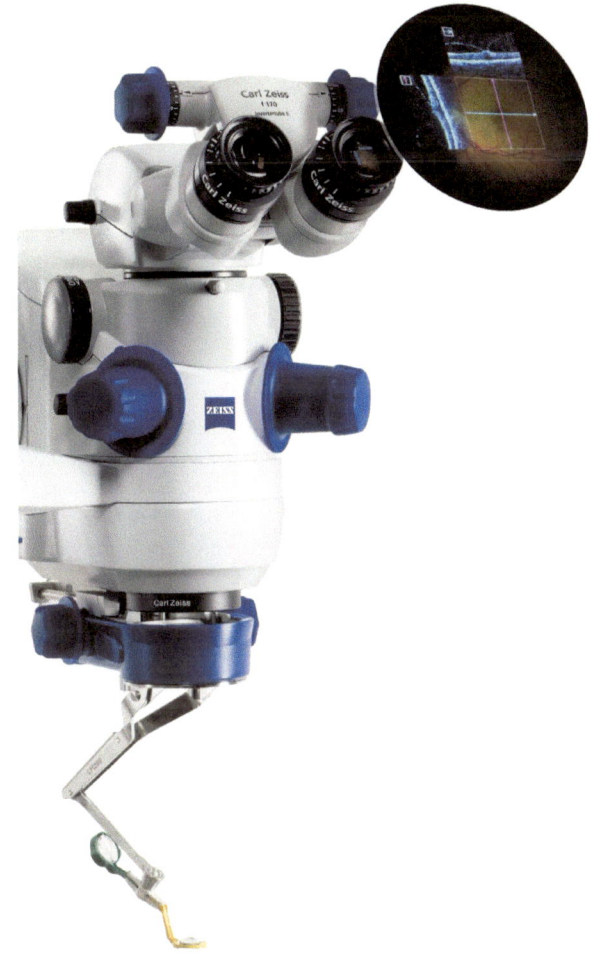

to reinvert the image. The field of view can be adjusted by changing the distance between the lens and the corneal surface [44]. The noncontact wide-angle viewing system does not require an assistant to hold the lens. The cornea must be coated with a viscoelastic material or be constantly irrigated to avoid corneal dehydration. Condensation on the lens, but this can be avoided with proper draping [39].

## Three-Dimensional Viewing

Recently, three-dimensional (3-D) viewing techniques for vitreoretinal surgery were introduced as an alternative to traditional viewing through microscope oculars. With 3-D viewing systems, images from the microsurgical field are displayed on a flat screen via a 3-D camera. The microscope head must still be positioned properly,

**Fig. 7.18** Early contact
lens for vitrectomy surgery

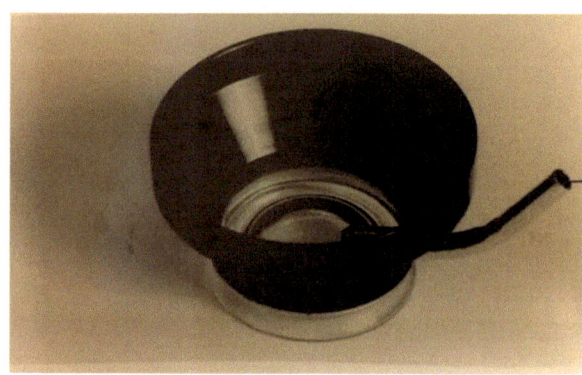

**Table 7.2** Wide angle viewing systems

| Contact | | | | Noncontact | | |
|---|---|---|---|---|---|---|
| System | Manufacturer | Magnification | Field of view | System | Manufacturer | Field of view |
| MiniQuad | Volk Optical | 0.48× | 106°/127° | Binocular Indirect Ophthalmoscopy (BIOM) HD Disposable Lens | Oculus | 130° |
| MiniQuad XL | Volk Optical | 0.39× | 112°/134° | Optic Fiber Free Intravitreal Surgery System (OFFISS) 120 D | Topcon | 130° |
| HRX | Volk Optical | 0.43× | 130°/150° | Merlin Wide Angle ASC Lens | Volk Optical | 120° |
| Landers Wide Field | Ocular | 0.38× | 130°/146° | RESIGHT 500/700 128 D | Carl Zeiss | 120° |
| Single Use Surgical Wide Field | Katena | 0.42× | 155° | Peyman-Wessels Landers (PWL) 132 D Upright Vitrectomy Lens | Ocular | 135° |
| A.V.I. Panoramic Viewing System | Advanced Visual Instruments (A.V.I.) | 0.48× | 130° | EIBOS 2 SPXL 132 D | Haag-Streit | 124° |

but visualization is independent of the oculars and requires the use of 3-D glasses for stereopsis. The single display allows multiple observers to view the 3-D surgical field. Through digital amplification of camera signals, lower illumination settings can be used, which can potentially reduce risks of phototoxicity [45]. 3-D viewing also has the potential to improve ergonomics compared to conventional binocular microsurgery [46]. The Ngenuity (Fig. 7.19, Alcon, 2016) is the only commercially available system currently.

**Fig. 7.19** Ngenuity 3-D
viewing system (Photo
courtesy of Alcon)

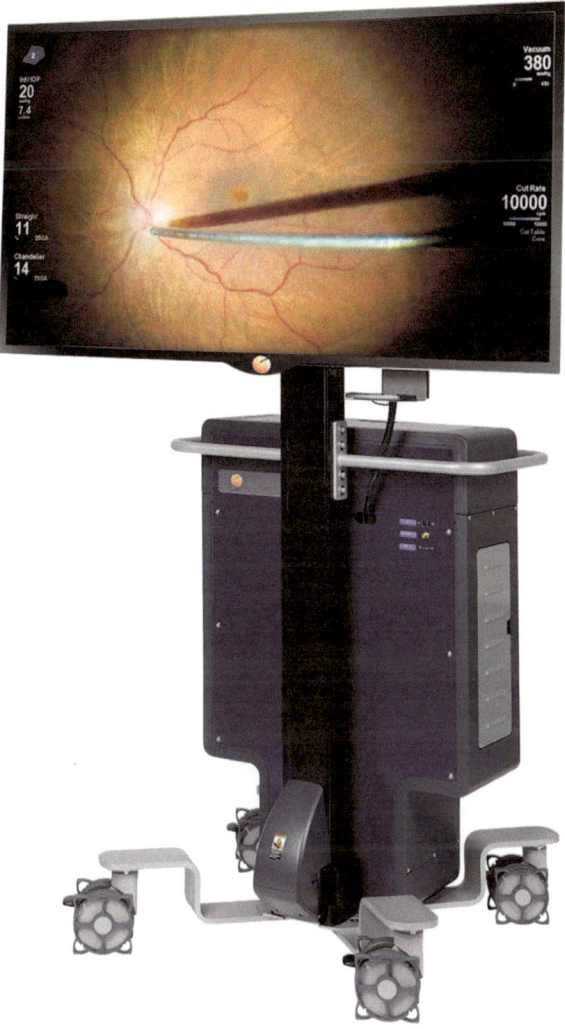

## *Illumination and Filters*

Initial vitrectomy was performed with coaxial light from the operating microscope
and later a modified slit-lamp affixed to the operating microscope (Fig. 7.20) [47].
In order to deliver intraocular illumination, Machemer and Parel placed fiberop-
tics around the VISC cutter (Fig. 7.21a) in 1974 and Peyman mounted a separate
fiberoptic light source attached to the vitrophage cutter in 1976 (Fig. 7.21b) [7,
48]. However, as early as 1974 the concept of separating the light source from the

**Fig. 7.20** Ophthalmic
surgical microscope
equipped with slit lamp
(Reproduced with
permission from Parel,
J-M., R. Machemer, and
W. Aumayr. "A New
Concept for Vitreous
Surgery: 5. An Automated
Operating Microscope."
*American journal of
ophthalmology* 77.2
(1974): 161–168)

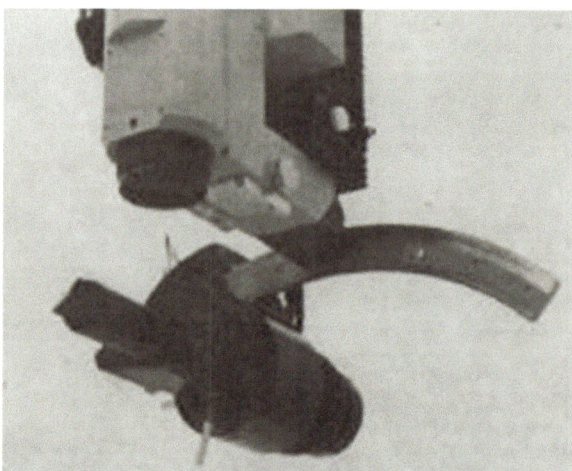

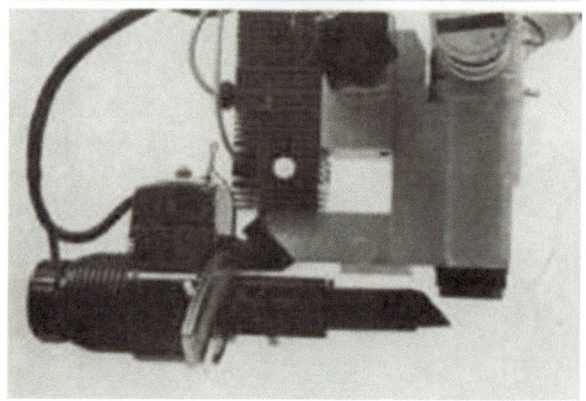

**Fig. 7.21** (**a**) Illuminated
VISC (Reproduced with
permission from Parel, J-M.,
R. Machemer, and
W. Aumayr. "A new concept
for vitreous surgery: 4.
Improvements in
instrumentation and
illumination." *American
journal of ophthalmology*
77.1 (1984): 6–12.) (**b**)
Illuminated vitrophage

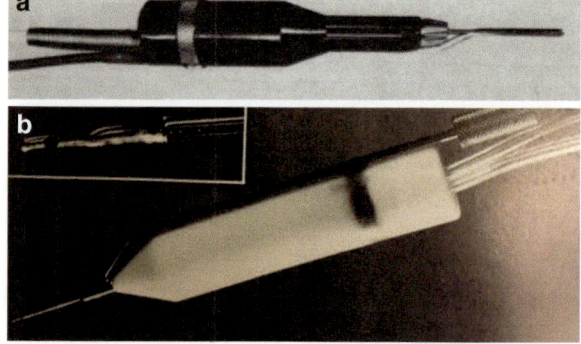

vitrector was introduced, by O'Malley and Heintz; this is currently standard practice for vitrectomy surgery [10]. The first light probes used halogen bulbs [49]. In order to improve illumination, xenon light sources were introduced. Theoretically the short wavelength of light emitted by xenon lamps could increase the rate of photochemical damage [50]. Light-emitting diode (LED) light sources coupled with smaller gauge instrumentation have the potential to allow reduction of the total amount retinal light exposure and can be used without a fiber [51]. A mercury vapor illuminator (Synergetics Inc., O'Fallon, Missouri, USA) was developed to provide powerful illumination and uses a dual-output pathway from one mercury vapor bulb with spherical reflectors adapted to generate homogenized illumination and sharpen the focus light spot. Spectral filters, also known as pass filters, have been introduced to eliminate hazardous wavelengths from the emission spectrum of light probes [52]. Many modern endoillumination devices have built in some variant of a yellow pass filter to screen lower wavelengths [50].

The structure of the light probes also determines the field of illumination. Straight light probes provide a field of view of 50–80°. Mid-field light probes provide a field of view of 90–110° [53–55]. Wide-angle light probes provide a field of view of up to 135–140°. Chandelier light sources illuminate from a greater distance than conventional light probes, reducing the risk of photochemical damage. Additionally, the use of chandeliers frees up the surgeon's hand from having to hold the light source and allows bimanual manipulation during surgery [56].

## Chromovitrectomy

Chromovitrectomy refers to the use of dyes during vitreoretinal surgery to aid in the identification of preretinal membranes or tissues [57]. The concept was introduced by Kazauki Kadonosono in 2000 when he reported the use of indocyanine green (ICG) to stain the internal limiting membrane (ILM) in macular hole surgery to improve ILM visualization and facilitate its removal [58]. However, suspected toxicity to the neuroretina and retinal pigment epithelium from ICG use has been reported and observed to be dependent upon the dye concentration, osmolarity of the solvent solutions, length of dye exposure time, and vitrectomy endolight illumination time [59]. Membrane Blue (trypan blue 0.15%, DORC, Zuidland, the Netherlands) is a dye that is FDA-approved for epiretinal membrane (ERM)/ILM peeling but is generally not as effective as ICG. Brilliant blue G is also used for this ERM/ILM peeling, but it is not FDA-approved for this indication. Triamcinolone acetonide is used to stain the vitreous to ensure complete removal of the vitreous during surgery and can stain ERMs, but is not FDA-approved [60]. Triesence® (Alcon, Fort Worth, TX, USA) is a preservative-free preparation of triamcinolone acetonide that is FDA-approved for intraocular use including use for vitreous visualization in intraocular surgery.

## Lensectomy and Phacoemulsification

Pars plana lensectomy or phacoemulsification from an anterior approach can be performed during or prior to vitrectomy when visualization of the fundus is limited due to dense cataract. Modern vitrectomy systems have the capability to perform pars plana vitrectomy as well as anterior segment phacoemulsification. However, many surgeons prefer to use pars plana lensectomy, especially when the crystalline lens is severely subluxated or dislocated, or there is retained lens material in the vitreous cavity. Historically pars plana lensectomy has been performed with the use of a 20 gauge fragmatome, requiring a conjunctival peritomy, a 20 gauge sclerotomy, and suture-closure of wounds [61–68]. Since the advent of smaller gauge transconjunctival vitrectomy, many retina surgeons use a combination of smaller gauge vitrectomy instrumentation and either enlarge one sclerotomy or create a separate sclerotomy for a larger gauge fragmatome instrument [69]. The Constellation Vision System (Alcon) uses a 20 gauge fragmatome, while both the EVA (DORC) and Stellaris PC/Elite (Bauch + Lomb) systems now have the option of a 23 gauge fragmatome for removal of lens material (Fig. 7.22) [70, 71]. The vitreous cutter can also be used for lens removal but this may require a longer time for dense cataract material.

## Instrumentation

The evolution of vitrectomy surgery and its applications is closely linked to the development of new instrumentation. While many retinal surgeons were key developers of various different instruments, Steve Charles has been one of the most influential developers of instruments and surgical techniques (Fig. 7.23).

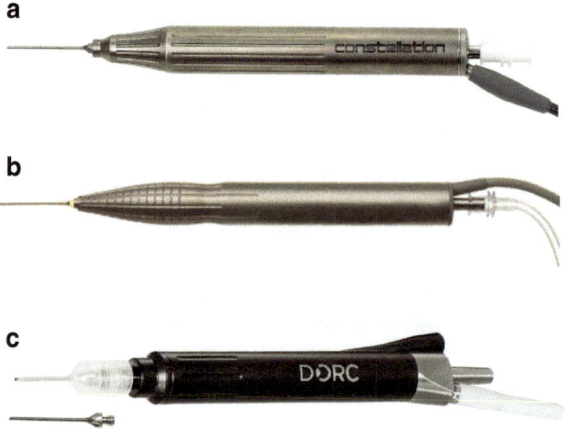

**Fig. 7.22** (**a**) Constellation 20 gauge fragmatome. (**b**) Bausch + Lomb 23 gauge fragmatome. (**c**) DORC 23 gauge phaco/fragmatome handpiece with fragmentation needle

**Fig. 7.23** Dr. Steven Charles who has developed multiple vitreoretinal surgical instruments and techniques

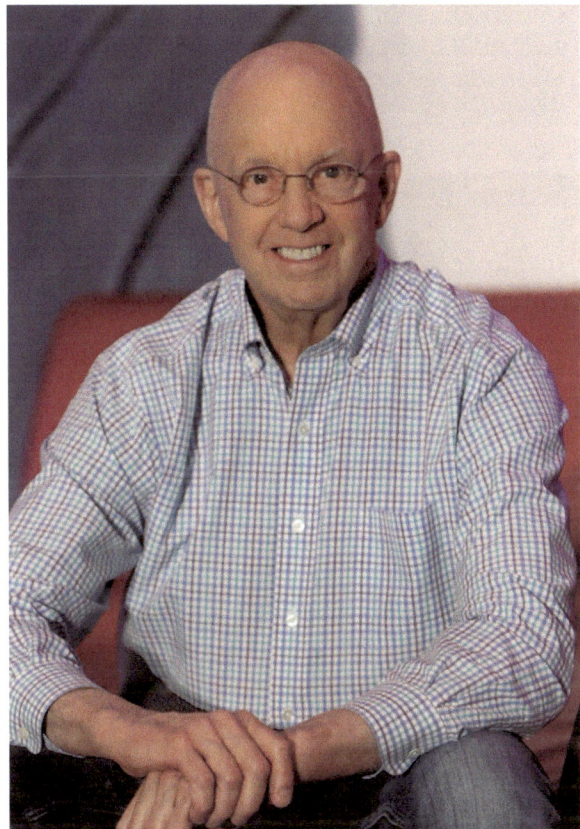

## Forceps

Various different forceps have been designed for different purposes in vitreoretinal surgery. Internal limiting membrane (ILM) forceps are designed with a small platform at the tip, which can be used to remove ILM through the pinch-peel technique or in combination with scrapers. Serrated forceps are designed to provide a stronger grip on tissues, for manipulation of thick and heavy membranes, such as those encountered in proliferative vitreoretinopathy or severe proliferative diabetic retinopathy. Micro-textured grasping forceps are designed to provide a strong grip on less thick or heavy membranes, while producing less tissue trauma [27].

## Membrane Scrapers

Bausch + Lomb has developed multiple membrane scrapers, including the Tano and variations on this device [72]. The Extendible Diamond Dusted Sweeper (DORC) is a similar membrane scraper to the Tano instrument. The FINESSE Flex Loop

(Alcon) is a nitinol flexible extendible loop scraper that can be used to create an edge to lift the ILM or an epiretinal membrane [73]. The force applied to the retina by the can be adjusted based upon whether the loop is partially or fully extended [74].

## Scissors

Horizontal scissors are used to cut retinal bands and tractional components near the retinal surface. Illuminated horizontal scissors are available from some manufacturers, which are useful during bimanual surgery and minimize the need for chandelier placement. Vertical scissors can have a sharp anterior edge to optimize close dissection, tissue segmentation, and delamination techniques. Vertical scissors are used in complex proliferative cases with multiplane tractional bands. Curved or angled scissors follow the contour of the eye to minimize retinal trauma and are better for segmentation and delamination [27, 74].

## Extrusion Cannulas

Soft-tip extrusion cannulas are useful to allow a more complete removal of fluid by enabling closer approach to the retinal tissue than the cutter. Newer soft-tip cannulas have retractable tips for greater ease with insertion through a valved cannula. Backflush cannulas allow for active and passive aspiration of fluid (not vitreous). Furthermore, the backflush feature can be used if retinal incarceration occurs at the tip and can be used to disperse blood settled on the retina [75, 76].

## Endolasers

Endolasers are used in vitreoretinal surgery to perform pan-retinal photocoagulation, laser to the edges of retinal breaks, cauterize bleeding vessels, ablate retinal and choroidal tumors, and perform endophotocyclocoagulation [77]. Early endolasers were straight, but newer endolasers with a curved tip are now available for easier access to the far periphery. Articulating endolasers allow continuously adjustable articulation up to 45° and improves access to the far periphery. The probe is semi-rigid, which makes insertion through a valved cannula easier. Illuminated laser probes are available in curved or extendable forms and can potentially improve peripheral viewing during laser and facilitate simultaneous depression and laser without the help of an assistant or the need for chandelier illumination. Aspirating laser probes provide the capacity for simultaneous endolaser and aspiration, which minimizes the need for instrument exchanges and potentially decreases total surgical time.

## *Diathermy*

The most common uses for diathermy in vitreoretinal surgery is to cauterize bleeding retinal vessels for hemostasis and to create drainage retinotomies. External diathermy application to a leaking sclerotomy has been reported effective in sealing the surgical wound [78–80].

## Perfluorocarbon Liquid

Stanley Chang (1987) introduced low viscosity fluorocarbons as an intraoperative adjunct during vitreous surgery for retinal detachments (Fig. 7.24) [81]. The high density and specific gravity of perfluorocarbon liquid allows reattachment of the retina and unrolling of retinal folds without having to use operating bed which enabled prone positioning of patients during the surgical repair (Fig. 7.25). Perfluorocarbon liquid can also prevent the need for a drainage retinotomy to drain subretinal fluid. For these reasons, perfluorocarbons have become used in the treatment of giant retinal tears and proliferative vitreoretinopathy. Additionally, the optical clarity of perfluorocarbon liquid allows for surgical manipulation beneath it, such as "floating" crystalline lens fragments off the macula for subsequent lensectomy. Its immiscibility with water provides a clear operating fluid in the setting of intraoperative hemorrhage. Perfluorocarbons are biologically inert, but evidence indicates that they are toxic when retained in the eye for longer periods of time [82]. Despite some concerns of toxicity, some studies have demonstrated benefit from using perfluorocarbon liquids as short term tamponade

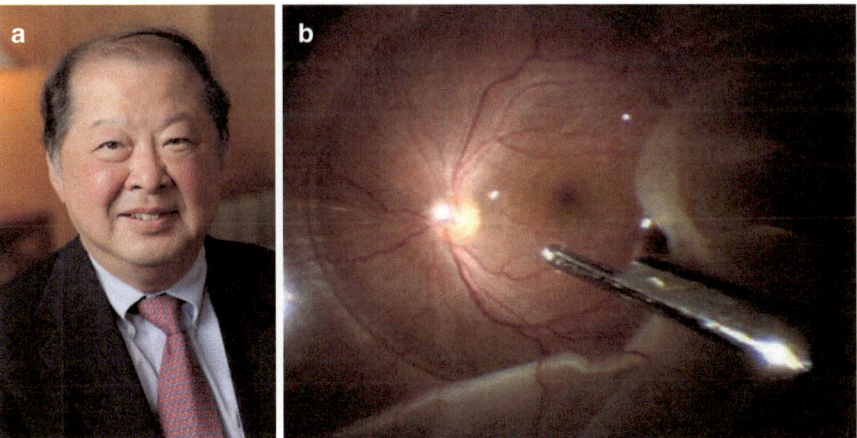

**Fig. 7.24** (**a**) Dr. Stanley Chang, the inventor of perfluorocarbon. (**b**) Perfluorocarbon used intraoperatively to flatten the retina

**Fig. 7.25** Inverted surgical bed used for vitreoretinal surgery

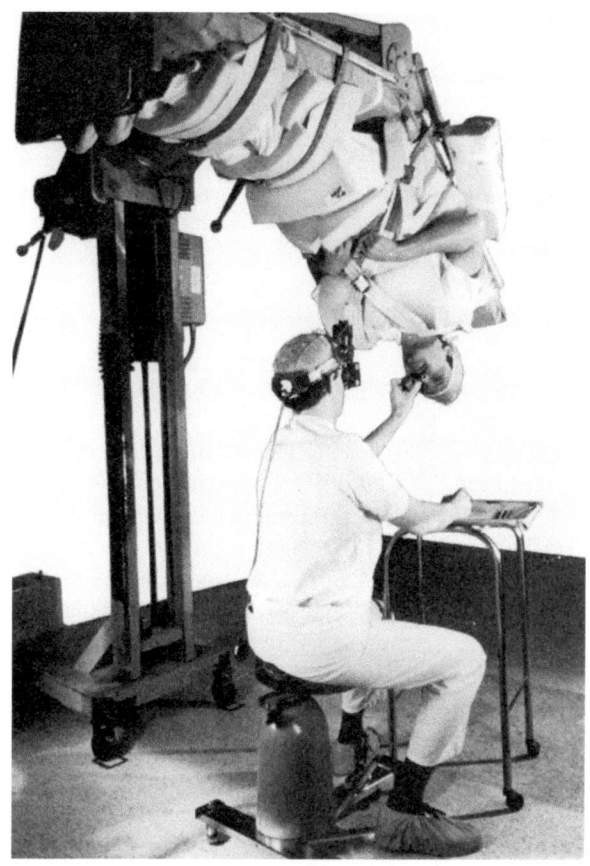

agents, ranging from 7 days to 3 months, in patients with inferior or complex retinal detachments [83–86]. Subretinal perfluorocarbon in the fovea is visually significant and generally requires removal.

## Subretinal Injections

Subretinal injections are performed for several indications. Subretinal tissue plasminogen activator (tPA) with or without air has been reported to displace submacular hemorrhage [87–93]. More recently, gene therapy through subretinal delivery of a viral vector has been performed effectively for with specific retinal dystrophies [94–97]. Luxturna (Voretigene neparvovec-rzyl, Spark Therapeutics Inc., Philadelphia, Pennsylvania, USA) is an FDA approved subretinal gene therapy for patients with inherited retinal disease due to mutations in both copies of the *RPE65* gene. Subretinal injection of human embryonic stem cell (HESC) and induced pluripotent stem cell (iPSC)-derived RPE cells/sheets for macular degeneration have

been performed in clinical trials [98–101]. There are multiple reusable and disposable small cannulas (as small as 41 gauge) that are available for subretinal injection
through trocars. New instruments are being developed to facilitate subretinal RPE
cell sheet delivery [102].

## Scleral Buckling

Scleral buckling (SB) can be used to treat primary rhegmatogenous retinal detachments, most commonly in phakic eyes [103]. Scleral buckling involves placement
of solid or porous silicone buckling elements—encircling, radial, or both—in order
to support equatorial or pre-equatorial breaks and reduce traction from the peripheral vitreous. The elements are either sutured to the sclera or placed through scleral
tunnels [104]. Once closure of the retinal breaks is achieved, the retinal pigment
epithelium pump removes subretinal fluid resulting in retinal reattachment [105,
106]. The breaks can be sealed with cryopexy and gas tamponade can be used to
aid retina reattachment. SB may be combined with PPV. A prospective randomized clinical trial of 681 eyes with medium complexity rhegmatogenous retinal
detachments showed that SB showed a benefit with regards to visual improvement
in phakic eyes, but PPV had a better anatomic outcome in pseudophakic patients
compared to SB [105]. In cases of proliferative vitreoretinopathy, the combination
allows support of the vitreous base and the ability to address membranes and/or
perform a retinectomy. One retrospective study found the combination of PPV and
SB to lead to better outcomes than PPV alone in retinal detachments that were at
risk to develop PVR [107].

Numerous intrascleral implants have been used in scleral buckling surgery,
including polyethylene, silicone, and gelatin implants. In 1985, episcleral hydrogel
implants (MIRAgel, MIRA Inc., Waltham, Massachusetts, USA) were introduced
as an alternative to silicone for treatment of rhegmatogenous retinal detachment.
The material was thought to have the potential to decrease risk of scleral erosion due
to its soft, pliable characteristics. However, after several years, it was discovered
that the hydrolytic degradation of the MIRAgel material caused progressive swelling of the explant and subsequent strabismus, ptosis, scleral erosion, conjunctivitis,
and infection [108]. These implants are no longer used.

In one study of 728 eyes that underwent scleral buckling, the incidence of erosion was analyzed based upon the type of implant used. The study found that erosion occurred in 62.3% of eyes with polyethylene tubes compared with 3.8% in eyes
with solid silicone implants with silicone circling bands. The use of solid silicone
implants and circling bands has greatly reduced the issue of implant erosion [109].

Chandelier-assisted SB uses chandelier endoillumination and a wide-angle fundus viewing system in lieu of an indirect ophthalmoscope. The advantages of this
technique are better visualization, improved ergonomics, and increased familiarity
for predominantly vitrectomy trained surgeons [110]. However, chandelier insertion
carries the risk of cataract from lens touch, and new breaks from vitreous traction

during eye manipulation [111, 112]. Use of an illuminated scleral depressor is a novel technique to improve localization of retinal breaks. This method uses a 20G light pipe with a bent tip as an illuminated scleral depressor to see the break in greater detail and screen suspect areas [110].

## Tamponade Agents

Tamponade agents are used to provide surface tension across retinal breaks in vitrectomy for rhegmatogenous retinal detachment repair. They prevent further fluid flow into the subretinal space until the retinopexy via photocoagulation or cryopexy provides a permanent seal. Gases and silicone oil (SO) are the most commonly used classes of tamponade agents. The use of tamponade agents for the treatment of retinal detachment was first described in 1911 by Joh Ohm who successfully treated two patients with intravitreal sterile air [113]. In 1962, Paul Cibis described the use of liquid silicone for the management of retinal detachment [114]. The use of inert expansile gas sulfur hexafluoride ($SF_6$) was described in 1973 by Edward Norton as a vitreous substitute [115].

Currently, the most common gas tamponades in the US are air, $SF_6$, and perfluoropropane ($C_3F_8$) [116]. Air is nonexpansile. $SF_6$ 100% expands two times over 1–2 days and $C_3F_8$ 100% expands about four times over 3–4 days [117]. Small volumes (0.5 $cm^3$ or less) of undiluted gas are generally used for pneumatic retinopexy. Diluted gas to fill the vitreous cavity is typically used for PPV at non-expansile concentrations ($SF_6$ 20% and $C_3F_8$ 14%). Gas tamponade agents resorb spontaneously from the vitreous cavity over an average period of 5–7 days for air, 2 weeks for $SF_6$ 20%, and 8 weeks for $C_3F_8$ [118].

The Silicone Study was a prospective multicenter randomized clinical trial that compared 1000 centistoke silicone oil to $SF_6$ 20% or $C_3F_8$ 14% in patients with retinal detachment associated with proliferative vitreoretinopathy, which reported that anatomic and visual outcomes after 1 year was significantly better with SO compared to $SF_6$ and not significantly different for SO compared to $C_3F_8$ [119]. A 6-year follow up of the Silicone Study reported that, among subjects whose macula was attached at 36 months, there were no significant anatomic or visual outcome differences among SO, $SF_6$, and $C_3F_8$ groups [119]. The European Vitreo-Retinal Society (EVRS) Retinal Detachment Study reported no significant difference in failure rate between tamponade with gas versus SO in patients with proliferative vitreoretinopathy [120].

In the USA, the most commonly used viscosities of silicone oils are 1000 and 5000 centistokes [121]. Due to the lower specific gravity of gases (0.001 g/mL) and silicone oils (0.97 g/mL) compared to vitreous (1.005–1.008 g/mL), these tamponade agents float in the vitreous cavity [122]. For this reason, gases and SO provide less effective tamponade for inferior breaks without a full fill of the vitreous cavity. Heavier-than-water tamponades, such as heavy silicone oils and perfluorocarbon liquids, are used as tamponade agents for inferior retinal breaks [123–127]. Heavy silicone oils are available for clinical use in many nations but not the United States.

## Postoperative Considerations and Complications

Over the years PPV has evolved with the development of smaller and faster vit-rectomy systems. Transconjunctival small-gauge instruments have provided the advantages of decreased operating time, self-sealing scleral wounds, decreased postoperative pain and inflammation, decreased astigmatism, and faster visual recovery over traditional 20 gauge instruments [128–132]. PPV and SB are now typically outpatient procedures with follow up 1 day after surgery. However, alter-native postoperative visits on the same day as surgery and 3 or more days after surgery have been reported [133, 134].

Overall, PPV has one of the lowest rates of endophthalmitis among intraocular surgical procedures [135]. As small-gauge transconjunctival PPV gained popularity, concerns arose about increased rates of endophthalmitis with 25 gauge transcon-junctival sutureless vitrectomy. A retrospective study in 2007 examined 8600 PPV patients and reported a 12-fold higher incidence of endophthalmitis in 25 gauge PPV compared to 20 gauge PPV [136]. However, later studies reported no signifi-cant difference in endophthalmitis rates between 20 gauge PPV and small incision vitrectomy [137, 138].

With regards to post-operative retinal detachment complications, a retrospec-tive study of 2432 vitrectomies reported a similar incidence of post-surgical retinal detachment after sutureless 23 gauge and 25 gauge PPV compared to 20 gauge PPV [139]. Another retrospective study of 4274 vitrectomies comparing intraoperative complications of 23 gauge versus 20 gauge PPV showed that 23 gauge PPV had a lower risk of choroidal hemorrhage and iatrogenic retinal tears compared to 20 gauge PPV, especially for eyes with rhegmatogenous retinal detachment [140].

Other post-operative complications of vitrectomy include cataract progression, cystoid macular edema, hypotony, and sympathetic ophthalmia [141, 142].

## Future Advancements in Vitreo-Retinal Surgery

Recent developments in vitreo-retinal surgery have led to advances in surgeon capa-bilities, visual outcomes, and patient safety. Robotic vitreo-retinal surgery is a rap-idly emerging technology within this domain. Early robotic vitreo-retinal surgical techniques have been aimed at tremor cancellation, improved precision, enhanced dexterity, force sensing and micron-scale distance sensing [143–147]. The use of robotics in vitreo-retinal surgery has been limited by the lack of broad clinical expe-rience among potential users and challenges to implementation.

Four-dimensional (4-D) OCT imaging has been introduced recently for use intraoperatively to provide enhanced visualization of volumetric tissue deforma-tion. It has been used in vitreo-retinal surgical cases for macular hold, ERM, myopic foveal schisis, diabetic macular edema, and retinal detachment. 4-D OCT imaging has the potential to provide enhanced intraoperative visualization from multiple perspectives, precise determination of instrument distance from the retina, and visualization of retinal contour deformation during and after surgical manipulation. This technology is presently limited by image quality and resolution [148].

## Summary

Vitreoretinal surgical techniques have evolved in the last 50 years largely due to the development and evolution of PPV. Developments include smaller gauge instrumentation, faster cut speeds, enhanced illumination techniques, microscopes, and perfluorocarbon liquids. These advancements have improved the safety and efficacy of vitrectomy and allowed surgeons to more effectively treat a wide variety of conditions, including complications of diabetic retinopathy, macular holes, and retinal detachments.

## References

1. Dodo T. Diapupillary resection of vitreous opacity. Nippon Ganka Gakkai Zasshi. 1955;59:1737–45.
2. Dodo T, Okuzawa Y, Baba N. [Trans-pupillary resection of vitreous body opacity]. Ganka. 1969;11(1):38–44.
3. Kasner D, Miller GR, Taylor WH, Sever RJ, Norton EW. Surgical treatment of amyloidosis of the vitreous. Trans Am Acad Ophthalmol Otolaryngol. 1968;72(3):410–8.
4. Machemer R, Buettner H, Norton EW, Parel JM. Vitrectomy: a pars plana approach. Trans Am Acad Ophthalmol Otolaryngol. 1971;75(4):813–20.
5. Machemer R. Reminiscences after 25 years of pars plana vitrectomy. Am J Ophthalmol. 1995;119(4):505–10.
6. Machemer R, Parel JM, Buettner H. A new concept for vitreous surgery. I. Instrumentation. Am J Ophthalmol. 1972;73(1):1–7.
7. Parel JM, Machemer R, Aumayr W. A new concept for vitreous surgery. 4. Improvements in instrumentation and illumination. Am J Ophthalmol. 1974;77(1):6–12.
8. Machemer R. A new concept for vitreous surgery. 2. Surgical technique and complications. Am J Ophthalmol. 1972;74(6):1022–33.
9. Peyman GA, Dodich NA. Experimental vitrectomy: instrumentation and surgical technique. Arch Ophthalmol. 1971;86(5):548–51.
10. O'Malley C, Heintz RM. Vitrectomy with an alternative instrument system. Ann Ophthalmol. 1975;7(4):585–8, 591–4.
11. Machemer R, Hickingbotham D. The three-port microcannular system for closed vitrectomy. Am J Ophthalmol. 1985;100(4):590–2.
12. de Juan E, Hickingbotham D. Refinements in microinstrumentation for vitreous surgery. Am J Ophthalmol. 1990;109(2):218–20.
13. Peyman GA. A miniaturized vitrectomy system for vitreous and retinal biopsy. Can J Ophthalmol. 1990;25(6):285–6.
14. Fujii GY, De Juan E, Humayun MS, Pieramici DJ, Chang TS, Awh C, et al. A new 25-gauge instrument system for transconjunctival sutureless vitrectomy surgery. Ophthalmology. 2002;109(10):1807–12; discussion 1813.

15. Fujii GY, De Juan E, Humayun MS, Chang TS, Pieramici DJ, Barnes A, et al. Initial experience using the transconjunctival sutureless vitrectomy system for vitreoretinal surgery. Ophthalmology. 2002;109(10):1814–20.
16. Eckardt C. Transconjunctival sutureless 23-gauge vitrectomy. Retina. 2005;25(2):208–11.
17. Oshima Y, Wakabayashi T, Sato T, Ohji M, Tano Y. A 27-gauge instrument system for transconjunctival sutureless microincision vitrectomy surgery. Ophthalmology. 2010;117(1):93–102.e2.
18. Machemer R, Norton EW. A new concept for vitreous surgery. 3. Indications and results. Am J Ophthalmol. 1972;74(6):1034–56.
19. Wilson D, Barr CC. Outpatient and abbreviated hospitalization for vitreoretinal surgery. Ophthalmic Surg. 1990;21(2):119–22.
20. Newsom RS, Wainwright AC, Canning CR. Local anaesthesia for 1221 vitreoretinal procedures. Br J Ophthalmol. 2001;85(2):225–7.
21. Huang JJ, Fogel S, Leavell M. Cost analysis in vitrectomy: monitored anesthesia care and general anesthesia. AANA J. 2001;69(2):111–3.
22. Wong DH. Regional anaesthesia for intraocular surgery. Can J Anaesth. 1993;40(7):635–57.
23. Celiker H, Karabas L, Sahin O. A comparison of topical or retrobulbar anesthesia for 23-gauge posterior vitrectomy. J Ophthalmol. 2014;2014:237028.
24. Trujillo-Sanchez GP, Gonzalez-De La Rosa A, Navarro-Partida J, Haro-Morlett L, Altamirano-Vallejo JC, Santos A. Feasibility and safety of vitrectomy under topical anesthesia in an office-based setting. Indian J Ophthalmol. 2018;66(8):1136–40.
25. Narendran V, Kothari AR, editors. Vitreoretinal surgery systems. In: Principles and practice of vitreoretinal surgery. 1st ed. Philadelphia: Jaypee Brothers Medical Publishers Ltd; 2014. p. 53–6.
26. Lai TYY. Machines and cutters: Stellaris PC. Dev Ophthalmol. 2014;54:8–16.
27. Charles S, Calzada J, Wood B, editors. 25-Gauge vitrectomy. In: Vitreous microsurgery. 5th ed. Philadelphia: Lippincott Williams & Wilkins; 2011. p. 103–11.
28. Mohamed S, Claes C, Tsang CW. Review of small gauge vitrectomy: progress and innovations. J Ophthalmol. 2017;2017:6285869.
29. Nagpal M, Paranjpe G, Jain P, Videkar R. Advances in small-gauge vitrectomy. Taiwan J Ophthalmol. 2012;2(1):6.
30. Osawa S, Oshima Y. 27-Gauge vitrectomy. Dev Ophthalmol. 2014;54:54–62.
31. Oellers P, Stinnett S, Hahn P. Valved versus nonvalved cannula small-gauge pars plana vitrectomy for repair of retinal detachments with Grade C proliferative vitreoretinopathy. Clin Ophthalmol. 2016;10:1001–6.
32. Oellers P, Stinnett S, Mruthyunjaya P, Hahn P. Small-gauge valved versus nonvalved cannula pars plana vitrectomy for retinal detachment repair. Retina. 2016;36(4):744–9.
33. Littmann H. [A new surgical microscope]. Klin Monatsblatter Augenheilkd Augenarztliche Fortbild. 1954;124(4):473–6.
34. Parel JM, Machemer R, Aumayr W. A new concept for vitreous surgery. 5. An automated operating microscope. Am J Ophthalmol. 1974;77(2):161–8.
35. Hattenbach L-O, Framme C, Junker B, Pielen A, Agostini H, Maier M. [Intraoperative real-time OCT in macular surgery]. Ophthalmologe. 2016;113(8):656–62.
36. Landers MB, Stefánsson E, Wolbarsht ML. The optics of vitreous surgery. Am J Ophthalmol. 1981;91(5):611–4.
37. Bovey EH, Gonvers M. A new device for noncontact wide-angle viewing of the fundus during vitrectomy. Arch Ophthalmol. 1995;113(12):1572–3.
38. Chalam KV, Shah VA. Optics of wide-angle panoramic viewing system-assisted vitreous surgery. Surv Ophthalmol. 2004;49(4):437–45.
39. Inoue M. Wide-angle viewing system. Dev Ophthalmol. 2014;54:87–91.
40. Chihara T, Kita M. New type of antidrying lens for vitreous surgery with a noncontact wide-angle viewing system. Clin Ophthalmol. 2013;7:353–5.
41. Ohji M, Tada E, Futamura H. Combining a contact lens and wide-angle viewing system for a wider fundus view. Retina. 2011;31(9):1958–60.

42. Ohno H. Combined use of high-reflective index vitrectomy meniscus contact lens and a non-contact wide-angle viewing system in vitreous surgery. Clin Ophthalmol. 2011;5:1109–11.
43. Shah VA, Chalam KV. Self-stabilizing wide-angle contact lens for vitreous surgery. Retina. 2003;23(5):667–9.
44. Mateo C, Burés-Jelstrup A. Contact versus noncontact wide-field viewing systems: why not have the best of both worlds? Retina. 2018;38(4):854–6.
45. Adam MK, Thornton S, Regillo CD, Park C, Ho AC, Hsu J. Minimal endoillumination levels and display luminous emittance during three-dimensional heads-up vitreoretinal surgery. Retina. 2017;37(9):1746–9.
46. Eckardt C, Paulo EB. Heads-up surgery for vitreoretinal procedures: an experimental and clinical study. Retina. 2016;36(1):137–47.
47. Machemer R. The development of pars plana vitrectomy: a personal account. Graefes Arch Clin Exp Ophthalmol. 1995;233(8):453–68.
48. Peyman GA. Improved vitrectomy illumination system. Am J Ophthalmol. 1976;81(1):99–100.
49. Sakaguchi H, Oshima Y. Considering the illumination choices in vitreoretinal surgery. Retin Physician. 2012;9:26–31.
50. Chow DR. The evolution of endoillumination. Dev Ophthalmol. 2014;54:77–86.
51. Koelbl PS, Lingenfelder C, Spraul CW, Kampmeier J, Koch FH, Kim YK, et al. An intraocular micro light-emitting diode device for endo-illumination during pars plana vitrectomy. Eur J Ophthalmol. 2019;29(1):75–81. https://doi.org/10.1177/1120672118757618.
52. Henrich PB, Valmaggia C, Lang C, Cattin PC. The price for reduced light toxicity: do endoilluminator spectral filters decrease color contrast during Brilliant Blue G-assisted chromovitrectomy? Graefes Arch Clin Exp Ophthalmol. 2014;252(3):367–74.
53. Witmer MT, Dugel PU. Machines and cutters: constellation. In: Oh H, Oshima Y, editors. Microincision vitrectomy surgery: emerging techniques and technology. New York: Karger Medical and Scientific Publishers; 2014. p. 1–7.
54. Lai TYY. Machines and cutters: Stellaris PC. In: Oh H, Oshima Y, editors. Microincision vitrectomy surgery: emerging techniques and technology. New York: Karger Medical and Scientific Publishers; 2014. p. 8–16.
55. Morales-Canton V, Kawakami-Campos PA. Machines and cutters: VersaVIT—potential and perspectives of office-based vitrectomy. In: Oh H, Oshima Y, editors. Microincision vitrectomy surgery: emerging techniques and technology. New York: Karger Medical and Scientific Publishers; 2014. p. 17–22.
56. Seider MI, Nomides REK, Hahn P, Mruthyunjaya P, Mahmoud TH. Scleral buckling with chandelier illumination. J Ophthalmic Vis Res. 2016;11(3):304–9.
57. Rodrigues EB, Meyer CH, Kroll P. Chromovitrectomy: a new field in vitreoretinal surgery. Graefes Arch Clin Exp Ophthalmol. 2005;243(4):291–3.
58. Kadonosono K, Itoh N, Uchio E, Nakamura S, Ohno S. Staining of internal limiting membrane in macular hole surgery. Arch Ophthalmol. 2000;118(8):1116–8.
59. Grisanti S, Altvater A, Peters S. Safety parameters for indocyanine green in vitreoretinal surgery. Dev Ophthalmol. 2008;42:43–68.
60. Al-Halafi AM. Chromovitrectomy: update. Saudi J Ophthalmol. 2013;27(4):271–6.
61. Margherio RR, Margherio AR, Pendergast SD, Williams GA, Garretson BR, Strong LE, et al. Vitrectomy for retained lens fragments after phacoemulsification. Ophthalmology. 1997;104(9):1426–32.
62. Ho SF, Zaman A. Clinical features and outcomes of pars plana vitrectomy in patients with retained lens fragments after phacoemulsification. J Cataract Refract Surg. 2007;33(12):2106–10.
63. Hansson LJ, Larsson J. Vitrectomy for retained lens fragments in the vitreous after phacoemulsification. J Cataract Refract Surg. 2002;28(6):1007–11.
64. Borne MJ, Tasman W, Regillo C, Malecha M, Sarin L. Outcomes of vitrectomy for retained lens fragments. Ophthalmology. 1996;103(6):971–6.
65. Scott IU, Flynn HW Jr, Smiddy WE, Murray TG, Moore JK, Lemus DR, et al. Clinical features and outcomes of pars plana vitrectomy in patients with retained lens fragments. Ophthalmology. 2003;110(8):1567–72.

66. Ho LY, Doft BH, Wang L, Bunker CH. Clinical predictors and outcomes of pars plana vitrectomy for retained lens material after cataract extraction. Am J Ophthalmol. 2009;147(4):587–594.e1.
67. Kadonosono K, Yamakawa T, Uchio E, Yanagi Y, Tamaki Y, Araie M. Comparison of visual function after epiretinal membrane removal by 20-gauge and 25-gauge vitrectomy. Am J Ophthalmol. 2006;142(3):513–5.
68. Chang C-J, Chang Y-H, Chiang S-Y, Lin L-T. Comparison of clear corneal phacoemulsification combined with 25-gauge transconjunctival sutureless vitrectomy and standard 20-gauge vitrectomy for patients with cataract and vitreoretinal diseases. J Cataract Refract Surg. 2005;31(6):1198–207.
69. Cho M, Chan RP. 23-gauge pars plana vitrectomy for management of posteriorly dislocated crystalline lens. Clin Ophthalmol. 2011;5:1737–43.
70. Arevalo JF, Berrocal MH, Arias JD, Banaee T. Minimally invasive vitreoretinal surgery: is sutureless vitrectomy the future of vitreoretinal surgery? J Ophthalmic Vis Res. 2011;6(2):136–44.
71. Shah GK, Ho VY. Vitrectomy platforms go to the next level. Retina Spec [Internet]. 2016. http://www.retina-specialist.com/article/noninfectious-uveitis-enriching-our-toolbox-1. [Cited 2018 Sept 17].
72. Kuhn F, Mester V, Berta A. The Tano Diamond Dusted Membrane Scraper: indications and contraindications. Acta Ophthalmol Scand. 1998;76(6):754–5.
73. Hsu J. Nitinol flex loop-assisted retrieval and sutureless intrascleral refixation of a dislocated intraocular lens implant. Retin Cases Brief Rep. 2018; E-pub before print.
74. Charles S, Calzada J, Wood B, editors. General posterior segment techniques. In: Vitreous microsurgery. 5th ed. Philadelphia: Lippincott Williams & Wilkins; 2011. p. 45–75.
75. Villegas V, Murray T. Know your retinal surgery toolbox. Retin Physician. 2018;15:24–9.
76. Charles S, Calzada J, Wood B, editors. Vitrectomy for retinal detachment. In: Vitreous microsurgery. 5th ed. Philadelphia: Lippincott Williams & Wilkins; 2011. p. 135–8.
77. Kuhn F. Endolaser. In: Kuhn F, editor. Vitreoretinal surgery: strategies and tactics [Internet]. Cham: Springer International Publishing; 2016. p. 263–76. https://doi.org/10.1007/978-3-319-19479-0_30. [Cited 2018 Sept 24].
78. Barak Y, Lee ES, Schaal S. Sealing effect of external diathermy on leaking sclerotomies after small-gauge vitrectomy: a clinicopathological report. JAMA Ophthalmol. 2014;132(7):891–2.
79. Reibaldi M, Longo A, Reibaldi A, Avitabile T, Pulvirenti A, Lippolis G, et al. Diathermy of leaking sclerotomies after 23-gauge transconjunctival pars plana vitrectomy: a prospective study. Retina. 2013;33(5):939–45.
80. Jusufbegovic D, Ozkok A, Schaal S. Intraoperative optical coherence tomography validates the immediate efficacy of external diathermy in sealing 25-gauge sclerotomy wounds. Retina. 2017;37(2):402–4.
81. Chang S. Low viscosity liquid fluorochemicals in vitreous surgery. Am J Ophthalmol. 1987;103(1):38–43.
82. Georgalas I, Ladas I, Tservakis I, Taliantzis S, Gotzaridis E, Papaconstantinou D, et al. Perfluorocarbon liquids in vitreoretinal surgery: a review of applications and toxicity. Cutan Ocul Toxicol. 2011;30(4):251–62.
83. Randolph JC, Diaz RI, Sigler EJ, Calzada JI, Charles S. 25-gauge pars plana vitrectomy with medium-term postoperative perfluoro-n-octane for the repair of giant retinal tears. Graefes Arch Clin Exp Ophthalmol. 2016;254(2):253–7.
84. Eiger-Moscovich M, Gershoni A, Axer-Siegel R, Weinberger D, Ehrlich R. Short-term vitreoretinal tamponade with heavy liquid following surgery for giant retinal tear. Curr Eye Res. 2017;42(7):1074–8.
85. Zhang Z, Wei Y, Jiang X, Zhang S. Surgical outcomes of 27-gauge pars plana vitrectomy with short-term postoperative tamponade of perfluorocarbon liquid for repair of giant retinal tears. Int Ophthalmol. 2018;38(4):1505–13.
86. Mikhail MA, Mangioris G, Best RM, McGimpsey S, Chan WC. Management of giant retinal tears with vitrectomy and perfluorocarbon liquid postoperatively as a short-term tamponade. Eye. 2017;31(9):1290–5.

87. Kamei M, Tano Y. Tissue plasminogen activator-assisted vitrectomy: surgical drainage of submacular hemorrhage. Dev Ophthalmol. 2009;44:82–8.
88. Vander JF. Tissue plasminogen activator irrigation to facilitate removal of subretinal hemorrhage during vitrectomy. Ophthalmic Surg. 1992;23(5):361–3.
89. Kamei M, Tano Y, Maeno T, Ikuno Y, Mitsuda H, Yuasa T. Surgical removal of submacular hemorrhage using tissue plasminogen activator and perfluorocarbon liquid. Am J Ophthalmol. 1996;121(3):267–75.
90. Moriarty AP, McAllister IL, Constable IJ. Initial clinical experience with tissue plasminogen activator (tPA) assisted removal of submacular haemorrhage. Eye. 1995;9(Pt 5):582–8.
91. Moisseiev E, Ben Ami T, Barak A. Vitrectomy and subretinal injection of tissue plasminogen activator for large submacular hemorrhage secondary to AMD. Eur J Ophthalmol. 2014;24(6):925–31.
92. Peyman GA, Nelson NC, Alturki W, Blinder KJ, Paris CL, Desai UR, et al. Tissue plasminogen activating factor assisted removal of subretinal hemorrhage. Ophthalmic Surg. 1991;22(10):575–82.
93. Lim JI, Drews-Botsch C, Sternberg P, Capone A, Aaberg TM. Submacular hemorrhage removal. Ophthalmology. 1995;102(9):1393–9.
94. Ghazi NG, Abboud EB, Nowilaty SR, Alkuraya H, Alhommadi A, Cai H, et al. Treatment of retinitis pigmentosa due to MERTK mutations by ocular subretinal injection of adeno-associated virus gene vector: results of a phase I trial. Hum Genet. 2016;135(3):327–43.
95. Testa F, Maguire AM, Rossi S, Pierce EA, Melillo P, Marshall K, et al. Three-year follow-up after unilateral subretinal delivery of adeno-associated virus in patients with Leber congenital Amaurosis type 2. Ophthalmology. 2013;120(6):1283–91.
96. Mühlfriedel R, Michalakis S, Garcia Garrido M, Biel M, Seeliger MW. Optimized technique for subretinal injections in mice. Methods Mol Biol. 2013;935:343–9.
97. Ikeda Y, Yonemitsu Y, Miyazaki M, Kohno R-I, Murakami Y, Murata T, et al. Stable retinal gene expression in nonhuman primates via subretinal injection of SIVagm-based lentiviral vectors. Hum Gene Ther. 2009;20(6):573–9.
98. Schwartz SD, Regillo CD, Lam BL, Eliott D, Rosenfeld PJ, Gregori NZ, et al. Human embryonic stem cell-derived retinal pigment epithelium in patients with age-related macular degeneration and Stargardt's macular dystrophy: follow-up of two open-label phase 1/2 studies. Lancet. 2015;385(9967):509–16.
99. da Cruz L, Fynes K, Georgiadis O, Kerby J, Luo YH, Ahmado A, et al. Phase 1 clinical study of an embryonic stem cell–derived retinal pigment epithelium patch in age-related macular degeneration. Nat Biotechnol. 2018;36(4):328.
100. Mandai M, Watanabe A, Kurimoto Y, Hirami Y, Morinaga C, Daimon T, et al. Autologous induced stem-cell–derived retinal cells for macular degeneration. N Engl J Med. 2017;376(11):1038–46.
101. Kashani AH, Lebkowski JS, Rahhal FM, Avery RL, Salehi-Had H, Dang W, et al. A bioengineered retinal pigment epithelial monolayer for advanced, dry age-related macular degeneration. Sci Transl Med. 2018;10(435):eaao4097.
102. Kamao H, Mandai M, Okamoto S, Sakai N, Suga A, Sugita S, et al. Characterization of human induced pluripotent stem cell-derived retinal pigment epithelium cell sheets aiming for clinical application. Stem Cell Rep. 2014;2(2):205–18.
103. Kuhn F, Aylward B. Rhegmatogenous retinal detachment: a reappraisal of its pathophysiology and treatment. Ophthalmic Res. 2014;51(1):15–31.
104. Gomaa AR, Elbaha SM. Applying sutureless encircling number 41 band and transscleral chandelier-assisted laser retinopexy for scleral buckling procedure. J Ophthalmol. 2017;2017:4671305.
105. Heimann H, Hellmich M, Bornfeld N, Bartz-Schmidt KU, Hilgers RD, Foerster MH. Scleral buckling versus primary vitrectomy in rhegmatogenous retinal detachment (SPR Study): design issues and implications. SPR Study report no. 1. Graefes Arch Clin Exp Ophthalmol. 2001;239(8):567–74.

106. Foster WJ, Dowla N, Joshi SY, Nikolaou M. The fluid mechanics of scleral buckling surgery for the repair of retinal detachment. Graefes Arch Clin Exp Ophthalmol. 2010;248(1): 31–6.
107. Storey P, Alshareef R, Khuthaila M, London N, Leiby B, DeCroos C, et al. Pars plana vitrectomy and scleral buckle versus pars plana vitrectomy alone for patients with rhegmatogenous retinal detachment at high risk for proliferative vitreoretinopathy. Retina. 2014;34(10):1945–51.
108. Crama N, Klevering BJ. The removal of hydrogel explants: an analysis of 467 consecutive cases. Ophthalmology. 2016;123(1):32–8.
109. Yoshizumi MO, Friberg T. Erosion of implants in retinal detachment surgery. Ann Ophthalmol. 1983;15(5):430–4.
110. Shanmugam PM, Ramanjulu R, Mishra KCD, Sagar P. Novel techniques in scleral buckling. Indian J Ophthalmol. 2018;66(7):909–15.
111. Hu Y, Si S, Xu K, Chen H, Han L, Wang X, et al. Outcomes of scleral buckling using chandelier endoillumination. Acta Ophthalmol (Copenh). 2017;95(6):591–4.
112. Imai H, Tagami M, Azumi A. Scleral buckling for primary rhegmatogenous retinal detachment using noncontact wide-angle viewing system with a cannula-based 25 G chandelier endoilluminator. Clin Ophthalmol. 2015;9:2103–7.
113. Ohm J. Über die Behandlung der Netzhautablösung durch operative Entleerung der subretinalen Flüssigkeit und Einspritzung von Luft in den Glaskörper [On the treatment of retinal detachment by surgical evacuation of subretinal fluid and injection of air into the vitreous]. Albrecht Von Graefes Arch Für Ophthalmol. 1911;79(3):442–50.
114. Cibis PA, Becker B, Okun E, Canaan S. The use of liquid silicone in retinal detachment surgery. Arch Ophthalmol. 1962;68:590–9.
115. Norton EW. Intraocular gas in the management of selected retinal detachments. Trans Am Acad Ophthalmol Otolaryngol. 1973;77(2):OP85–98.
116. Mohamed S, Lai TY. Intraocular gas in vitreoretinal surgery. Hong Kong J Ophthalmol. 2010;14(1):8–13.
117. Kreissig I. The perfluorocarbon gases. In: A practical guide to minimal surgery for retinal detachment. 1st ed. Stuttgart: Thieme; 2000. p. 129–32.
118. Williamson TH. Principles of internal tamponade. In: Vitreoretinal surgery [Internet]. 2nd ed. Berlin: Springer; 2013. p. 61–87. //www.springer.com/us/book/9783642318719. [Cited 2018 Sept 16].
119. Abrams GW, Azen SP, McCuen BW, Flynn HW, Lai MY, Ryan SJ. Vitrectomy with silicone oil or long-acting gas in eyes with severe proliferative vitreoretinopathy: results of additional and long-term follow-up. Silicone Study report 11. Arch Ophthalmol. 1997;115(3):335–44.
120. Adelman RA, Parnes AJ, Sipperley JO, Ducournau D, European Vitreo-Retinal Society (EVRS) Retinal Detachment Study Group. Strategy for the management of complex retinal detachments: the European vitreo-retinal society retinal detachment study report 2. Ophthalmology. 2013;120(9):1809–13.
121. Foster WJ. Vitreous substitutes. Expert Rev Ophthalmol. 2008;3(2):211–8.
122. Cazabon S, Hillier RJ, Wong D. Heavy silicone oil: a "novel" intraocular tamponade agent. Optom Vis Sci. 2011;88(6):772–5.
123. Rizzo S, Romagnoli MC, Genovesi-Ebert F, Belting C. Surgical results of heavy silicone oil HWS-45 3000 as internal tamponade for inferior retinal detachment with PVR: a pilot study. Graefes Arch Clin Exp Ophthalmol. 2011;249(3):361–7.
124. Er H. Primary heavy silicone oil usage in inferior rhegmatogenous retinal detachment. Ophthalmologica. 2010;224(2):122–5.
125. Levasseur SD, Schendel S, Machuck RWA, Dhanda D. High-density silicone oil Densiron-68 as an intraocular tamponade for primary inferior retinal detachments. Retina. 2013;33(3):627–33.
126. Reza AT. Postoperative Perfluro-N-Octane tamponade for complex retinal detachment surgery. Bangladesh Med Res Counc Bull. 2014;40(2):63–9.

127. Sigler EJ, Randolph JC, Calzada JI, Charles S. Pars plana vitrectomy with medium-term postoperative perfluoro-N-octane for recurrent inferior retinal detachment complicated by advanced proliferative vitreoretinopathy. Retina. 2013;33(4):791–7.
128. Rizzo S, Genovesi-Ebert F, Murri S, Belting C, Vento A, Cresti F, et al. 25-gauge, sutureless vitrectomy and standard 20-gauge pars plana vitrectomy in idiopathic epiretinal membrane surgery: a comparative pilot study. Graefes Arch Clin Exp Ophthalmol. 2006;244(4):472–9.
129. Khan MA, Kuley A, Riemann CD, Berrocal MH, Lakhanpal RR, Hsu J, et al. Long-term visual outcomes and safety profile of 27-gauge pars plana vitrectomy for posterior segment disease. Ophthalmology. 2018;125(3):423–31.
130. Tayyab H, Khan AA, Sadiq MAA, Karamat I. Comparison of 23 gauge transconjunctival releasable suture vitrectomy with standard 20 gauge vitrectomy. Pak J Med Sci. 2018;34(2):328–32.
131. Xia F, Jiang Y-Q. Clinical outcomes of 23-gauge vitrectomy may be better than 20-gauge vitrectomy for retinal detachment repair. Mol Vis. 2015;21:893–900.
132. Ho J, Grabowska A, Ugarte M, Muqit MM. A comparison of 23-gauge and 20-gauge vitrectomy for proliferative sickle cell retinopathy—clinical outcomes and surgical management. Eye (Lond). 2018;32(9):1449–54.
133. Ho VY, Shah GK. Short-and long-term outcomes of vitreoretinal surgeries with deferred first postoperative visits at day 3 or later. J Vitreoretinal Dis. 2017;1(2):126–32.
134. Ringeisen AL, Parke DW. Reconsidering the postoperative day 0 visit for retina surgery. Ophthalmic Surg Lasers Imaging Retina. 2018;49(9):e52–6.
135. Rahmani S, Eliott D. Postoperative endophthalmitis: a review of risk factors, prophylaxis, incidence, microbiology, treatment, and outcomes. Semin Ophthalmol. 2018;33(1):95–101.
136. Kunimoto DY, Kaiser RS, Wills Eye Retina Service. Incidence of endophthalmitis after 20-and 25-gauge vitrectomy. Ophthalmology. 2007;114(12):2133–7.
137. Scott IU, Flynn HW Jr, Acar N, Dev S, Shaikh S, Mittra RA, et al. Incidence of endophthalmitis after 20-gauge vs 23-gauge vs 25-gauge pars plana vitrectomy. Graefes Arch Clin Exp Ophthalmol. 2011;249(3):377–80.
138. Wu L, Berrocal MH, Arévalo JF, Carpentier C, Rodriguez FJ, Alezzandrini A, et al. Endophthalmitis after pars plana vitrectomy: results of the Pan American Collaborative Retina Study Group. Retina. 2011;31(4):673–8.
139. Rizzo S, Belting C, Genovesi-Ebert F, di Bartolo E. Incidence of retinal detachment after small-incision, sutureless pars plana vitrectomy compared with conventional 20-gauge vitrectomy in macular hole and epiretinal membrane surgery. Retina. 2010;30(7):1065–71.
140. Neffendorf JE, Gupta B, Williamson TH. Intraoperative complications of patients undergoing small-gauge and 20-gauge vitrectomy: a database study of 4,274 procedures. Eur J Ophthalmol. 2017;27(2):226–30.
141. Gass JD. Sympathetic ophthalmia following vitrectomy. Am J Ophthalmol. 1982;93(5):552–8.
142. Gupta OPI, Weichel ED, Regillo CD, Fineman MS, Kaiser RS, Ho AC, et al. Postoperative complications associated with 25-gauge pars plana vitrectomy. Ophthalmic Surg Lasers Imaging. 2007;38(4):270–5.
143. Roizenblatt M, Edwards TL, Gehlbach PL. Robot-assisted vitreoretinal surgery: current perspectives. Robot Surg. 2018;5:1–11.
144. Gonenc B, Handa J, Gehlbach P, Taylor RH, Iordachita I. A comparative study for robot assisted vitreoretinal surgery: micron vs. the steady-hand robot. IEEE Int Conf Robot Autom. 2013;2013:4832–7.
145. Balicki M, Xia T, Jung MY, Deguet A, Vagvolgyi B, Kazanzides P, Taylor R. Prototyping a hybrid cooperative and tele-robotic surgical system for retinal microsurgery. MIDAS J. 2011; E-pub Dec 2011.
146. Gonenc B, Handa J, Gehlbach P, Taylor RH, Iordachita I. Design of 3-DOF force sensing micro-forceps for robot assisted vitreoretinal surgery. Conf Proc IEEE Eng Med Biol Soc. 2013;2013:5686–9.

147. Edwards TL, Xue K, Meenink HCM, Beelen MJ, Naus GJL, Simunovic MP, et al. First-in-human study of the safety and viability of intraocular robotic surgery. Nat Biomed Eng. 2018;2:649–56.
148. Carrasco-Zevallos OM, Keller B, Viehland C, Shen L, Seider MI, Izatt JA, et al. Optical coherence tomography for retinal surgery: perioperative analysis to real-time four-dimensional image-guided surgery. Invest Ophthalmol Vis Sci. 2016;57(9):OCT37–50.

# Chapter 8
# Clinical Updates and Recent Developments in Neuro-Ophthalmology

Amrita-Amanda D. Vuppala and Neil R. Miller

## Updates in Diagnostic Criteria/Clinical Presentation

The ability to diagnose efficiently and accurately neuro-ophthalmic conditions is imperative to guiding timely intervention. In this section, we introduce new neuro-ophthalmic diagnoses and review updates to the diagnostic criteria for previously described conditions. These updates are intended to guide clinicians in accurate examination, identification and management of commonly encountered neuro-ophthalmic conditions. The updates are outlined by subspecialty to help the reader think in terms of a differential diagnosis for conditions with similar presentations.

### *Updates in Neuro-immunology*

Perhaps one of the most exciting areas in neuro-ophthalmology at the present time are neuro-ophthalmic diagnoses pertaining to neuro-immunology. Over the years, with the invention of magnetic resonance imaging (MRI) and the discovery of new antibodies, two of the most well-known autoimmune conditions causing optic neuritis, multiple sclerosis (MS) and neuromyelitis optica (NMO), were delineated as separate entities. The diagnostic criteria for these conditions include guidelines for clinical and imaging features as well as serum and cerebrospinal fluid (CSF) testing. Revisions to these criteria have been designed to increase the sensitivity and

A.-A. D. Vuppala
University of Nebraska Medical Center, Omaha, NE, USA
e-mail: amritaamanda.vuppala@unmc.edu

N. R. Miller (✉)
Johns Hopkins University School of Medicine, Baltimore, MD, USA
e-mail: nrmiller@jhmi.edu

specificity for diagnosis; the most recent criteria for MS and NMO are described below. The mystery remains as to why some patients with clinical presentations similar to MS or NMO are seronegative. More recently, the clinical significance of previously described antibodies including those to myelin oligodendrocyte glyco-protein (MOG) and glial fibrillary acidic protein (GFAP) have been identified as separate, unique pathologies with presentations that may present with optic neuritis and clinically may appear to be similar to MS and/or NMO. This section will review the current literature regarding these new antibodies, the associated clinical presen-tations and the recommended medical management.

## Multiple Sclerosis (MS)

Multiple Sclerosis (MS) is a well-known inflammatory demyelinating disease and is the single most common cause of disability in young adults, with age at onset strongly influencing the course of progression [1]. In the 1970s, when MS was first being diagnosed, there were no treatment options, and diagnosis was limited to autopsy and direct tissue examination [2]. Since then, our ability to diagnose MS has changed dramatically with the use of MRI in 2001 and subsequent updates in the clinical diagnostic criteria. In the same way, disease-modifying therapies (DMTs) have multiplied, with over a dozen DMTs currently approved worldwide over the past 25 years [2]. With an improved ability to delay or halt clinical progression, the need to diagnose and treat patients with MS earlier has become paramount [3].

The McDonald Criteria for diagnosing MS were first established in 2001 [4] but have been revised many times over the last 17 years, resulting in an increase in the number of patients diagnosed with the condition. The most recent revision of the McDonald Criteria for diagnosing MS occurred in 2017 [5]. This revision included three major changes. The first was related to the inclusion of symptomatic supraten-torial, infratentorial and spinal cord lesions on MRI to meet the criteria for dissemi-nation of lesions; previously, only asymptomatic lesions could be used. Second, if enhancing and non-enhancing lesions are found on an MRI at one point in time, this can be considered dissemination in time. Finally, a patient meeting the criteria for a clinically isolated syndrome may be diagnosed with MS if oligoclonal bands are present in the cerebrospinal fluid [5, 6].

## Neuromyelitis Optica (NMO)

NMO is a rare autoimmune disease of the central nervous system (CNS) that pri-marily affects the spinal cord and optic nerves, leading to optic neuritis and lon-gitudinally extending transverse myelitis. Onset is typically in the third to fourth decade of life. There is a strong female predominance with a female:male ratio as high as 9–10:1 [7]. Clinical attacks may be recurrent as is the case with MS and anti-MOG disease (see below); however, unlike MS and anti-MOG disease, it may take only one attack of NMO-related optic neuritis and transverse myelitis to leave a patient blind and paraplegic. In other words, the disability risk with NMO is extremely high [8]. It was not until 2004 when NMO-IgG was identified as a specific marker autoantibody that can be used to distinguish MS from NMO [9]. These autoantibodies target the most abundant water channel in the CSF: aquaporin-4 (AQP4), located on the astrocytic foot processes of the blood-brain barrier [10]. Over time, it was discovered that the range of clinical presentations associated with AQP4 autoimmunity was much broader than just optic neuritis and longitudinally extending transverse myelitis [10, 11]. Subsequently, Wingerchuck et al. outlined new criteria and described NMO spectrum disorder (NMOSD). The new criteria take into account the serum status of AQP4-IgG (present, absent or unknown) and add additional requirements for patients with absent or unknown AQP4-IgG status. These requirements include specific core clinical characteristics of optic neuritis, acute myelitis, area postrema syndrome, acute brainstem syndrome, symptomatic narcolepsy or acute diencephalic syndrome and/or symptomatic cerebral syndrome with typical brain lesions. There also are additional MRI requirements for this group of patients [12].

New information regarding AQP4 antibody status and its relation to prognosis also has become available. A large, retrospective cohort study evaluating the efficacy of immunotherapy in NMOSD suggests that several factors, including age, antibody status and the presence of previous attacks, may predict further attacks in patients diagnosed and treated for NMOSD [8]. Indeed, the presence of AQP4 in the serum of patients with NMOSD may predict future recurrent disease as opposed to patients with seronegative presentations of NMOSD who are more likely to have a monophasic course [13].

## Myelin Oligodendrocyte Glycoprotein (MOG-IgG)

Myelin oligodendrocyte glycoprotein (MOG) is a glycoprotein that is expressed on the outer membrane of myelin. This glycoprotein is specifically found within the CNS, including the brain, optic nerves and spinal cord [14]. MOG antibodies bind to extracellular glycoprotein on the myelin sheath and to oligodendrocytes [15]. First identified in the 1990s, MOG antibodies initially were identified in patients with relapsing autoimmune illness who were presumed to have MS [16, 17]. After studies revealed low sensitivity of MOG in larger MS populations, skepticism arose regarding the validity of MOG-IgG as a reliable biomarker for MS [18]. Shortly thereafter, MOG-IgG was identified in several pediatric cases of acute disseminated encephalomyelopathy (ADEM) and by 2011, the first report of MOG antibodies in NMOSD was reported [19]. Recent studies have concluded that the presence of MOG-IgG antibodies in a patient with an acute neurologic syndrome is indicative of an entity separate from both MS and NMO [20, 21]. In one study, it was stated that up to 42% of NMOSD patients who tested negative for AQP4 worldwide tested positive for MOG-IgG [14]. In another study, MOG-IgG was found in 20% of patients with a demyelinating illness that did not fit the criteria for MS or NMOSD [6].

The clinical manifestations of patients presenting with MOG-IgG are extremely variable. Perhaps because of this, several studies have reported different findings in regards to age and sex predilections as well clinical phenotype for MOG-IgG disease. MOG-IgG likely affects both men and woman equally or has a very slight female predominance and age of onset is 20–30 years of age [22, 23]. Clinically, the majority of MOG-IgG patients present with optic neuritis, with or without other accompanying neurologic symptoms. The optic neuritis may be unilateral; however, simultaneous bilateral optic neuritis can occur and may occur with higher frequency than in NMOSD [21]. Anti-MOG antibody-related optic neuritis attacks may be recurrent, with the reported number of attacks ranging from one to eight [23]. Patients who develop anti-MOG antibody-related optic neuritis tend to have an anterior optic neuritis: the fundus exam typically reveals optic disc swelling, sometimes with associated flame hemorrhages (Fig. 8.1).

Other neurologic manifestations include atypical cerebral inflammatory lesions (that may have been characterized as relapsing steroid-responsive autoimmune encephalitis in the past), ADEM, atypical MS or CNS vasculitis. Aseptic meningitis and pseudotumor cerebri (PTC)-like presentations (with elevated opening pressure) also have been reported [24]. Finally, patients with anti-MOG-IgG-associated disease are more likely to have seizures and encephalitis as part of the presentation compared with patients with AQP4-IgG-associated disease [20].

Data from several cohorts suggest that both visual and neurological outcome are favorable in the majority of cases of MOG-IgG disease; only a small number of patients are left with severe visual deficits, cognitive impairment or are wheelchair bound [22]. Phenotype at onset may predict long-term outcome including likeli-

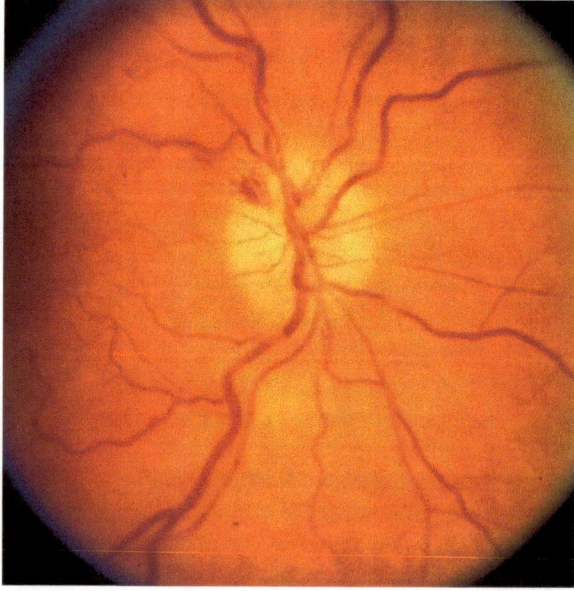

**Fig. 8.1** Right optic disc of a patient with MOG-IgG-associated anterior optic neuritis. Note diffuse swelling associated with a single flame-shaped hemorrhage

**Fig. 8.2** T1-weighted, post-contrast axial MRI of a patient with bilateral, simultaneous anti-MOG antibody-related optic neuritis. Note marked enhancement of the orbital portions of both optic nerves. This is not typical of the findings in idiopathic or MS-related optic neuritis

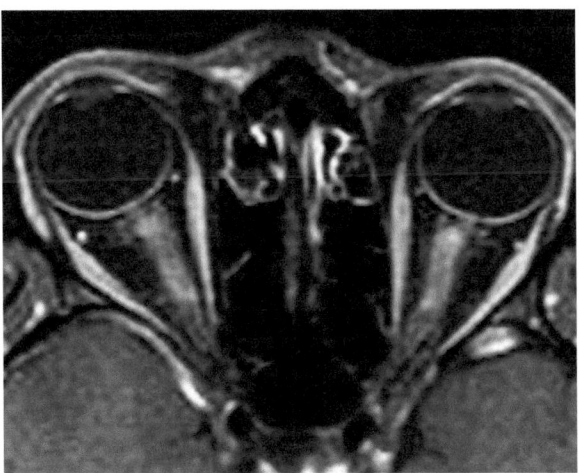

hood for relapse; however, a large number prospective studies will be needed to determine if this is the case [22]. CSF studies in the majority of cases reveal a pleocytosis that may be mild (>5 white blood cells) to significant (≥50 white blood cells), and the CSF protein concentration may be increased.

Neuroimaging findings in patients with anti-MOG antibody-related optic neuritis include a long enhancing segment of the optic nerve including its orbital and intracranial portions (Fig. 8.2).

Some patients have perineural enhancement with extension of the enhancement into the surrounding orbital tissues [3]. In a cohort of 246 patients with recurrent optic neuritis, no patient with positive MOG-IgG showed MS-like MRI lesions [21].

In general, treatment of patients with anti-MOG antibody-related disease with systemic corticosteroids provides rapid and robust clinical improvement; however, relapse upon withdrawal of steroids is not uncommon [25]. Thus, it is recommended that treatment include a prolonged steroid taper to minimize chances of an early relapse from steroid withdrawal and that close monitoring be performed once the steroids are discontinued [14]. The finding of optical coherence (OCT) retinal nerve fiber layer (RNFL) changes in patients with anti-MOG antibody-associated transverse myelitis who have not experienced an attack of acute optic neuritis supports the need for early and sustained immunosuppression [26].

**Glial Fibrillary Acidic Protein (GFAP)**

GFAP auto-antibody-positive meningoencephalitis is a newly described entity for which the clinical phenotype has been described in only a small number of patients. The presentation may be subacute or chronic and is characterized by encephalitis or meningoencephalitis accompanied by bilateral optic disc swelling at initial presentation, although some variations in this presentation have been observed [27].

The cause for the bilateral optic disc swelling is unknown; however, the majority of patients do not have an elevated opening pressure on lumbar puncture. The underlying pathophysiology for GFAP autoantibody-positive meningoencephalitis is unknown but may be related to venous inflammation based on fluorescein angiography showing prominent venular leakage in one patient with this entity and the presence of radial perivascular enhancement on MRI in several patients [27]. Knock-out studies of GFAP in mice revealed local impairment in the blood brain barrier and disruption in normal white matter architecture with late onset CNS dysmyelination [28]. Patients with GFAP antibody-related neurologic disease typically have evidence of inflammation and GFAP-IgG in their CSF.

GFAP antibody-positive neurologic disease tends to be very steroid responsive, with the majority of patients showing improvement in their optic disc swelling and MRI lesions after a course of high-dose intravenous corticosteroid treatment followed by a prolonged oral steroid taper. The optic disc swelling in these patients has been reported to be visually asymptomatic, although arcuate visual field deficits after treatment and resolution have been observed [27]. It is not yet known if GFAP-IgG occurs in isolation or if it co-exists with other demyelinating diseases such as MS and NMO.

## Recurrent Optic Neuritis

MS previously was recognized as a major cause of recurrent optic neuritis [21]; however, more recently, the glial antibodies AQP4 and MOG-IgG also have been recognized as important contributors. AQP4 IgG has been reported to be present in the serum in 8.3–25% of patients with recurrent optic neuritis [29, 30]. In addition, it is known that patients with anti-MOG antibody-associated optic neuritis tend to experience recurrent attacks. One cross-sectional cohort study of 246 patients with recurrent optic neuritis reported that one-third of all patients had a positive glial antibody (either MOG-IgG or AQP4) [21]. The same study concluded that that AQP4-IgG seropositivity predicts a worse visual outcome than MOG-IgG seropositivity, double seronegativity (ie, idiopathic recurrent optic neuritis), or MS. Interestingly, although the relapse rate of recurrent optic neuritis is higher in MOG-IgG-positive patients compared with patients with MS and NMO, the visual prognosis is better [21, 31]. Recurrent optic neuritis may behave differently in the glial antibody diseases compared with MS-related recurrent optic neuritis. Although recurrent optic neuritis in patients with MS tends to attack the same optic nerve that initially was affected, glial antibody-associated recurrent optic neuritis appears to be randomly distributed between the two optic nerves [32].

Chronic relapsing inflammatory optic neuropathy (CRION) is a recurrent optic neuritis that is steroid responsive and is a rare cause of subacute and recurrent painful vision loss unrelated to demyelinating or connective tissue disease [33]. This diagnosis should be made with extreme caution and only after extensive testing and imaging. In the previously discussed cohort of 246 patients with recurrent optic neuritis (see above), 4/14 patients with CRION tested positive for MOG-IgG, whereas no patient tested positive for AQP4 or had an MS-like phenotype. Patients with recurrent optic neuritis who have negative MOG-IgG and AQP4 but who also do not fulfill criteria for MS pose a diagnostic and management challenge, especially as the probability of permanent vision loss is higher in this group compared with MS or MOG-IgG-positive patients. Unfortunately, there are no specific treatment recommendations for this subset of patients. Most are treated with systemic corticosteroids, with other immunosuppressive agents used when necessary.

## Conclusion and Recommendations

The differentiation of these various entities causing optic nerve and CNS inflammation and demyelination remains crucial due to the difference in optimum treatment approach and both visual and neurological outcomes. Especially in the case of MS and NMO, incorrect management can potentially lead to worsening of the disease course. At this time, our recommendation would be to start with the diagnostic criteria for MS and NMO. If the presentation is atypical or does not fulfill the above criteria, proceed with MOG testing. MOG testing has a 98.5% specificity but 1.5% of healthy controls testing positive for MOG-IgG [34]. The sensitivity for MOG testing is much lower, ranging from 5% in MOG to about 36% in ADEM cases [14]. International guidelines for diagnosis and testing in MOG were published in 2018 and recommend testing for MOG-IgG in patients in whom at least minimal clinical criteria are met. The minimal criteria include an attack of optic neuritis, transverse myelitis or brainstem lesion; objective evidence of a demyelinating process detected by MRI or optical coherence tomography (OCT); and other typical findings of MOG-IgG disease, including a longitudinally extensive lesion in the optic nerve or spinal cord [35]. These guidelines also give recommendations for "red flags" if the result comes back positive in atypical presentations.

Complete neuro-ophthalmologic evaluation, MRI brain and orbits (and in appropriate cases cervical and thoracic spine) with and without contrast and optical coherence tomography also should be performed for all patients. Treatment appropriate for the diagnosis should be initiated early.

In regards to monitoring, we recommend that all of these patients be followed with OCT. Optic neuritis causes substantial retinal damage and vision loss independent of the underlying disease. Ganglion cell/internal plexiform layer damage begins close to clinical onset and, thus, the structure-function correlations between OCT and vision make OCT an important tool for monitoring acute optic neuritis [36]. The utility of OCT to differentiate among MS, NMOSD, and anti-MOG antibody-related optic nerve disease is still poorly understood. Various studies have presented controversial results including equal RNFL thinning in both anti-MOG-IgG and AQP4-related disease [37, 38], increased thinning of the RNFL in AQP4 compared with MOG disease [39]. A recent study showed RNFL thinning to be similar in MS, MOG, and idiopathic optic neuritis [36].

## *Neuro-Degenerative Diseases*

### Parkinson Disease

The clinical diagnosis of Parkinson disease (PD) emphasizes the motor manifestations and cardinal signs of tremor, bradykinesia, rigidity and postural instability. Perhaps because of this, visual signs and symptoms have been under-recognized. In fact, non-motor symptoms, including visual complaints, impact a patient's quality of life significantly and may predict progression and disease outcomes [40].

Ophthalmic findings in PD are likely related to the loss of dopaminergic neurons with accumulation of alpha synuclein in the retina [41], or related to a disturbance of cortical visual processing from intracranial loss of dopaminergic neurons and accumulation of alpha synuclein. Visual impairment has been suggested as a marker for early diagnosis of PD [42] and can be recognized by neuro-ophthalmic exam. Thus, the role of a neuro-ophthalmologist is very important in the early identification of PD and other parkinsonian presentations. Below is a summary of the visual problems seen in PD with clinical implications and influence of levodopa therapy.

**Color Vision**—Color vision deficiencies have been reported in PD patients who are not treated with a dopaminergic drug [43]. The gold standard test for assessing color deficiencies is the Farnsworth-Munsell 100 Hue Test; however the results are influenced by cognitive difficulties and motor deficits [44, 45]. Interestingly, color vision impairment also is present in patients with Rapid Eye Movement (REM) sleep behavior disorder (RBD), an early manifestation of alpha synucleinopathies, In the case of RBD, color vision deficiency is a risk factor for disease conversion to PD [46] and also may predict rapid disease progression [44]. Patients with the LRRK2 gene mutation of PD have more color impairments compared with patients with idiopathic PD [47]. Levodopa therapy may improve color vision in PD patients [48].

**Visual Contrast Sensitivity**—PD patients may experience problems with contrast sensitivity in relation to both static and moving stimuli [49]. Worsening contrast sensitivity is related to disease progression [50] and is partly reversible with levodopa therapy [51, 52].

**Saccades**—Patients with PD often make hypometric reflexive (visually guided) and voluntary (memory-based) saccades [53, 54]. Clinically, instead of making accurate saccades to a target, the patient makes several small saccadic movements to reach it [55]. Such patients also may have difficulty initiating memory-guided saccades [56] and performing anti-saccades [57, 58]. The amplitude of voluntary more than reflexive saccades is reduced with PD disease progression [54], whereas the latency of visually guided saccades worsens in early disease stages but then stabilizes [54]. Levodopa therapy has little to no effect on changing saccadic amplitude. Although levodopa may shorten the latency for voluntary saccades, it also prolongs the latency of reflexive saccades [54].

**Smooth Pursuit Eye Movements**—Smooth pursuit may be impaired in healthy elderly patients in general [59] but also in patients of all ages with PD [60, 61]. Reduced pursuit gain has been identified in early and untreated patients with PD [62]. The efficacy of dopaminergics in improving smooth pursuit is unclear, with some authors suggesting improved pursuit gain [59, 63] and others finding no improvement [64].

**Convergence Insufficiency**—Reduced convergence amplitude is a common finding in PD [65, 66]. Such patients often have horizontal binocular diplopia when attempting near tasks such as reading and sewing. Convergence amplitude and near point of convergence measurements are better when evaluated in PD patients during the "on" state compared to the "off" state, possibly suggesting that dopaminergic therapy may be useful for this symptom [67]. Other patients may benefit from convergence exercises, converging (base-in) prisms, extraocular muscle surgery, or simply occluding the lower portion of one of their spectacle lens with tape.

**Stereopsis**—PD patients with abnormal stereopsis show worse motor functions, supported by higher scores on the unified PD rating scale (UPDRS) compared with PD patients with abnormal stereopsis [40]. Depth perception deficits correlate with color deficiencies in patients with PD [68]. Stereopsis impairment in PD has been associated with a faster cognitive decline [69] and suggests disease progression [68]. It is also a predictor for dementia in PD patients at 24 months [69].

Ocular findings in PD for which there are no data regarding the utility in determining progression or prognosis include square-wave jerks and ocular tremor (ocular oscillations in antiphase to the direction of a head tremor during fixation) [70]. Visual hallucinations in PD previously were thought to correlate with levodopa therapy; however, minor hallucinations have been reported in PD patients naive to levodopa therapy and in premotor phases of PD as well [71]. Because visual hallucinations have been associated with abnormalities in color vision and contrast sensitivity [72], they may suggest disease progression and also may reflect impending dementia or even impending psychosis later in the course of the disease [40]. Nevertheless, caution is warranted in attributing visual hallucinations to worsening disease, as they may be a medication side effect.

**Progressive Supranuclear Palsy (PSP)**

In 2017, the Movement Disorder Society put forth a new set of recommendations for diagnostic criteria of PSP [73]. These criteria identified four functional domains, with ocular motor dysfunction being one of the four along with postural instability, akinesia and cognitive dysfunction. The ocular motor domain refers to several clinical findings related to eye movements, including vertical supranuclear gaze palsy, slowed velocity of vertical saccades, frequent macro square-wave jerks and apraxia of eyelid opening. Although definitive diagnosis of PSP requires pathology, the new PSP criteria suggest categories for probable, possible and suggestive PSP based on clinical features alone. By identifying these eye movement abnormalities, neuro-ophthalmologists can play an important role in helping to facilitate the early diagnosis of PSP. However, it also should be emphasized that many patients with pathologically confirmed PSP do not have eye movement abnormalities early in their disease course. Thus, the lack of eye movement abnormalities does not exclude the diagnosis of PSP [74].

## Space Flight-Associated Neuro-Ocular Syndrome (SANS)

Both subjective and objective changes in visual function with associated structural changes in the optic nerve are recognized to occur in astronauts spending long periods of time in space. Previously described as visual impairment and intracranial pressure (VIIP) syndrome, scientists at the National Aeronautics and Space Exploration Administration (NASA) have more recently termed this phenomenon "spaceflight-associated neuro-ocular syndrome" (SANS). Clinical findings associated with this syndrome include optic disc swelling of varying severity (unilateral and/or bilateral), flattening of the posterior globe, refractive error (hyperopic shifts), choroidal and retinal folds and nerve fiber layer (NFL) infarcts with cotton-wool spots and, rarely, hemorrhages [75, 76]. Patients with SANS have structural changes that can be appreciated on various imaging studies including MRI, ultrasonography and OCT. For example, globe flattening may be appreciated on MRI on earth and by ultrasound in space, and OCT reveals changes in the NFL.

The pathophysiology for SANS is unclear. Lumbar punctures performed on a few astronauts with persistent optic disc swelling after their return to earth from long-duration space flight reveal mildly elevated opening pressures (22–28.5 cm $H_2O$), suggesting that the optic disc swelling represents papilledema, similar to that observed in patients with terrestrial pseudotumor cerebri (PTC). However, the demographics are quite dissimilar in that SANS occurs in non-obese, middle-aged men rather than obese young women of child-bearing age. In addition, SANS often is characterized by asymmetric disc swelling whereas most patients with PTC have symmetric disc swelling. Another difference is that choroidal folds are commonly seen in SANS and often are associated with very mild optic disc swelling, whereas choroidal folds are an uncommon finding in PTC and usually are associated with significant disc swelling. Thus, although raised ICP may be a factor in some cases of SANS, the most widely accepted mechanism for SANS is prolonged exposure to a microgravity environment, with resultant microgravity fluid shifts and jugular venous distention [75, 77, 78]. Another suggested mechanism for SANS includes compartmentalization of CSF within the orbital subarachnoid space; however, this hypothesis has not been confirmed. The role of lymphatics and venous flow is unknown.

Ongoing efforts to understand the pathophysiology of SANS include the use of OCT and OCTA to study structural changes in the optic nerve, retinal tissue and choroid. ICP measurements thus far have been limited to pre- or post-flight terrestrial lumbar punctures. Researchers currently are trying to find a way to measure the ICP inflight using various techniques [79].

## Updates on Toxic and Nutritional Optic Neuropathies

Toxic-nutritional optic neuropathies (TNON) may occur in the setting of various offending agents including medications, poisonous environmental exposures, illicit substances, metabolic derangements and nutritional deficiencies [80]. The classic clinical presentation for this group of optic neuropathies includes subacute, progressive, bilateral, painless vision loss. Visual field testing often reveals bilateral central and cecocentral scotomas due to loss of the papillomacular bundle [81]. Patients also may experience significant deficient of color vision and contrast sensitivity. Depending on when in the course of the optic neuropathy the patient is evaluated, the optic discs may appear normal, there may be mild optic disc swelling and hyperemia that mimic that sometimes seen in patients with Leber Hereditary Optic Neuropathy (LHON), or the optic discs may be pale, particularly temporally [82]. The mechanism of injury is at least in some of these cases is thought to be related to disruption of normal physiologic processes in the retinal ganglion cells and synapses in the afferent visual pathway [83]. This hypothesis has been confirmed by recent OCT studies showing thinning of the retinal ganglion cell/inner plexiform layer in patients with toxic optic neuropathies [84]. It is important to note that some patients have a combination of insults; e.g., both a toxic process and a nutritional deficiency, resulting in a compounding injury to the optic nerve. This is referred to as a toxic-nutritional optic neuropathy (TNON). Many TNONs share a mechanism of injury similar to that which produces mitochondrial optic neuropathies, particularly LHON, and, thus, careful evaluation should include testing for LHON in the appropriate clinic setting, such as those patients who do not improve or worsen despite repletion of the deficient nutrient or cessation of the toxic substance [85].

## Toxins

The most commonly reported causes of toxic optic neuropathies include methanol, ethylene glycol and toluene [85]. Methanol toxicity typically occurs in patients consuming alcoholic beverages that contain excessive methanol rather than ethanol. Toxicity in this setting is related to the accumulation of toxic metabolites (formaldehyde and formic acid), leading to metabolic acidosis and cellular dysfunction. Acute demyelination of the optic nerve secondary to toxic formic acid may cause axon degeneration [86]. Treatment includes hemodialysis, ethanol and fomepizole. These antidotes are meant to inhibit alcohol dehydrogenase. The problem with ethanol is that it is not readily available in developing countries, and given the pharmacokinetics of ethanol, it is difficult to maintain adequate plasma concentrations. Serial monitoring of ethanol levels is required. Ethanol also may cause liver injury and hypoglycemia. There is no evidence for superiority of ethanol versus fomepizole in the treatment of methanol toxicity; however, fomepizole may have fewer adverse effects despite being very expensive [87, 88]. It has been suggested that treatment with steroids (IV methylprednisolone) may inhibit the demyelination process caused by methanol and also may prevent blindness and retinal atrophy [89]; however, this is a controversial issue and has not been proven in clinical trials [90]. There is also recent research suggesting that erythropoietin (EPO) may be useful for methanol poisoning, with reports of improved visual acuity after treatment with IV recombinant human EPO, but this, too, remains unsubstantiated by prospective clinical trials [91].

## Medication-Induced

As novel oral and injectable pharmacologic agents emerge for various disease processes, the need to monitor for visual and ocular side effects becomes increasingly important. Medication-induced optic neuropathies typically are related to the dose of the offending agent and the length of time the patient was consuming it. We briefly review some updates in the literature for various medications and provide a table for commonly encountered medications causing optic neuropathy by category (Table 8.1).

Although it was previously thought that ethambutol causes an optic neuropathy at high doses (25 mg/kg/day), recent reports suggest that an optic neuropathy may occur at lower doses closer to the recommended dose of 15 mg/kg/day. Particularly in patients with renal dysfunction, progressive visual field deficits have been reported, even in the setting of concurrent hemodialysis [93]. Aside from immediate cessation of the medication, there are no new treatments for ethambutol-induced optic neuropathy. Rigorous monitoring with visual acuity, visual fields, color vision, and OCT thus remain important. In particular, it has been suggested that assessment of the thickness of the retinal ganglion cell/inner plexiform layer (rather than the peripapillary retinal nerve fiber layer) can be used to diagnose ethambutol-induced optic neuropathy at its earliest stage [94].

Linezolide is an antibiotic used to treat complicated, multidrug-resistant, grampositive skin infections and pneumonia. It is generally well tolerated when used for up to 28 days [95]; however, it is known to cause a bilateral optic neuropathy in some patients. Dempsey et al. recently suggest a new screening protocol for linezolid use in adult patients, with screening beginning within 1 month after initiating linezolid, followed by a subsequent evaluation every 30–60 days beginning 3 months from initiation if needed for long-term use [96].

Amiodarone is a commonly used antiarrhythmic drug used to treat atrial fibrillation in cardiac patients around the world. Amiodarone-associated optic neuropathy (AAON) is a somewhat controversial diagnosis in that most patients receiving amiodarone have significant cardiac disease as well as other vascular risk factors for NAION, which AAON mimics. The difference between the two conditions is that AAON tends to be bilateral and mild, with optic disc swelling resolving over

**Table 8.1** Commonly encountered medications causing optic neuropathy

| Antimycobacterials/antimicrobials | Ethambutol, Isoniazid, Linezolid, Ciprofloxacin, Cimetidine, Chloramphenicol, Erythromycin, Streptomycin, Dapsone, Quinine, Clioquinol |
|---|---|
| Antidepressants | Pheniprazine |
| Reversal agents | Disulfiram |
| Chemotherapeutic agents | Methotrexate, Cisplatin, Carboplatin, Vincristine, cyclosporine, tamoxifen, Infliximab, Clomiphene |
| Cardiovascular medications | Amiodarone, PDE-5 inhibitors, Blood pressure medications causing hypotension such as amlodipine may cause bilateral optic neuropathy [92] |

4–6 months, whereas NAION tends to be unilateral, ranges in severity of optic disc swelling from mild to severe, and generally resolves in 6–11 weeks [97]. The exact mechanism of injury is unclear, although ultrastructural changes within in the optic nerve axons and disruption of axoplasmic flow have been suggested [98]. Most cases of AAON occur within the first year of taking the medication. Thus, it is recommended that patients undergo regular evaluations during the first year of treatment, followed by annual evaluations thereafter [99]. Treatment is cessation of the medication, assuming that there are other cardiac regimens available for the patient. Thus, the decision regarding management of patients with presumed AAON should be made in conjunction with the patient's cardiologist.

Phosphodiesterase-5 (PDE-5) inhibitors, including sildenafil, tadalafil, and vardenafil, commonly are used to treat erectile dysfunction and pulmonary arterial hypertension in both the pediatric and adult populations. Although it is clear that some patients taking PDE-5 inhibitors can develop an optic neuropathy, it is unclear if there is a cause-and-effect relationship. Favoring such a relationship are the fact that PDE-5 inhibitors are vasodilators and, thus, may cause systemic hypotension. Also, several challenge cases have been reported [100]. Finally, a study involving 102 centers found a twofold increased risk of an acute NAION-like optic neuropathy occurring within five half-lives of the use of a PDE-5 inhibitor compared with use in a prior time period [101] and a similar multicenter study involving 279 men reported similar results [102]. On the other hand, a retrospective cohort study of four million male patients prescribed PDE-5 inhibitors showed no difference in the rate of development of an optic neuropathy compared with published rates of NAION [103]. In addition, a pharmaco-epidemiological nested case-control study in which 1109 cases of NAION were matched to 1,237,900 controls found no significant association with the use of PDE-5 inhibitors [104]. Having said this, there was a report of the development of an acute optic neuropathy in a child using sildenafil for chylothorax [105]. Other visual side effects of PDE-5 inhibitors include dose-dependent, reversible color vision problems (cyanopsia) and photophobia [106].

**Nutritional Deficiencies**

Nutritional optic neuropathies often are considered a subset of toxic optic neuropathies, with the clinical presentation being very similar; i.e., bilateral, subacute, and characterized by central or cecocentral scotomas. True nutritional optic neuropathies are rare and occur more commonly in developing countries. In the Western world, nutritional deficiencies often occur in the setting of chronic alcoholism, following bariatric surgery, and even in patients with severe depression resulting in a poor diet. Once identified, replacing the deficient nutrient and removing other offending agents may result in visual improvement, assuming that the patient does not have contributing genetic factors or other toxic insults [82] or that there has not been irreversible damage to the optic nerves. Vitamins B12, B1 (thiamine), and B2 (riboflavin), as well as folic acid (particularly in chronic alcoholics) and copper are commonly encountered deficiencies that can produce an optic neuropathy. Deficiencies in zinc and other fat-soluble vitamins (A, D, E) may also be seen, particularly after gastric bypass surgery, and have the potential to result in various neuropathies, including optic neuropathy [107]. When determining if a vitamin deficiency is the cause of an optic neuropathy, the clinical history is of critical importance. Vitamin levels in the serum may not be reliable in all cases. In particular, serum vitamin B12 levels may be falsely normal due to B12 binding transcobalamin [85], and red blood cell folate is a better indicator of folate levels than serum folate [108].

### The Role of Alcohol and Tobacco

Patients who consume large quantities of alcohol are, as noted above, at risk for developing a bilateral optic neuropathy [83]. Although previously termed "tobacco-alcohol amblyopia," this term is inappropriate. Firstly, the pathology is related to optic nerve injury and, thus, is not an "amblyopia" [109]. Secondly, there is absolutely no evidence to suggest cigarette smoking causes an optic neuropathy in otherwise healthy individuals who do not also consume alcohol heavily. In fact, the bilateral optic neuropathy that occurs in patients who abuse alcohol almost always is due not to the toxic effects of the alcohol (unless the individual is consuming methanol, see above) but to the vitamin deficencies that occur when alcohol abusers do not have an appropriate diet. Treatment thus is alcohol cessation combined with vitamin and folate supplementation. As in the case of other toxic and nutritional deficiencies, the prognosis for visual recovery is good it the diagnosis is made and treatment is commenced before irreversible damage to the optic nerve occurs.

## *Glaucoma and the Role of Cerebrospinal Fluid Pressure*

Primary open-angle glaucoma (POAG) is a leading cause of blindness worldwide [110]. Although elevated intraocular pressure (IOP) is commonly encountered and can be modified, not all patients with what appears to be typical POAG have elevated IOP [111]. Accordingly, other mechanisms for optic nerve damage that is consistent with POAG have been hypothesized. In particular, the role of CSF flow on the optic nerve in patients with so-called "normal-tension glaucoma" (NTG) has been raised. Three main mechanisms have been proposed to describe the role of ICP in NTG: (1) a barotraumatic phenomenon, (2) failure of CSF dynamics and (3) ocular glymphatic system dysfunction.

The barotraumatic theory of NTG hypothesizes that low ICP causes a clinical picture of glaucoma by inducing a high pressure gradient across the lamina cribrosa, ultimately damaging the optic nerve head [111]. Several studies using swept-source OCT indicate that the lamina cribrosa is the principal site where retinal ganglion cell axon insult occurs [112]. The lamina cribrosa provides structural and functional support to retinal ganglion cell axons as they go through the high-pressure environment in the eye to the low-pressure environment of the subarachnoid space surrounding the orbital optic nerve [113]. It is postulated that significant pressure changes in the intraocular space or the subarachnoid space has a potential to bio-mechanically injure the nerve through deformation of the laminar and optic nerve head biomechanics.

Another proposed mechanism for NTG includes that of failed CSF flow dynamics. The theory in this case is that low ICP leads to inadequate clearance of toxic substances from the CSF, causing optic nerve damage [114]. It is well-known that CSF circulation and turnover play an important role in the elimination of toxic substances from the CNS [115]. Because CSF turnover rate is directly proportional to the formation but inversely related to the volume, decreased CSF production may lead to decreased CSF turnover and, thus, allow for accumulation of biologically highly active toxic substances and ultimate neurotoxicity [110].

The third and most common proposed mechanism used to explain the development of what appears to be typical glaucomatous field and disc changes despite normal IOP involves the ocular glymphatics. The ocular glymphatic system consists of channels around the optic nerve and retina through which CSF is recirculated and neurotoxic metabolites are cleared. These channels have been found paravascularly, around the central retinal vein and central retinal artery [116]. A paravascular channel of the optic nerve has also been suggested and confirmed in studies of the optic nerves of mice [117]. It has been suggested that CSF flow along the perivascular space surrounding the central retinal artery into the anterior optic nerve and retina and then back along the perivascular space surrounding the central retinal vein into the subarachnoid space surrounding the optic nerve removes potentially toxic metabolites. If ICP is too low, CSF flow may stop or decline due to an increased pressure barrier. This, in turn, hinders paravascular flow from the optic nerve to retina, resulting in suppression of the glymphatic fluid system and toxin accumulation followed by glaucomatous optic neuropathy [110].

# Updates in Imaging

## New Imaging Sign in Multiple Sclerosis

The most recent imaging criteria by the Magnetic Resonance Imaging in MS (MAGNIMS) committee was published in 2015 [118]. Although brain MRI is a very sensitive test for diagnosing MS as well as for monitoring disease activity and treatment response, MRI spine is less sensitive [119, 120]. The typical MRI findings in MS include the presence of multiple focal white matter lesions and three or more of these lesions should involve the periventricular white matter [121]. In addition, however, an addition MRI sign, the central vein sign, has been suggested to differentiate MS from MS mimics [122, 123]. Pathologically, white matter lesions in MS correspond with inflammatory infiltrates that develop around venules. Using susceptibility-based MRI sequences, the association between brain white matter venules and perivenular lesions can be visualized. It has been found that the

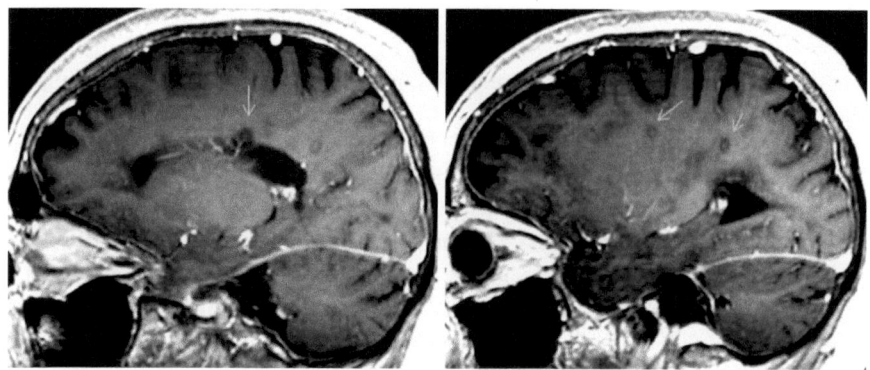

**Fig. 8.3** T2-FLAIR sequence showing the central vein sign in periventricular lesions in a patient with multiple sclerosis (Both images courtesy of Dr. David Poage, MD)

proportion of MS lesions with a central vein is high [122, 124] and when compared against other pathologies including CNS vasculopathies, the high frequency of perivenular lesions on MRI is pathologically specific for MS and, thus, important for improving the accuracy with which MS can be diagnosed [122, 123] (Fig. 8.3). It is important to note that the frequency of the central vein sign is the same for 1.5 and 3 T MRI machines and can be applied across the various phenotypes of MS [122].

## *Imaging Updates in Giant Cell Arteritis (GCA)*

Evidence-based recommendations for imaging in GCA (and other large vessel disease such as Takayasu Arteritis) were suggested by the European League against Rheumatism in May 2018 [125]. In particular, the League recommended that imaging with ultrasonography, MRI or both should be performed in patients in whom GCA is suspected, followed by temporal artery biopsy if the diagnosis is still in question after imaging and clinical examination. Imaging should be performed as early as possible after the initiation of therapy as glucocorticoid use may reduce the sensitivity of imaging [126, 127]. Ultrasonography is recommended as the first imaging test of choice in patients with GCA and predominantly cranial symptoms. The League specifically recommended imaging of the superficial temporal and axillary arteries; however, other authors also have included examination of the carotid, vertebral, occipital and subclavian arteries when possible [128]. The two imaging findings seen on ultrasound in patients with GCA include the "hypoechoic halo" and the "compression sign." The halo sign is due to homogenous, hypoechoic vessel wall thickening that is delineated toward the luminal side and visible in longitudinal and transverse planes [129]. The hypoechoic halo is thought to represent inflammation of the vessel wall. This sign was found to have a sensitivity of 77% and specificity of 96% in a systemic literature review where data was pooled from 43

**Fig. 8.4** High-resolution, T1-weighted, post-contrast MRI showing vascular mural enhancement in a patient with biopsy-proven giant cell arteritis (arrows). Note the central arterial flow void and the ragged infiltrative appearance around it. (Image courtesy of Dr. Andrew G. Lee and colleagues)

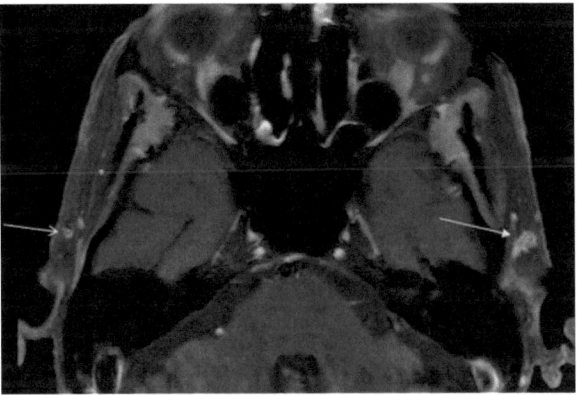

different studies [130]. The compression sign refers to continued visibility of the hypoechoic vessel wall while the ultrasound probe is used to apply pressure to the artery. This sign has been found to have a sensitivity of 77–79% and a specificity of 100% [125, 131]. In the event that ultrasound is inconclusive or simply is not available, the League recommended high-resolution scalp MRI of the cranial arteries—specifically, the temporal and occipital arteries—to assess for mural inflammation manifesting as mural contrast enhancement and arterial wall thickening (Fig. 8.4) [125]. One prospective cohort study of 170 patients with suspected GCA found MRI to be 93.6% sensitive and 77.9% specific in diagnosing patients with GCA [132]. It should be noted, however, that accurate identification of abnormal ultrasonographic and MRI findings is highly dependent on the individual performing the study in the case of ultrasound and on the individual interpreting the study in both cases. Other authors have raised the question as to what to do when imaging shows inflammation but temporal artery biopsy at the same location is negative. To date, there is no recommendation for how to handle this situation [128, 133].

New consensus criteria for the classification and diagnosis of GCA is expected to come out in 2019 via the Diagnostic and Classification Criteria in Vasculitis Study (DCVAS) and will replace the initial criteria created by the American College of Rheumatology in 1990s [134].

## Updates in Testing and Diagnostic Modalities

### *Myasthenia Gravis (MG) Antibodies (MuSK and LRP4)*

MG is an autoimmune disorder in which antibodies, primarily those to acetylcholine receptors, result in disruption of neuronal transmission at the neuromuscular junction. Clinical symptoms include skeletal muscle weakness and fatigability [135]. Ocular myasthenia gravis (OMG) refers to isolated involvement of the extraocular muscles and typically presents as double vision, ptosis, or both.

Approximately 60% of patients with MG have ptosis and/or diplopia at onset, and almost all patients with MG experience ocular symptoms at some point during their disease course [136]. In some cases, it is difficult to make the diagnoses of OMG based on clinical examination alone due to the potential for OMG to mimic ocular motor nerve palsies or brainstem motility deficits (eg, internuclear ophthalmoplegia) or even an ocular myopathy [137]. When the diagnosis cannot be made from the examination alone, the role of serum antibodies becomes important. For decades, antibody testing in MG was limited to the acetylcholine binding, blocking and modulating antibodies, with the binding antibody being the most frequently detected in both ocular and systemic MG [137]; however, although the presence of an elevated acetylcholine receptor antibody is highly specific for diagnosing OMG, these antibodies are typically positive in only half of all patients presenting with OMG [138]. This is in stark contrast to cases of generalized MG where seropositivity is reported to be as high as 85–90% [139–141]. Now, two new antibodies, LDL-related receptor-related protein 4 (LRP4) and Muscle-specific tyrosine kinase antibodies (MuSK) have been identified that may help to increase the diagnostic sensitivity of OMG.

LRP4 antibodies are thought to play a role in maintenance of the neuromuscular junction. During formation of the neuromuscular junction, LRP4 binds with agrin to form a complex that promotes acetylcholine receptor clustering and differentiation on the postsynaptic membrane by activation of MuSK. LRP4 antibodies have been found in 1–5% of all patients with MG and 7–33% of patients who are negative for acetylcholine antibodies and MuSK [136, 142, 143]. LRP4 positivity is more common in women than men and is associated with a mild disease course with only rare escalation to myasthenic crisis. Most importantly for the ophthalmologist, it can be present in patients with isolated ocular symptoms [136, 144–146]. The prevalence of OMG is similar in patients with acetylcholine antibodies and LRP4 antibodies [147]. Thus, an assay for LRP4 antibodies should be performed in patients for whom OMG is highly suspected but in whom acetylcholine receptor antibodies are negative [137].

MuSK antibodies cause a reduction in the postsynaptic density of acetylcholine receptors by binding to an extracellular domain [143, 148]. MuSK antibodies are present in 1–10% of all patients with MG [149, 150], with higher prevalence in the female gender and patients of Mediterranean descent [139, 145]. From 20 to 40% of patients with generalized MG but negative acetylcholine receptor antibodies will test positive for MuSK [143, 148]; however, they are rarely found in patients with OMG. One study found MuSK antibodies in only three of 82 patients with OMG [151, 152]. Nevertheless, in patients with MuSK-positive OMG, the ocular manifestations appear to be more symmetric and less fluctuating than typical MG [152]. Given the low diagnostic yield of MuSK in isolated OMG, it is recommended that this testing be reserved for patients with suspected MG despite negative acetylcholine receptor and LRP4 antibody testing [137]. A positive assay for MuSK antibody in patients with OMG has been associated with a high risk for early generalization [152, 153].

## Optical Coherence Tomography (OCT)

The use of OCT has rapidly escalated over the years since its initial invention in the 1990s [154]. This increased usage is directly correlated with improved knowledge of how OCT can be used for diagnosis and monitoring of various ophthalmic and neurologic conditions. By providing high-resolution structural information about the retina and optic nerve, OCT has become an imaging procedure that is routinely performed in ophthalmology clinics worldwide. Below, we review OCT findings in various neuro-ophthalmic disorders.

OCT can be useful in discerning the etiology of an optic neuropathy in a patient with glaucoma and other comorbidities. Glaucomatous optic neuropathy typically causes thinning in the superior and inferior quadrants of the disc, with temporal sparing, whereas many non-glaucomatous optic neuropathies tend to affect the papillomacular nerve fiber bundle, ultimately causing more temporal thinning in addition to super or inferior thinning [155]. In a patient presenting with an optic neuropathy and no visual acuity or field change, thinning on the OCT may be the only indication that there has been damage to the optic nerve.

### OCT in Optic Disc Elevation

Measurement of the RNFL by OCT may be useful in patients with PTC or other etiologies of disc swelling such as non-arteritic anterior ischemic optic neuropathy (NAION) to monitor improvement of the thickened RNFL [156] (Fig. 8.5). In addition, assessment of the position of the lamina cribrosa (bowed out vs bowed in) may be useful in differentiating local swelling from papilledema. Finally, in patients who present with an apparently elevated disc, OCT may help differentiate true disc swelling from congenital elevation (eg, pseudopapilledema). No change in OCT for several months after initial examination may provide reassurance that the disc elevation is congenital rather than acquired.

### OCT in Neurodegenerative Disease

Thinning of the RNFL and the ganglion cell/inner plexiform layer has been reported in various neurodegenerative diseases such as Alzheimer disease (AD), PD, Mild Cognitive impairment syndrome, and MS.

Alzheimer Disease: Although it has been established that there is some thinning of the RNFL in patients with AD and that progressive thinning correlates with disease progression, it is unclear if a specific quadrant of the nerve or specific layer of the retina is particularly susceptible [157] (Fig. 8.6). In OCT studies in patients with AD, the AD was not confirmed with pathology, thus giving room for similar diagnoses like vascular dementia or other dementia subtypes to be included, confounding the reported findings [157]. The future of OCT in patients with dementia is to learn

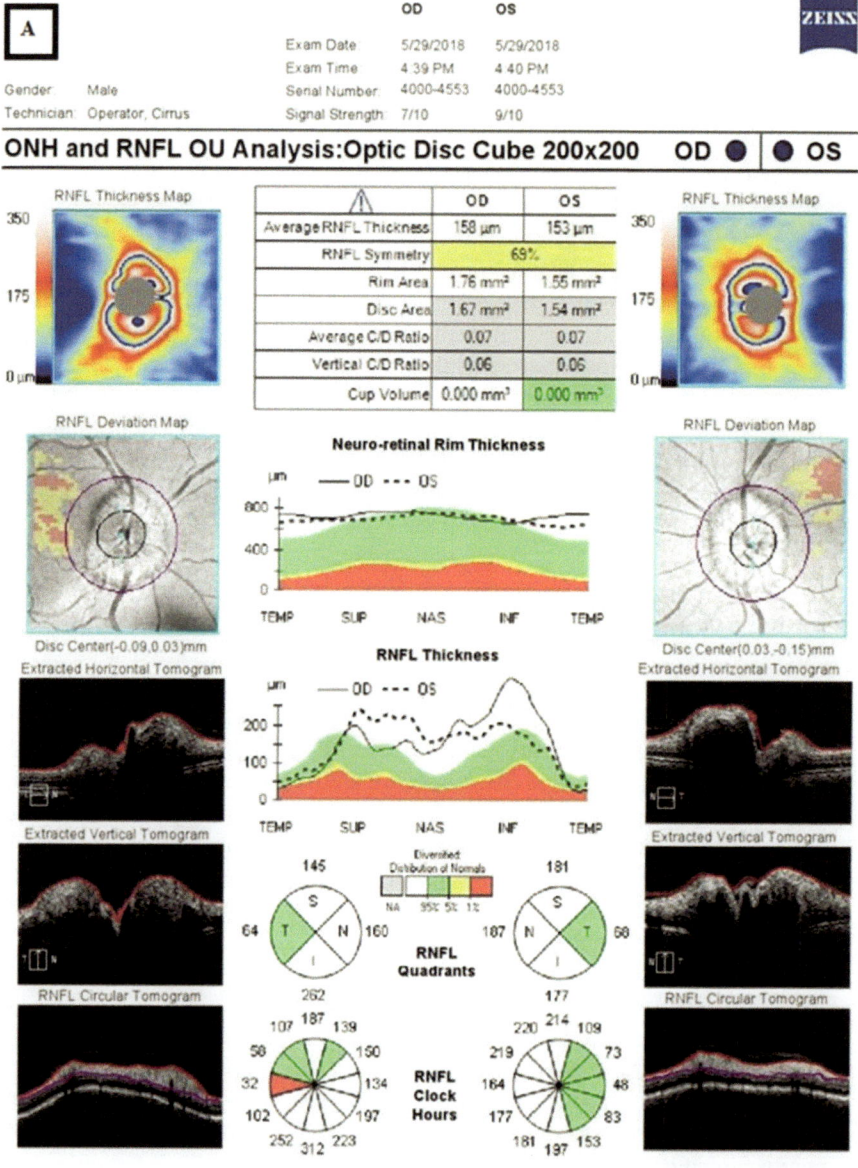

**Fig. 8.5** OCT in optic disc elevation before (**a**) and after (**b**) treatment with Diamox (Acetazolamide). The coinciding fundus photos showing significant papilledema before treatment (**c**), with improvement after treatment (**d**) are also shown

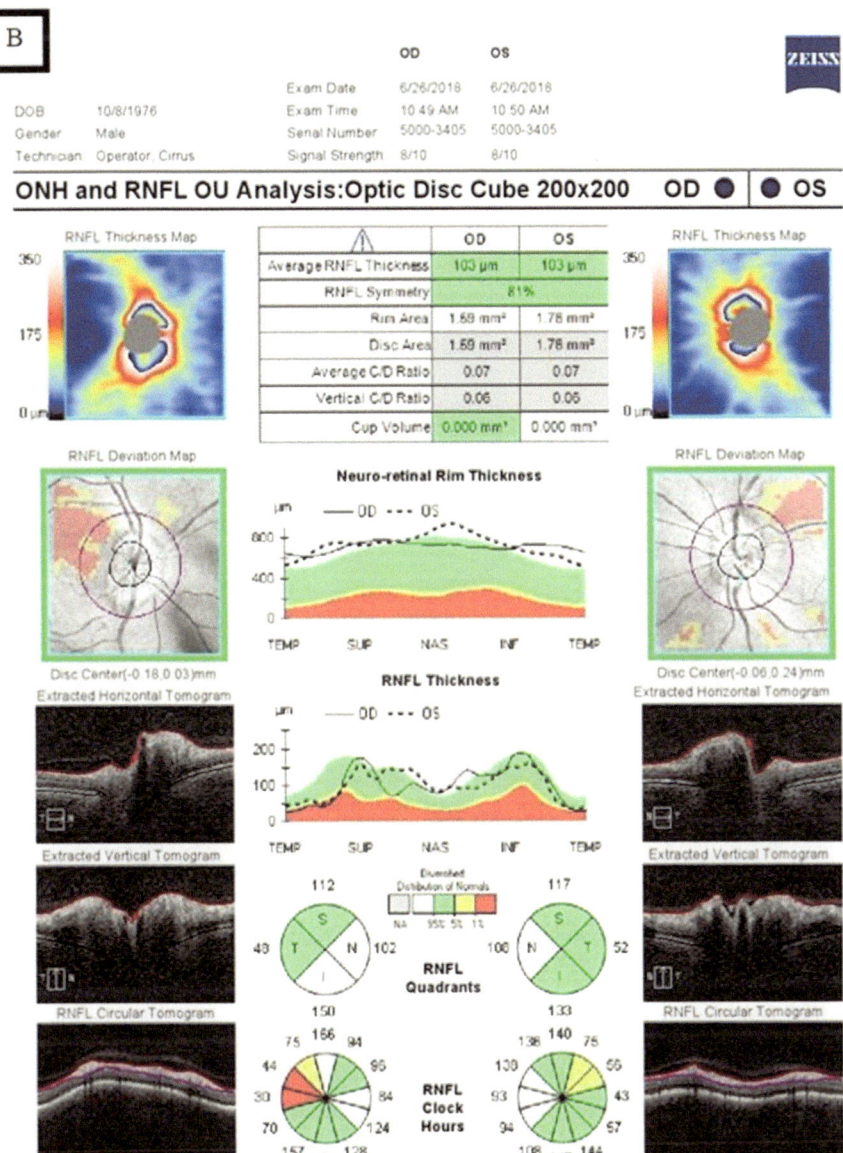

**Fig. 8.5** (continued)

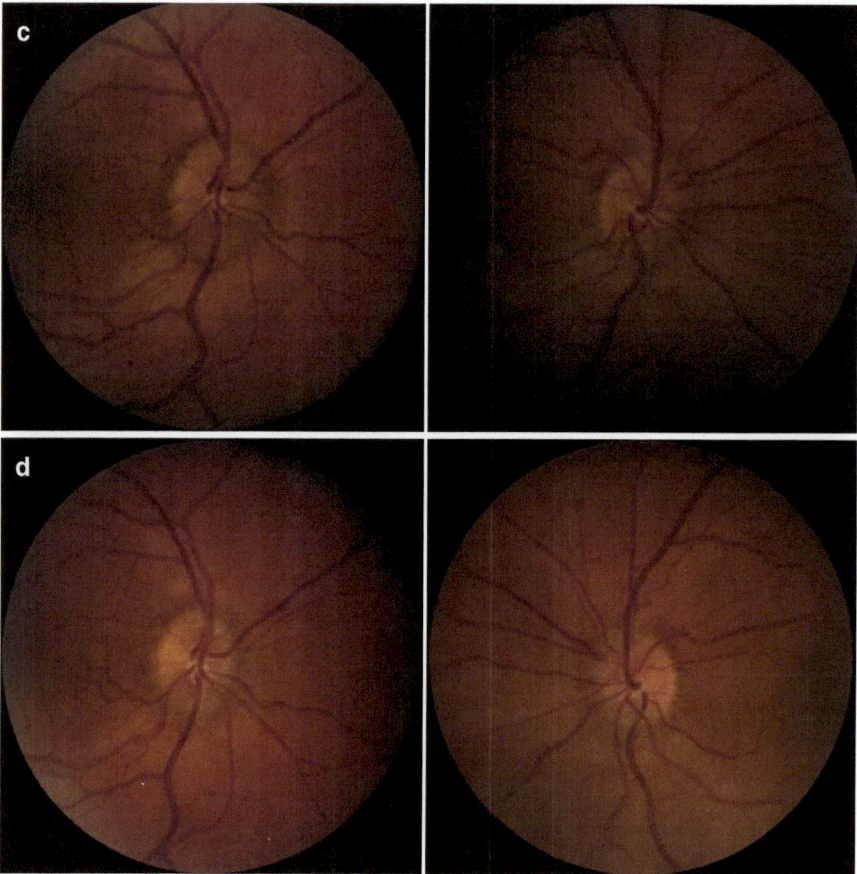

**Fig. 8.5** (continued)

if specific retinal or optic nerve changes point to a specific etiology. If this proves to be the case, it will allow OCT to be used as a diagnostic tool for patients with cognitive impairment.

MS: RNFL thinning and resultant optic nerve atrophy is a well-known and accepted marker of disease burden in patients with MS, even in cases in which there is no reported history of prior optic neuritis [158, 159]. There also have been reports of reduced macular volume at baseline without any reduction in RNFL thickness in patients with MS [160] as well as reduced central foveal area, all suggesting involvement of outer retinal layers [161]. OCT thus has become an important monitoring tool for MS and other etiologies of optic neuritis, helping to determine progression, prognosis, and need for modification of therapy. Its utility to differentiate MS from NMO, MOG and GFAP autoantibody disease remains poorly understood.

PD: Some studies have shown thinning of the RNFL contralateral to the side of motor symptoms in patients with PD [162], although this finding is controversial as there are other studies that have not shown thinning [163, 164]. Nevertheless, macular retinal thickness and the total macular volumes are reduced in PD, and the degree of macular thinning may correlate with disease progression and severity [165, 166], although further studies are needed to confirm this finding. Increased choroidal thickness on OCT was also observed in PD patients compared with unaffected controls [167]. The significance of this finding is unclear.

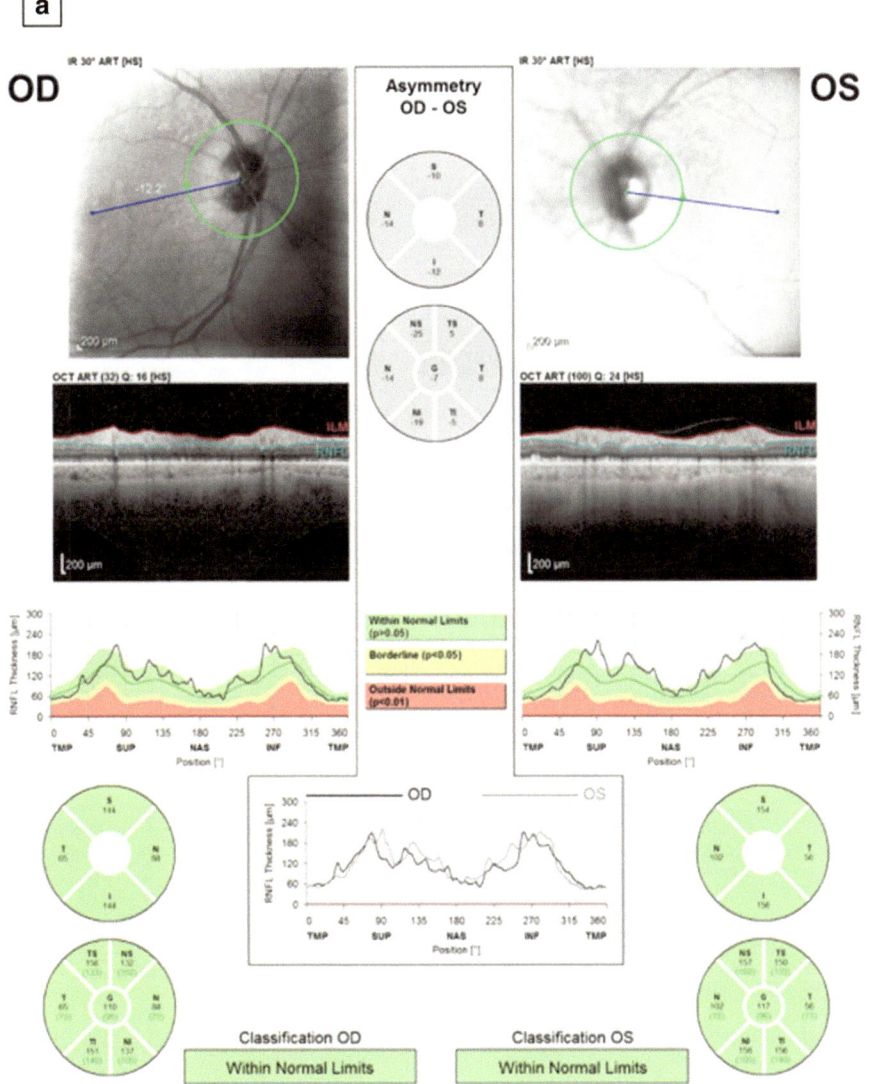

**Fig. 8.6** OCT in a patient with mild/moderate Alzheimer disease (AD). Compared with the OCT from a normal individual (**a**), the OCT in a patient with AD (**b**) shows mild but definite thinning of the peripapillary retinal nerve fiber layer in both the right and left eyes. (Images courtesy of Dr. Elizabeth Couser)

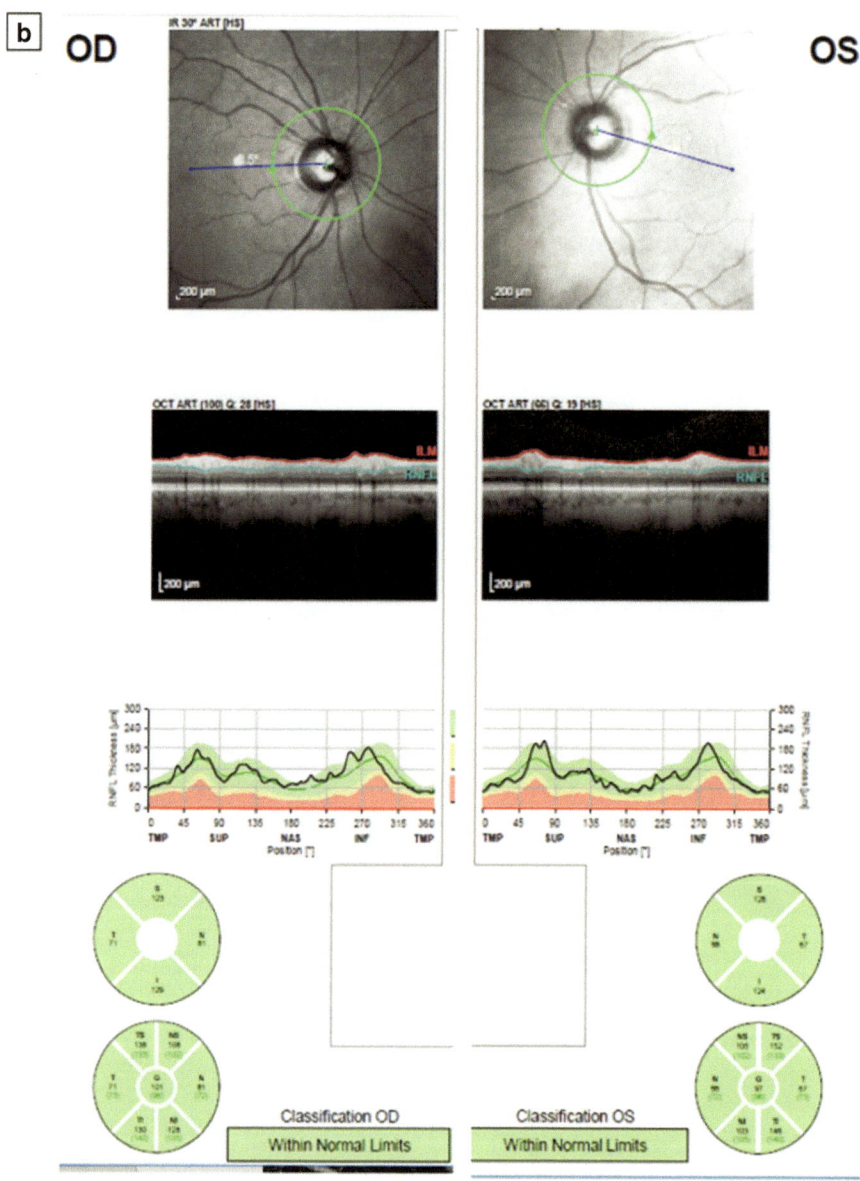

**Fig. 8.6** (continued)

## *Optical Coherence Tomography Angiography (OCTA)*

The addition of angiography to standard OCT (OCTA) has become a new area of interest in the evaluation of patients with optic neuropathies as well as neurologic conditions since it was introduced commercially in 2014 [168]. Although Doppler

OCT has been used to measure retinal blood flow in the past, it assesses only the axial component of blood flow velocity and is not sensitive to the slow, transverse blood flow in retinal, choroidal, and optic disc capillary networks as is possible with OCTA [169]. OCTA provides a three-dimensional motion-contrasted, cross-sectional image that is produced by the backscattering of light in the retinal vascular and neurosensory tissue as moving red blood cells are contrasted against static neurosensory tissue. Because OCTA uses the intrinsic contrast of moving red blood cells, no dye is needed [168]. The benefit is that one may obtain quantitative information about retinal vasculature using a non-invasive test. It also has been suggested that the imaging resolution obtained by these photos are "histology level" [170]. Clinical applications of OCTA in relation to neuro-ophthalmic conditions are discussed below:

## OCTA in Optic Neuropathies

Decreased peripapillary capillary density that correlates with RNFL thinning has been found using OCTA in patients with optic neuropathies. Although this may seem like an obvious observation in patients with ischemic optic neuropathies where circulation is the direct cause of the insult, decreased peripapillary capillary density also has been identified in patients with optic neuritis, traumatic optic neuropathy, autoimmune optic neuritis, compressive optic neuropathy (chiasmal compression) and Leber hereditary of optic neuropathy (LHON). In these cases, although ischemia is not the underlying cause, it has been suggested that optic nerve injury leads to subsequent RNFL loss with associated decrease in capillary flow. The suggested mechanism is that chronic injury to an optic nerve leads to a reduction in the number of nerve fibers that results in a decrease in metabolic demand and subsequent reduced capillary blood flow. The decreased peripapillary capillary density is a secondary consequence [171]. Clinically, OCTA may be helpful in differentiation of various etiologies of chronic optic neuropathy. Significant and profound peripapillary capillary loss relative to RNFL thinning may suggest an ischemic etiology such as anterior arteritic ischemic optic neuropathy (AAION) or NAION as opposed to, for example, optic neuritis (Fig. 8.7). Other causes of optic nerve compression and injury including chiasmal compression and optic disc drusen have been found to have decreased retinal perfusion on OCTA [171]. Studies are still lacking to determine if OCTA can be used to determine etiologies of optic neuropathy in an acute setting. Data regarding the influence of optic disc swelling on the measurements in OCTA remain poorly described.

## OCTA in Multiple Sclerosis

OCTA of the optic disc has revealed reduced flow index and vessel density in eyes of patients with MS, with and without a prior history of optic neuritis compared with normal subjects [172, 173]. Reports regarding macular OCTA changes in MS are inconsistent and inconclusive [174].

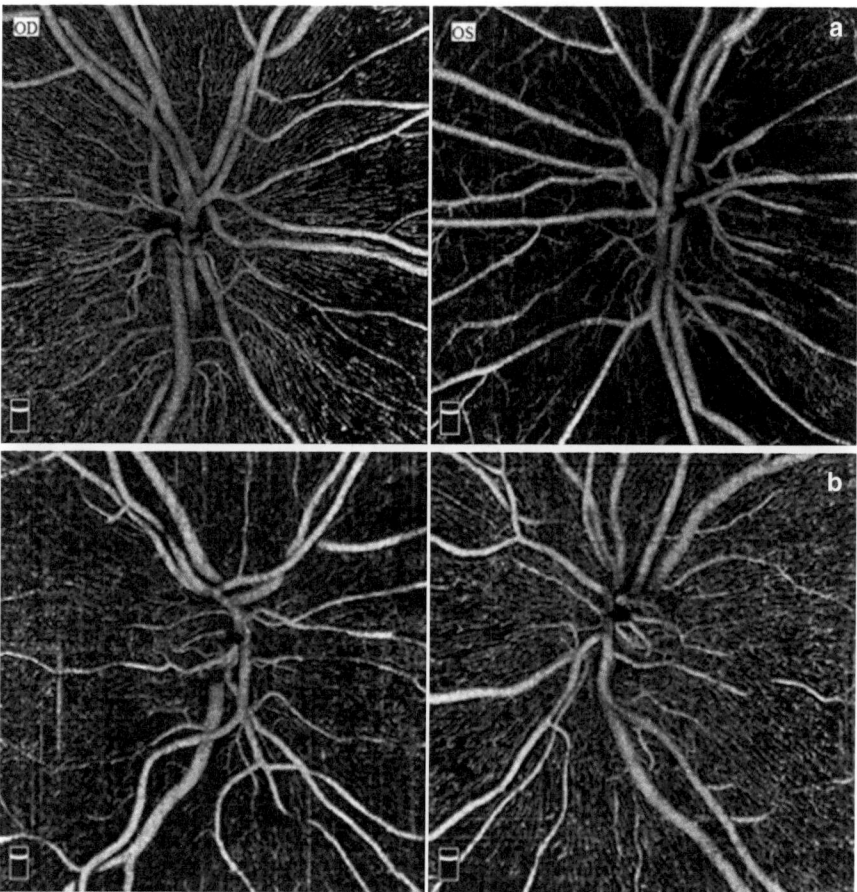

**Fig. 8.7** OCTA in non-arteritic ischemic optic neuropathy (NAION) in the **left eye** (**a**) and in chronic optic neuritis involving the **right eye** (**b**). Note that there is reduction in the disc and peripapillary vessel density in both pathologies. Although there is a reduction in peripapillary vascular density in all optic neuropathies, significant and profound peripapillary capillary loss relative to RNFL thinning may suggest an ischemic etiology. (Images courtesy of Dr. Amanda Henderson)

## OCTA in LHON

In some patients, OCTA has shown peripapillary telangiectatic blood vessels that were not visualized with fluorescein angiography [175]. A recent small study of six patients with LHON evaluated with OCTA (total 12 eyes) concluded that the peripapillary microvascular network in these patients is very abnormal, thus suggesting that there may be a contribution of microangiopathy to the vision loss in this population [176]. More recently, a study of optic nerve head and macular OCTAs in 15 patients with LHON (20 eyes compared with 20 controls) showed that changes in superficial and deep capillary plexi occur nasal and inferior to the optic disc, corresponding with the papillomacular bundle [177] (Fig. 8.8). The same study showed a significant correlation between reduction in the superficial capillary plexus vessel

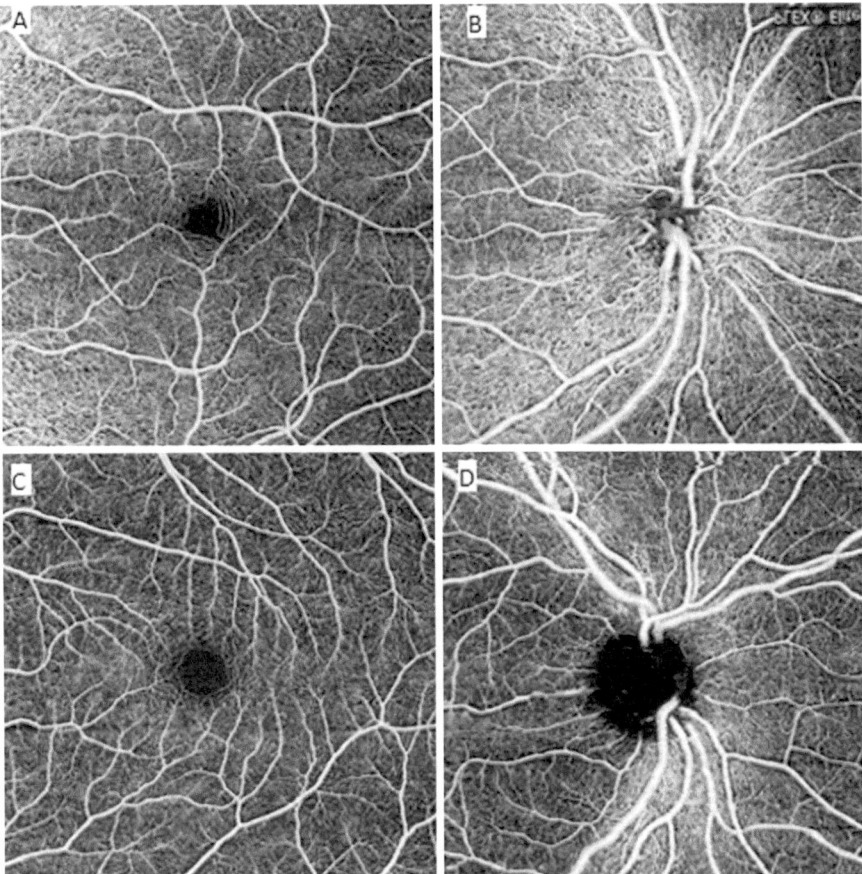

**Fig. 8.8** OCTA of the macula (**a**) and optic nerve head (**b**) in a 27-year-old woman with acute genetically proven LHON (11,778 mutation) 4 weeks after symptom onset. Note the increased perfusion of the vessels at the disc and macula, particularly on the nasal aspect which corresponds to the papillomacular bundle. This is in contrast to the OCTA in chronic LHON (6 months after symptom onset), where there is microvascular drop out in the macula (**c**) and atrophy of the superficial plexus of the optic disc (**d**). Pictures (**c**) and (**d**) are from a 15-year-old boy with LHON associated with the 14,484 mutation. (Images courtesy of Dr. Alfredo Sadun and Dr. William Sultan)

density an severity of vision loss measured by visual acuity. Of note, the authors also found no association between OCT-assessed structural changes (thinning of the retinal nerve fiber or ganglion cell layers) and best-corrected visual acuity.

## Updates in Treatment

Unfortunately, large-number, prospective, controlled studies are significantly lacking for many of the treatment and management updates in neuro-ophthalmology. Below we review several of the updated recommendations for various neuro-ophthalmic problems that are based primarily on systemic reviews and meta-analyses, with a few exceptions.

## *Treatment in Giant Cell Arteritis*

Giant Cell Arteritis (GCA) is a vasculitis that affects medium-to-large vessels and is an important cause of acute vision loss in neuro-ophthalmic patients over the age of 50. Previously, GCA was diagnosed by clinical examination, serum inflammatory markers (erythrocyte sedimentation rate, C-reactive protein, and platelets), and temporal artery biopsy (the gold standard for diagnosis). Although temporal artery biopsies may be used to may confirm the presence of GCA, a negative biopsy does not definitively exclude it due to the potential for inflammatory lesions to skip certain arteries or segments [128, 178].

Despite our increased ability to recognize GCA, treatment continues to be a challenge. For decades, management of GCA was limited to long courses of steroids and immunosuppressants that have debilitating side effects and do not secure a good outcome. In a landmark clinical trial, the GiACTA Trial, the drug tocilizumab was identified as the first non-corticosteroid agent with good efficacy for management of GCA [179]. Tocilizumab is an IL-6 inhibitor that works by reducing and inhibiting acute phase reactants contributing to inflammation. In the GiACTA trial, 251 patients with newly diagnosed or relapsed GCA were treated with either tocilizumab and steroids or placebo and steroids. This study was a double-blind, randomized controlled trial. The patients were divided in a 2:1:1:1 ratio among the following treatment regimens: weekly subcutaneous tocilizumab (162 mg) plus a 26-week prednisone taper, every-other-week subcutaneous tocilizumab (162 mg) and 26-week prednisone taper; weekly placebo +26-week prednisone taper and weekly placebo +52-week prednisone taper. Tocilizumab exhibited a marked steroid-sparing effect with a higher rate of sustained remission at 52 weeks compared with placebo. Of note, weekly dosing of tocilizumab was superior to every-other-week dosing. Overall, the cumulative prednisone dose in the tocilizumab group was significantly less than the amount used in the placebo group. No patient treated with weekly tocilizumab developed any permanent visual deficits, and quality of life measures were improved with tocilizumab compared with placebo. Tocilizumab was approved by the FDA in 2017, shortly after completion of this trial. The downside for the use of tocilizumab is that at this time, long-term follow-up is lacking for its use in GCA. Also, the high cost of this medication has led some physicians to resort to this medication only in cases where patients cannot tolerate long-term corticosteroid treatment or have failed corticosteroid treatment [128]. Of note, and in line with the new recommendations above regarding imaging in GCA, 46% of the patients in the GiACTA trial were diagnosed based on positive imaging rather than temporal artery biopsy. It should also be noted that although tocilizumab clearly has efficacy as an add-on treatment for GCA, no studies have been performed in which it has been used as a first-line treatment.

Abatacept is a CTLA-4 inhibitor that has been shown to be effective in GCA. In a small, randomized, placebo-controlled trial, 41 patients were treated with an induction course of abatacept 10 mg/kg intravenous with a 28-week prednisone taper. The patients were then divided into two groups, one of which went on to receive monthly treatment with abatacept and the other, placebo. The abatacept group showed a statistically higher rate of relapse-free survival (48% compared with 31%). One patient from the abatacept group had a visual event related to GCA that occurred 28 weeks after the initial induction [180].

## Ocrelizumab in Multiple Sclerosis

In March 2017, the FDA approved the drug ocrelizumab for the treatment for multiple sclerosis. This medication is the first to be approved for primary progressive MS and also is the first monoclonal antibody approved for use in secondary progressive MS. Ocrelizumab is an anti-CD20 antibody that has been evaluated in phase II and III trials and found to lower disability progression and improve radiologic and relapse-related outcomes compared with placebo in patients with MS [181].

## Treatment for Optic Pathway Gliomas and Optic Nerve Sheath Meningiomas

### Optic Pathway Gliomas

Falsini et al. performed a randomized, double-masked, phase II clinical trial in 17 patients with optic pathway gliomas and stable visual function and imaging [182]. Patients received either a 10-day course of 0.5 mg murine nerve growth factor (NGF) or placebo (10 NGF/8 placebo). Patients were evaluated clinically (visual acuity, visual field), by imaging (OCT, MRI), and by electrophysiological testing (visual evoked potentials and photopic negative responses) before therapy and at 15, 30, 90, and 180 days after therapy. There were no adverse effects from the treatment and all patients who received NGF showed statistically significant improvements in all parameters.

### Optic Nerve Sheath Meningiomas

It has become increasingly clear that the appropriate management of an optic nerve sheath meningioma (ONSM) for patients who require intervention because of progressive visual loss is stereotactic fractionated or conformal radiation therapy (FCRT). Pandit et al. performed a retrospective chart review with prospective follow-up of adult patients treated with FCRT for primary ONSM at four academic medical centers between 1995 and 2007 with ≥10 years of follow-up after treatment [183]. They identified 16 patients with mean post-treatment follow-up of 14.6 years; (range: 10.5–20.7 years). The mean age at symptom onset was 47.6 years (range: 36–60 years). FCRT was performed at a mean of 2.3 years after symptom onset (range: 0.2–14.0 years). At last follow-up, visual acuity had improved or stabilized in 14 of the 16 (88%) patients, and 11 (69%) had retained or achieved ≥20/40. Mean deviation on automated perimetry remained stable ($-14.5$ dB pre-treatment vs. $-12.2$ dB at last follow-up; $p = 0.68$; $n = 10$). Two (11%) patients had persistent pain, proptosis, or diplopia, compared with seven (44%) pre-treatment ($p = 0.11$). Two (13%) patients developed radiation retinopathy more than 6 months after completion of therapy, one (50%) of whom had worse VA compared with pre-treatment. No patient developed tumor involvement or radiation damage in the fellow eye. Based on these findings, the authors concluded that FCRT stabilizes or improves visual function in most patients with primary ONSM and is associated with a low risk of significant ocular sequelae. We agree that this treatment should be considered instead of surgery in patients with primary ONSM who require intervention because of significant or progressive visual loss.

## Leber Hereditary Optic Neuropathy (LHON)

LHON is a well-known mitochondrial disorder and is an important cause of hereditary optic nerve-related permanent vision loss. LHON should be suspected in a young male with subacute vision loss and a maternal family history of similar vision loss [184]. Clinical examination findings are similar to those of other mitochondrial optic neuropathies and include variably reduced visual acuity, impaired color vision, and central or cecocentral scotomas. At onset, the optic discs may appear normal or hyperemic with telangiectatic vessels on the disc surface and in the peripapillary region. Eventually, optic disc pallor occurs that usually is more profound temporally than nasally Diagnosis is confirmed by gene testing for one of the three most common mitochondrial DNA mutations: 11778G>A/MT-ND4, 3460G>A/MT-ND1 and 14484T>C/MT-ND6. These three mutations account for about 90% of cases, however, if this screen is negative and there is a high suspicion for LHON based on the clinical picture, entire mitochondrial genome sequencing should be pursued to identify other rare mutations [144, 184].

There currently is no consistently beneficial treatment for LHON. The drug idebenone is the main intervention for preventing visual deterioration in LHON when administered in the acute or subacute phase of the disorder. More recent treatment options being evaluated are adeno-associated viral vector-based gene therapy and mitochondrial replacement therapy.

### Idebenone

LHON is the first mitochondrial disease for which a treatment has been approved by the European Medicine Agency. The approved treatment is idebenone which has been used empirically since 1992 [185]. Idebenone is a short-chain benzoquinone with antioxidant properties. It carries mitochondrial electrons to complex III of the mitochondrion and directly promotes ATP production, ultimately activating ganglion cells of the retina with resulting visual recovery [186]. The therapeutic benefit of idebenone has been evaluated through a placebo-controlled randomized clinical trial [187] and a large retrospective case series [186]. In 2016, an international consensus statement on the clinical and therapeutic management in LHON was put forth by a panel of world experts [184]. The consensus recommendation for therapeutic management in LHON is to initiate idebenone as soon as possible at a dose of 900 mg/day in patients with symptom onset of less than 1 year and to continue the treatment for 1 year. They panel did not find evidence to suggest the use of idebenone in patients with chronic disease.

## Gene Therapy

The mutations generated in LHON affect mitochondrial genome complex I of the electron transport chain and typically involve a single amino acid exchange [188]. The goal of gene therapy in LHON is to replace the missing protein product. In the case of the LHON 11778G>A mutation, this pertains to missing ND4 (mitochondrial encoded NADH:ubiquinone oxidoreductase core subunit 4). Genetically modified adeno-associated viral vectors (AAV2) have been developed to deliver a mitochondrial ND4 gene construct either into the mitochondrial matrix compartment [189] or into the nuclear genome [190] to compensate for the 11778G>A mutation [191]. It has yet to be determined if these modified ND4 subunits will integrate smoothly into complex 1 and be stable enough to allow the electron transport chain to run efficiently [192]; however, preliminary data from clinical trials have supported the safety of AAV2-based gene therapy vectors and have found some visual improvement in eyes treated by intravitreal injection of the vector [193–195]. Clinical trials to establish efficacy are ongoing.

## Mitochondrial Replacement Therapy (MRT)

MRT is being studied with the goal of completely replacing mutated mitochondria with normal mitochondria to prevent maternal transmission of mitochondrial DNA mutations. This is done by reproductive technologies that allow for uncoupling of the mitochondrial DNA from nuclear DNA [196] such that only the mitochondrial part of the DNA comes from a donor [197]. Parental nuclear material is transferred into a mitochondrial donor zygote carrying wild-type mitochondrial DNA to minimize or eliminate carryover of mutant DNA. Preliminary results are promising and may pave the way for eliminating the transmission of mutated maternal mitochondrial DNA in the future [196, 198].

## *Visual Restoration Therapy*

The reported number of patients suffering from vision loss after stroke, either hemorrhagic or ischemic, ranges from 45 to 92% in the acute setting and from 8 to 25% chronically [199–201]. Although both efferent and afferent pathways may be affected by stroke, homonymous hemianopia is the most common visual field deficit occurring after stroke [200, 202]. Homonymous hemianopias often are debilitating, leaving a patient symptomatic for years [199]. Although 50% of patients with homonymous hemianopia from a stroke may show some degree of improvement, complete resolution is seen in only 8–12% of patients [201].

The benefit of several types of proposed visual rehabilitation after stroke continues to be a controversial topic of discussion among ophthalmologists and neurologists. Proposed interventions for visual restoration include the use of prisms to expand the area of good vision, saccadic exploration to explore the blind hemifield, and restorative therapy to bring attention to the border between the seeing and non-seeing area in an effort to increase the area of vision [202]. Unfortunately, none of the prospective studies evaluating these interventions has been double blind and controlled, and the results have been inconclusive. For example, in patients who have undergone visual restoration therapy, there is no correlation between improvement in visual field and improved ability to perform daily activities. Some patients have reported improved daily activities despite no change in their field defect and some patients with an apparent visual field improvement has reported no improvement in their ability to perform daily activities. In addition, even when patients have reported improvement in quality of life, when asked to draw what they perceive to be the area of their scotoma after visual restoration therapy, there was no statically significant change in the area of vision loss when compared with what was drawn at baseline [203]. On the other hand, functional MRI and magnetoencephalography studies performed after visual stimulation activities (although without a control) have suggested there may be some plasticity contributing to visual recovery and visual training; however, the utility of these imaging findings in the absence of evidence to support retinotopic reorganization is limited [202, 204, 205].

Researchers have suggested various theoretical mechanisms for apparent visual recovery. These mechanisms include activation of uninjured but suboptimally activated occipital cortex, bypassing damaged cortex, changes in neuronal chemistry and sprouting of new connections to name a few [206–208]. Alternatively, it has been suggested that the apparent visual recovery is actually due to unstable fixation. It is hoped that with an increased theoretical understanding of visual rehabilitation, new and reliable clinical therapies are on the horizon.

## *Endovascular Intervention Updates*

Neuro endovascular intervention has become important in the world of neuro-ophthalmology due to intersections in management [209]. This intersection includes strokes, aneurysms, CNS vasculitis, and venous sinus stenting for pseudotumor cerebri (PTC) to name a few. Neuroendovascular intervention provides an additional avenue to aid in diagnosis and management of vision-related problems; however, the treatment itself may cause adverse visual events in some cases. Below we review a few of the scenarios where neuro-ophthalmology and neuro-intervention intersect.

**Aneurysms**

Aneurysms are a common cause of neuro-ophthalmic referrals. Common complaints related to aneurysm compression or rupture include double vision from ocular motor nerve palsy, pupillary changes, visual pathway disorders and compressive chiasmopathy or optic neuropathy [210]. Compression of the structures that comprise the afferent and efferent visual pathways suggests a large and probably unstable aneurysm, the diagnosis and treatment of which is crucial in preventing major permanent visual and/or neurological deficits as well as death [210]. As neuroendovascular intervention evolves as a treatment for aneurysms at risk for rupture, it is important that ophthalmologists and neurologists understand the mechanism of treatment and the potential adverse effects. Neuroendovascular aneurysmal repair involves endoluminal reconstruction. This refers to the use of a stenting devise to redirect flow away from an aneurysmal sac or outpouching while endothelial ingrowth around the stent leads to remodeling of the vessel lumen. In cases where a stent may not be appropriate, usually determined by aneurysm architecture, detachable platinum coils may be used to embolize the aneurysm outpouching [209]. Figure 8.9 below provides an example of a coiled aneurysm, before and after coiling. Adverse events from endovascular treatment include headaches, problems related to compression from mass effect of the thrombosed aneurysm, and intraprocedural rupture [209]. Aneurysms located near the skull base have been noted to swell often which causes stretching of the dura and pain. In one case report, mass effect from a repaired anterior cerebral artery aneurysm caused optic tract edema with unilateral vision loss and a homonymous field cut [211]. In this case, the patient was treated with high-dose steroids with near-complete recovery. A meta-analysis of 13 retrospective studies encompassing 477 patients compared visual outcomes of aneurysm repair by surgical clipping with endovascular coiling [210]. Complete recovery after each procedure reached 78% in the surgical group versus 44% in the endovascular group. Similar findings were observed when comparing recovery rate specifically for cranial neve palsies. Surgical intervention also results in improvement of visual field deficits from anterior visual pathway compression. It must be emphasized, however, that surgical intervention is associated with higher complication rates, longer stays in the intensive care unit, and higher hospital costs compared with endovascular intervention. Decision for neurovascular versus surgical approach is highly influenced by location (experience of the operator in a high volume versus low volume institution) and aneurysm architecture.

Griessenauer et al. treated 127 consecutive patients with 160 ophthalmic segment aneurysms using flow diverters [212]. In this cohort, complete occlusion of the aneurysm was observed in 90 of 101 (89%) cases with a mean follow-up of 18 months. Of ten patients with visual symptoms, one had immediate improvement in visual function. Among 117 patients without visual symptoms, two (1.6%) experienced visual impairment following treatment. There was no mortality related to the procedure, but, in addition to the two patients who experienced visual impairment post-procedure, two developed a permanent neurological deficit (hemiplegia). Based on their experience in this large series, the authors concluded that treatment of ophthalmic segment aneurysms with flow diversion is a safe and effective procedure compared with clipping. Several of the same authors participated in a two-center retrospective cohort study of consecutively treated ophthalmic segment aneurysms that compared stent-assisted coil embolization with flow diversion [213]. Sixty-two aneurysms were treated with stent-coiling and 106 were treated with flow diversion. The authors found that stent-coiling and flow diversion were equally effective in treating these aneurysms and that there were no significant differences in procedural complications or in angiographic, functional, or visual outcomes. In fact, in this series, no patient with stent-coiling had a permanent visual complication whereas only one patient in the flow diversion series had permanent visual loss.

For the efferent visual system, the issue relates to third nerve palsy recovery after treatment of ruptured and unruptured internal carotid-posterior communicating (PCom) aneurysms. [214] described the effect of endovascular treatment of 34 patients with third nerve palsy associated with a ruptured PCom aneurysm. At 6-month follow-up, 21 (61.8%) had experienced complete recovery of their palsy whereas 8 (23.5%) had incomplete recovery. The mean time to resolution was 24.5 days. As might be expected, there was a trend toward complete recovery among patients with an initially incomplete palsy. No patient in this series had post-operative worsening of an incomplete palsy. Hall et al. described the effect of treatment of unruptured PCom aneurysms on resolution of third nerve palsy [215]. These authors reported their experience with 15 patients and provided a narrative review of 179 patients from 31 case reports or cohort studies. Based on their experience and literature review, they concluded that surgical clipping was associated with a higher rate of recovery than was endovascular treatment. Again, patients who presented with a complete palsy had a lower rate of recovery than did those with a partial palsy.

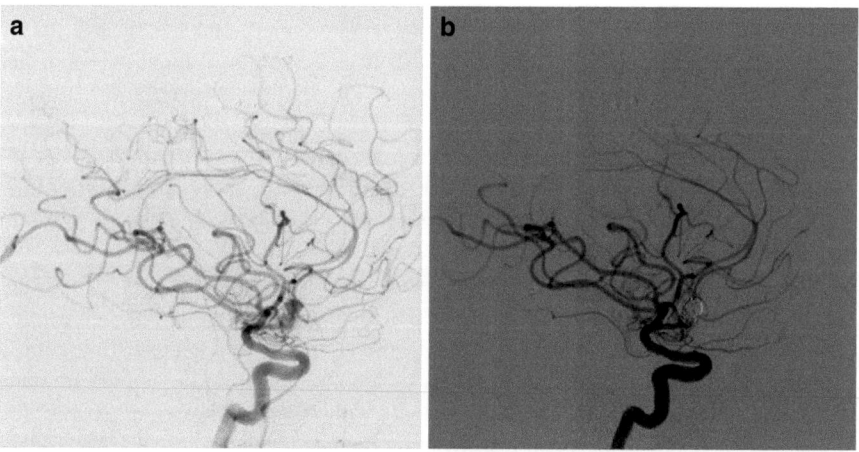

**Fig. 8.9** Cather angiogram imaged showing an Anterior communicating artery aneurysm, (**a**) before and (**b**) after coiling. After coiling, there may be compression of neighboring brain tissue or blood vessels from the coil mass. (Pictures courtesy of Dr. Michael Pichler, MD)

## Venous Sinus Stenting in Primary Pseudotumor Cerebri (PTC)

Various institutions across the world have begun implementing venous sinus stenting as a therapy for medically refractory pseudotumor cerebri (PTC) and, in some cases, first-line therapy (Fig. 8.10). Liu et al. described ten patients with PTC and venous sinus stenosis with an elevated gradient across the region of stenosis (30.0 ± 13.2 mmHg) and elevated ICP (42.2 ± 15.9 mmHg) for whom medical therapy had failed and who subsequently underwent venous sinus stenting [216]. Following stent placement, all patients had resolution of the stenosis and gradient (1 ± 1 mmHg). More importantly, however, the authors monitored ICP throughout the procedure and noted an immediate decrease in ICP following placement of the stent (17.0 ± 8.3 mmHg) with a further decrease overnight. This publication and another by Matloob et al. confirm the immediate effects of venous sinus stenting on ICP in this group of patients [217]. Another prospective observational study that consisted of 13 patients with venous sinus stenosis, visual field changes, and medically refractory, medically intolerant or fulminant PTC also concluded that venous sinus stenting is a safe and immediately effective method of reducing intracranial pressure (ICP) in PTC [218]. This study also reported improvement in headache and other associated symptoms of PTC, as well as reduction or resolution of papilledema, resolution of RNFL thickness, and improvement in visual field as measured by mean deviation using automated perimetry. A number of other series with smaller groups of patients also have reported successful stenting and resolution of increased ICP and associated symptoms [219]. Several recent retrospective literature reviews, systematic reviews and meta-analyses of patients undergoing venous sinus stenting for medically refractory PTC conclude that stenting has high technical success and low complication rates in appropriately selected patients [220–222]. Recommendations on the appropriate selection of patients also have been suggested based on literature review [222]. This obviously is an important consideration for those patients who present with evidence of optic nerve dysfunction and for whom a decision must be made regarding performing immediate optic nerve sheath decompression, and/or drainage of cerebrospinal fluid.

Despite the enthusiasm for venous sinus stenting for patients with PTC and venous sinus stenosis, a recent single-center case series of 41 patients studied clinical, radiological and manometric outcomes 120 days after venous sinus stenting [223]. Although the results from this study supported prior findings of reduced venous sinus pressure and lower complication rates compared with shunting at 120 days, at least 20% of the patients developed restenosis and only 63.3% of patients showed improvement or resolution of papilledema. This raises a question regarding the long-term viability and clinical outcomes of venous sinus shunting. Ultimately, prospective, randomized controlled studies designed to assess long-term outcomes and complications of stenting for PTC will be required to determine if venous sinus stenting provides sufficient long-term benefit to become the procedure of choice in patients with PTC and venous sinus stenosis.

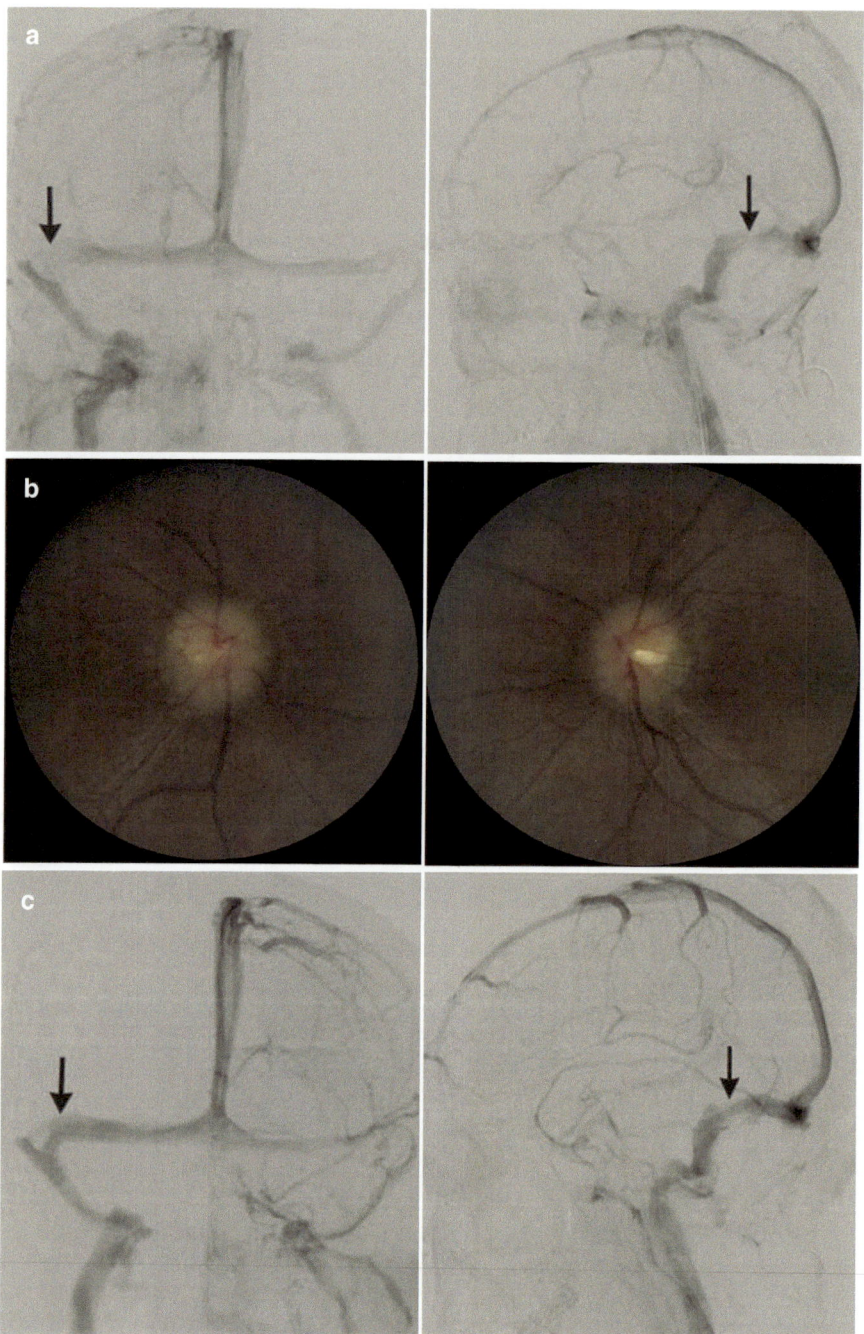

**Fig. 8.10** Fundus photos and coinciding MR venogram images in a patient with Pseudotumor Cerebri and venous sinus stenosis; (**a**) venous sinus stenosis seen on MR venogram; (**b**) fundus photos showing papilledema prior to sinus stenting; (**c**) venous sinus now open after endovascular stenting; (**d**) improved papilledema

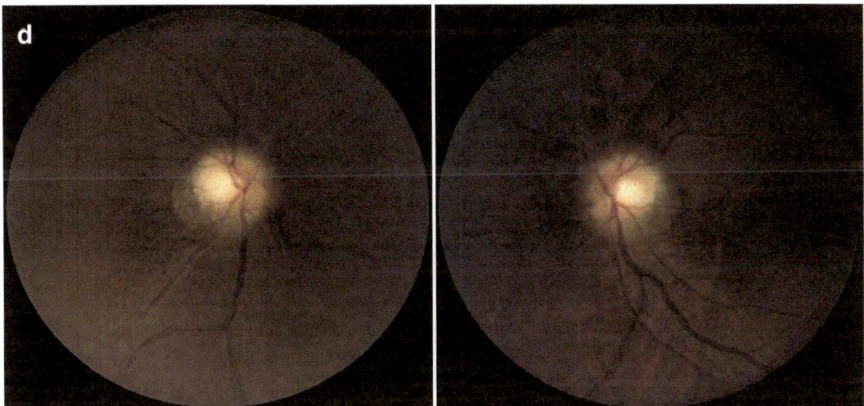

**Fig. 8.10**  (continued)

# References

1. Oost W, Talma N, Meilof JF, Laman JD. Targeting senescence to delay progression of multiple sclerosis. J Mol Med. 2018;96(11):1153–66. https://doi.org/10.1007/s00109-018-1686-x.
2. Bove RM, Hauser SL. Diagnosing multiple sclerosis: art and science. Lancet Neurol. 2018;17(2):109–11. https://doi.org/10.1016/S1474-4422(17)30461-1.
3. Zabad RK, Stewart R, Healey KM. Pattern recognition of the multiple sclerosis syndrome. Brain Sci. 2017;7(10):E138. https://doi.org/10.3390/brainsci7100138.
4. McDonald WI, Compston A, Edan G, Goodkin D, Hartung HP, Lublin FD, et al. Recommended diagnostic criteria for multiple sclerosis: guidelines from the International Panel on the diagnosis of multiple sclerosis. Ann Neurol. 2001;50(1):121–7.
5. Thompson AJ, Banwell BL, Barkhof F, Carroll WM, Coetzee T, Comi G, et al. Diagnosis of multiple sclerosis: 2017 revisions of the McDonald criteria. Lancet Neurol. 2018;17(2):162–73. https://doi.org/10.1016/s1474-4422(17)30470-2.
6. Seay M, Galetta S. Glial fibrillary acidic protein antibody: another antibody in the multiple sclerosis diagnostic mix. J Neuroophthalmol. 2018;38(3):281–4. https://doi.org/10.1097/wno.0000000000000689.
7. Bizzoco E, Lolli F, Repice AM, Hakiki B, Falcini M, Barilaro A, et al. Prevalence of neuro-myelitis optica spectrum disorder and phenotype distribution. J Neurol. 2009;256(11):1891–8. https://doi.org/10.1007/s00415-009-5171-x.
8. Stellmann JP, Krumbholz M, Friede T, Gahlen A, Borisow N, Fischer K, et al. Immunotherapies in neuromyelitis optica spectrum disorder: efficacy and predictors of response. J Neurol Neurosurg Psychiatry. 2017;88(8):639–47. https://doi.org/10.1136/jnnp-2017-315603.
9. Lennon VA, Wingerchuk DM, Kryzer TJ, Pittock SJ, Lucchinetti CF, Fujihara K, et al. A serum autoantibody marker of neuromyelitis optica: distinction from multiple sclerosis. Lancet. 2004;364(9451):2106–12. https://doi.org/10.1016/s0140-6736(04)17551-x.
10. Jarius S, Wildemann B, Paul F. Neuromyelitis optica: clinical features, immunopathogenesis and treatment. Clin Exp Immunol. 2014;176(2):149–64. https://doi.org/10.1111/cei.12271.
11. Jung JS, Preston GM, Smith BL, Guggino WB, Agre P. Molecular structure of the water channel through aquaporin CHIP. The hourglass model. J Biol Chem. 1994;269(20):14648–54.

12. Wingerchuk DM, Banwell B, Bennett JL, Cabre P, Carroll W, Chitnis T, et al. International consensus diagnostic criteria for neuromyelitis optica spectrum disorders. Neurology. 2015;85(2):177–89. https://doi.org/10.1212/WNL.0000000000001729.
13. Ketelslegers IA, Modderman PW, Vennegoor A, Killestein J, Hamann D, Hintzen RQ. Antibodies against aquaporin-4 in neuromyelitis optica: distinction between recurrent and monophasic patients. Mult Scler. 2011;17(12):1527–30. https://doi.org/10.1177/1352458511412995.
14. Narayan R, Simpson A, Fritsche K, Salama S, Pardo S, Mealy M, et al. MOG antibody disease: a review of MOG antibody seropositive neuromyelitis optica spectrum disorder. Mult Scler Relat Disord. 2018;25:66–72. https://doi.org/10.1016/j.msard.2018.07.025.
15. Brunner C, Lassmann H, Waehneldt TV, Matthieu JM, Linington C. Differential ultrastructural localization of myelin basic protein, myelin/oligodendroglial glycoprotein, and 2',3'-cyclic nucleotide 3'-phosphodiesterase in the CNS of adult rats. J Neurochem. 1989;52(1):296–304.
16. Berger T, Rubner P, Schautzer F, Egg R, Ulmer H, Mayringer I, et al. Antimyelin antibodies as a predictor of clinically definite multiple sclerosis after a first demyelinating event. N Engl J Med. 2003;349(2):139–45. https://doi.org/10.1056/NEJMoa022328.
17. Reindl M, Linington C, Brehm U, Egg R, Dilitz E, Deisenhammer F, et al. Antibodies against the myelin oligodendrocyte glycoprotein and the myelin basic protein in multiple sclerosis and other neurological diseases: a comparative study. Brain. 1999;122(11):2047–56. https://doi.org/10.1093/brain/122.11.2047.
18. Kuhle J, Pohl C, Mehling M, Edan G, Freedman MS, Hartung H-P, et al. Lack of association between antimyelin antibodies and progression to multiple sclerosis. N Engl J Med. 2007;356(4):371–8. https://doi.org/10.1056/NEJMoa063602.
19. Mader S, Gredler V, Schanda K, Rostasy K, Dujmovic I, Pfaller K, et al. Complement activating antibodies to myelin oligodendrocyte glycoprotein in neuromyelitis optica and related disorders. J Neuroinflammation. 2011;8(1):184. https://doi.org/10.1186/1742-2094-8-184.
20. Hamid SM, Whittam D, Saviour M, et al. Seizures and encephalitis in myelin oligodendrocyte glycoprotein igg disease vs aquaporin 4 igg disease. JAMA Neurol. 2018;75(1):65–71. https://doi.org/10.1001/jamaneurol.2017.3196.
21. Jitprapaikulsan J, Chen JJ, Flanagan EP, Tobin WO, Fryer JP, Weinshenker BG, et al. Aquaporin-4 and myelin oligodendrocyte glycoprotein autoantibody status predict outcome of recurrent optic neuritis. Ophthalmology. 2018;125(10):1628–37. https://doi.org/10.1016/j.ophtha.2018.03.041.
22. Zhou Y, Jia X, Yang H, Chen C, Sun X, Peng L, et al. Myelin oligodendrocyte glycoprotein (MOG) antibody-associated demyelination: comparison between onset phenotypes. Eur J Neurol. 2019;26(1):175–83. https://doi.org/10.1111/ene.13791.
23. Chen JJ, Flanagan EP, Jitprapaikulsan J, Lopez-Chiriboga ASS, Fryer JP, Leavitt JA, et al. Myelin oligodendrocyte glycoprotein antibody (MOG-IgG)-positive optic neuritis: clinical characteristics, radiologic clues and outcome. Am J Ophthalmol. 2018;195:8–15. https://doi.org/10.1016/j.ajo.2018.07.020.
24. Narayan RN. Atypical anti-MOG syndrome with aseptic meningoencephalitis and pseudotumor cerebri-like presentations. Mult Scler Relat Disord. 2018;27:30–3. https://doi.org/10.1016/j.msard.2018.10.003.
25. Chalmoukou K, Alexopoulos H, Akrivou S, Stathopoulos P, Reindl M, Dalakas MC. Anti-MOG antibodies are frequently associated with steroid-sensitive recurrent optic neuritis. Neurol Neuroimmunol Neuroinflamm. 2015;2(4):e131. https://doi.org/10.1212/NXI.0000000000000131.
26. Pandit L, Mustafa S, Nakashima I, Takahashi T, Kaneko K. MOG-IgG-associated disease has a stereotypical clinical course, asymptomatic visual impairment and good treatment response. Mult Scler J Exp Transl Clin. 2018;4(3):2055217318787829. https://doi.org/10.1177/2055217318787829.
27. Chen JJ, Aksamit AJ, McKeon A, Pittock SJ, Weinshenker BG, Leavitt JA, et al. Optic disc edema in glial fibrillary acidic protein autoantibody-positive meningoencephalitis. J Neuroophthalmol. 2018;38(3):276–81. https://doi.org/10.1097/wno.0000000000000593.

28. Liedtke W, Edelmann W, Bieri PL, Chiu FC, Cowan NJ, Kucherlapati R, et al. GFAP is necessary for the integrity of CNS white matter architecture and long-term maintenance of myelination. Neuron. 1996;17(4):607–15.
29. Matiello M, Lennon VA, Jacob A, Pittock SJ, Lucchinetti CF, Wingerchuk DM, et al. NMO-IgG predicts the outcome of recurrent optic neuritis. Neurology. 2008;70(23):2197–200. https://doi.org/10.1212/01.wnl.0000303817.82134.da.
30. Benoilid A, Tilikete C, Collongues N, Arndt C, Vighetto A, Vignal C, et al. Relapsing optic neuritis: a multicentre study of 62 patients. Mult Scler. 2014;20(7):848–53. https://doi.org/10.1177/1352458513510223.
31. Peng Y, Liu L, Zheng Y, Qiao Z, Feng K, Wang J. Diagnostic implications of MOG/AQP4 antibodies in recurrent optic neuritis. Exp Ther Med. 2018;16(2):950–8. https://doi.org/10.3892/etm.2018.6273.
32. Lotan I, Hellmann MA, Benninger F, Stiebel-Kalish H, Steiner I. Recurrent optic neuritis—different patterns in multiple sclerosis, neuromyelitis optica spectrum disorders and MOG-antibody disease. J Neuroimmunol. 2018;324:115–8. https://doi.org/10.1016/j.jneuroim.2018.09.010.
33. Saini M, Khurana D. Chronic relapsing inflammatory optic neuropathy. Ann Indian Acad Neurol. 2010;13(1):61–3. https://doi.org/10.4103/0972-2327.61280.
34. Peschl P, Bradl M, Hoftberger R, Berger T, Reindl M. Myelin oligodendrocyte glycoprotein: deciphering a target in inflammatory demyelinating diseases. Front Immunol. 2017;8:529. https://doi.org/10.3389/fimmu.2017.00529.
35. Jarius S, Paul F, Aktas O, Asgari N, Dale RC, de Seze J, et al. MOG encephalomyelitis: international recommendations on diagnosis and antibody testing. J Neuroinflammation. 2018;15(1):134. https://doi.org/10.1186/s12974-018-1144-2.
36. Soelberg K, Specovius S, Zimmermann HG, Grauslund J, Mehlsen JJ, Olesen C, et al. Optical coherence tomography in acute optic neuritis: a population-based study. Acta Neurol Scand. 2018;138(6):566–73. https://doi.org/10.1111/ane.13004.
37. Peng A, Kinoshita M, Lai W, Tan A, Qiu X, Zhang L, et al. Retinal nerve fiber layer thickness in optic neuritis with MOG antibodies: a systematic review and meta-analysis. J Neuroimmunol. 2018;325:69–73. https://doi.org/10.1016/j.jneuroim.2018.09.011.
38. Pache F, Zimmermann H, Mikolajczak J, Schumacher S, Lacheta A, Oertel FC, et al. MOG-IgG in NMO and related disorders: a multicenter study of 50 patients. Part 4: afferent visual system damage after optic neuritis in MOG-IgG-seropositive versus AQP4-IgG-seropositive patients. J Neuroinflammation. 2016;13(1):282. https://doi.org/10.1186/s12974-016-0720-6.
39. Stiebel-Kalish H, Lotan I, Brody J, Chodick G, Bialer O, Marignier R, et al. Retinal nerve fiber layer may be better preserved in MOG-IgG versus AQP4-IgG optic neuritis: a cohort study. PLoS One. 2017;12(1):e0170847. https://doi.org/10.1371/journal.pone.0170847.
40. Turcano P, Chen JJ, Bureau BL, Savica R. Early ophthalmologic features of Parkinson's disease: a review of preceding clinical and diagnostic markers. J Neurol. 2018. https://doi.org/10.1007/s00415-018-9051-0.
41. Gelb DJ, Oliver E, Gilman S. Diagnostic criteria for parkinson disease. Arch Neurol. 1999;56(1):33–9. https://doi.org/10.1001/archneur.56.1.33.
42. Diederich NJ, Pieri V, Hipp G, Rufra O, Blyth S, Vaillant M. Discriminative power of different nonmotor signs in early Parkinson's disease. A case-control study. Mov Disord. 2010;25(7):882–7. https://doi.org/10.1002/mds.22963.
43. Buttner T, Kuhn W, Muller T, Patzold T, Heidbrink K, Przuntek H. Distorted color discrimination in 'de novo' parkinsonian patients. Neurology. 1995;45(2):386–7.
44. Bertrand JA, Bedetti C, Postuma RB, Monchi O, Genier Marchand D, Jubault T, et al. Color discrimination deficits in Parkinson's disease are related to cognitive impairment and white-matter alterations. Mov Disord. 2012;27(14):1781–8. https://doi.org/10.1002/mds.25272.
45. Regan BC, Freudenthaler N, Kolle R, Mollon JD, Paulus W. Colour discrimination thresholds in Parkinson's disease: results obtained with a rapid computer-controlled colour vision test. Vis Res. 1998;38(21):3427–31.

46. Postuma RB, Gagnon JF, Bertrand JA, Genier Marchand D, Montplaisir JY. Parkinson risk in idiopathic REM sleep behavior disorder: preparing for neuroprotective trials. Neurology. 2015;84(11):1104–13. https://doi.org/10.1212/wnl.0000000000001364.
47. Marras C, Schule B, Munhoz RP, Rogaeva E, Langston JW, Kasten M, et al. Phenotype in parkinsonian and nonparkinsonian LRRK2 G2019S mutation carriers. Neurology. 2011;77(4):325–33. https://doi.org/10.1212/WNL.0b013e318227042d.
48. Buttner T, Kuhn W, Patzold T, Przuntek H. L-Dopa improves colour vision in Parkinson's disease. J Neural Transm Park Dis Dement Sect. 1994;7(1):13–9.
49. Ming W, Palidis DJ, Spering M, McKeown MJ. Visual contrast sensitivity in early-stage Parkinson's disease. Invest Ophthalmol Vis Sci. 2016;57(13):5696–704. https://doi.org/10.1167/iovs.16-20025.
50. Hutton JT, Morris JL, Elias JW, Varma R, Poston JN. Spatial contrast sensitivity is reduced in bilateral Parkinson's disease. Neurology. 1991;41(8):1200–2.
51. Bodis-Wollner I, Marx MS, Mitra S, Bobak P, Mylin L, Yahr M. Visual dysfunction in Parkinson's disease. Loss in spatiotemporal contrast sensitivity. Brain. 1987;110(Pt 6):1675–98.
52. Bulens C, Meerwaldt JD, Van der Wildt GJ, Van Deursen JB. Effect of levodopa treatment on contrast sensitivity in Parkinson's disease. Ann Neurol. 1987;22(3):365–9. https://doi.org/10.1002/ana.410220313.
53. Blekher T, Weaver M, Rupp J, Nichols WC, Hui SL, Gray J, et al. Multiple step pattern as a biomarker in Parkinson disease. Parkinsonism Relat Disord. 2009;15(7):506–10. https://doi.org/10.1016/j.parkreldis.2009.01.002.
54. Terao Y, Fukuda H, Ugawa Y, Hikosaka O. New perspectives on the pathophysiology of Parkinson's disease as assessed by saccade performance: a clinical review. Clin Neurophysiol. 2013;124(8):1491–506. https://doi.org/10.1016/j.clinph.2013.01.021.
55. DeJong JD, Jones GM. Akinesia, hypokinesia, and bradykinesia in the oculomotor system of patients with Parkinson's disease. Exp Neurol. 1971;32(1):58–68.
56. Crawford T, Goodrich S, Henderson L, Kennard C. Predictive responses in Parkinson's disease: manual keypresses and saccadic eye movements to regular stimulus events. J Neurol Neurosurg Psychiatry. 1989;52(9):1033–42.
57. Lueck CJ, Tanyeri S, Crawford TJ, Henderson L, Kennard C. Antisaccades and remembered saccades in Parkinson's disease. J Neurol Neurosurg Psychiatry. 1990;53(4):284–8.
58. Briand KA, Strallow D, Hening W, Poizner H, Sereno AB. Control of voluntary and reflexive saccades in Parkinson's disease. Exp Brain Res. 1999;129(1):38–48.
59. Zackon DH, Sharpe JA. Smooth pursuit in senescence. Effects of target acceleration and velocity. Acta Otolaryngol. 1987;104(3–4):290–7.
60. White OB, Saint-Cyr JA, Tomlinson RD, Sharpe JA. Ocular motor deficits in Parkinson's disease. II. Control of the saccadic and smooth pursuit systems. Brain. 1983;106(Pt 3):571–87.
61. Shibasaki H, Tsuji S, Kuroiwa Y. Oculomotor abnormalities in Parkinson's disease. Arch Neurol. 1979;36(6):360–4.
62. Gibson JM, Pimlott R, Kennard C. Ocular motor and manual tracking in Parkinson's disease and the effect of treatment. J Neurol Neurosurg Psychiatry. 1987;50(7):853–60.
63. Bares M, Brazdil M, Kanovsky P, Jurak P, Daniel P, Kukleta M, et al. The effect of apomorphine administration on smooth pursuit ocular movements in early Parkinsonian patients. Parkinsonism Relat Disord. 2003;9(3):139–44.
64. Waterston JA, Barnes GR, Grealy MA, Collins S. Abnormalities of smooth eye and head movement control in Parkinson's disease. Ann Neurol. 1996;39(6):749–60. https://doi.org/10.1002/ana.410390611.
65. Nowacka B, Lubinski W, Honczarenko K, Potemkowski A, Safranow K. Ophthalmological features of Parkinson disease. Med Sci Monit. 2014;20:2243–9. https://doi.org/10.12659/msm.890861.
66. Racette BA, Gokden MS, Tychsen LS, Perlmutter JS. Convergence insufficiency in idiopathic Parkinson's disease responsive to levodopa. Strabismus. 1999;7(3):169–74.

67. Almer Z, Klein KS, Marsh L, Gerstenhaber M, Repka MX. Ocular motor and sensory function in Parkinson's disease. Ophthalmology. 2012;119(1):178–82. https://doi.org/10.1016/j.ophtha.2011.06.040.
68. Sun L, Zhang H, Gu Z, Cao M, Li D, Chan P. Stereopsis impairment is associated with decreased color perception and worse motor performance in Parkinson's disease. Eur J Med Res. 2014;19:29. https://doi.org/10.1186/2047-783x-19-29.
69. Kwon KY, Kang SH, Kim M, Lee HM, Jang JW, Kim JY, et al. Nonmotor symptoms and cognitive decline in de novo Parkinson's disease. Can J Neurol Sci. 2014;41(5):597–602. https://doi.org/10.1017/cjn.2014.3.
70. Kaski D, Saifee TA, Buckwell D, Bronstein AM. Ocular tremor in Parkinson's disease is due to head oscillation. Mov Disord. 2013;28(4):534–7. https://doi.org/10.1002/mds.25342.
71. Pagonabarraga J, Martinez-Horta S, Fernandez de Bobadilla R, Perez J, Ribosa-Nogue R, Marin J, et al. Minor hallucinations occur in drug-naive Parkinson's disease patients, even from the premotor phase. Mov Disord. 2016;31(1):45–52. https://doi.org/10.1002/mds.26432.
72. Diederich NJ, Goetz CG, Raman R, Pappert EJ, Leurgans S, Piery V. Poor visual discrimination and visual hallucinations in Parkinson's disease. Clin Neuropharmacol. 1998;21(5):289–95.
73. Hoglinger GU, Respondek G, Stamelou M, Kurz C, Josephs KA, Lang AE, et al. Clinical diagnosis of progressive supranuclear palsy: the movement disorder society criteria. Mov Disord. 2017;32(6):853–64. https://doi.org/10.1002/mds.26987.
74. Respondek G, Levin J, Hoglinger GU. Progressive supranuclear palsy and multiple system atrophy: clinicopathological concepts and therapeutic challenges. Curr Opin Neurol. 2018;31(4):448–54. https://doi.org/10.1097/wco.0000000000000581.
75. Lee AG, Mader T, Gibson C, Brunstetter TJ, Tarver W. Space flight-associated neuro-ocular syndrome (SANS). Eye (Lond). 2018;32(7):1164–7.
76. Mader TH, Gibson CR, Pass AF, Kramer LA, Lee AG, Fogarty J, et al. Optic disc edema, globe flattening, choroidal folds, and hyperopic shifts observed in astronauts after long-duration space flight. Ophthalmology. 2011;118(10):2058–69. https://doi.org/10.1016/j.ophtha.2011.06.021.
77. Mader TH, Gibson CR, Otto CA, Sargsyan AE, Miller NR, Subramanian PS, et al. Persistent asymmetric optic disc swelling after long-duration space flight: implications for pathogenesis. J Neuroophthalmol. 2017;37(2):133–9. https://doi.org/10.1097/wno.0000000000000467.
78. Arbeille P, Fomina G, Roumy J, Alferova I, Tobal N, Herault S. Adaptation of the left heart, cerebral and femoral arteries, and jugular and femoral veins during short- and long-term head-down tilt and spaceflights. Eur J Appl Physiol. 2001;86(2):157–68. https://doi.org/10.1007/s004210100473.
79. Lerner DJ, Chima RS, Patel K, Parmet AJ. Ultrasound guided lumbar puncture and remote guidance for potential in-flight evaluation of VIIP/SANS. Aerosp Med Hum Perform. 2019;90(1):58–62. https://doi.org/10.3357/amhp.5170.2019.
80. Wasinska-Borowiec W, Aghdam KA, Saari JM, Grzybowski A. An updated review on the most common agents causing toxic optic neuropathies. Curr Pharm Des. 2017;23(4):586–95. https://doi.org/10.2174/1381612823666170124113826.
81. Miller NR, Subramanian P, Patel V. Walsh & Hoyt's clinical neuro-ophthalmology: the essentials. Philadelphia: Lippincott Williams & Wilkins; 2015. p. 325–7.
82. Jefferis JM, Hickman SJ. Treatment and outcomes in nutritional optic neuropathy. Curr Treat Options Neurol. 2019;21(1):5. https://doi.org/10.1007/s11940-019-0542-9.
83. Chiotoroiu SM, Noaghi M, Stefaniu GI, Secureanu FA, Purcarea VL, Zemba M. Tobacco-alcohol optic neuropathy—clinical challenges in diagnosis. J Med Life. 2014;7(4):472–6.
84. Vieira LM, Silva NF, Dias dos Santos AM, dos Anjos RS, Pinto LA, Vicente AR, et al. Retinal ganglion cell layer analysis by optical coherence tomography in toxic and nutritional optic neuropathy. J Neuroophthalmol. 2015;35(3):242–5. https://doi.org/10.1097/wno.0000000000000229.
85. Wang MY, Sadun AA, Chan JW. Nutritional and toxic optic neuropathies. In: Chan JW, editor. Optic nerve disorders: diagnosis and management. New York: Springer; 2014. p. 177–207.

86. Nurieva O, Hubacek JA, Urban P, Hlusicka J, Diblik P, Kuthan P, et al. Clinical and genetic determinants of chronic visual pathway changes after methanol—induced optic neuropathy: four-year follow-up study. Clin Toxicol (Phila). 2019;57(6):387–97. https://doi.org/10.1080/15563650.2018.1532083.

87. Grzybowski A, Kanclerz P. Progressive chronic retinal axonal loss following acute methanol-induced optic neuropathy: four-year prospective cohort study. Am J Ophthalmol. 2018;195:246–7. https://doi.org/10.1016/j.ajo.2018.08.019.

88. Beatty L, Green R, Magee K, Zed P. A systematic review of ethanol and fomepizole use in toxic alcohol ingestions. Emerg Med Int. 2013;2013:638057. https://doi.org/10.1155/2013/638057.

89. Abrishami M, Khalifeh M, Shoayb M, Abrishami M. Therapeutic effects of high-dose intravenous prednisolone in methanol-induced toxic optic neuropathy. J Ocul Pharmacol Ther. 2011;27(3):261–3. https://doi.org/10.1089/jop.2010.0145.

90. Kowalski T, Verma J, Greene SL, Curtin J. Methanol toxicity: a case of blindness treated with adjunctive steroids. Med J Aust. 2019;210(1):14–5.e1. https://doi.org/10.5694/mja2.12040.

91. Pakdel F, Sanjari MS, Naderi A, Pirmarzdashti N, Haghighi A, Kashkouli MB. Erythropoietin in treatment of methanol optic neuropathy. J Neuroophthalmol. 2018;38(2):167–71. https://doi.org/10.1097/wno.0000000000000614.

92. Kao R, Landry Y, Chick G, Leung A. Bilateral blindness secondary to optic nerve ischemia from severe amlodipine overdose: a case report. J Med Case Rep. 2017;11(1):211. https://doi.org/10.1186/s13256-017-1374-4.

93. Scoville BA, De Lott LB, Trobe JD, Mueller BA. Ethambutol optic neuropathy in a hemodialysis patient receiving a guideline-recommended dose. J Neuroophthalmol. 2013;33(4):421–3. https://doi.org/10.1097/wno.0000000000000075. https://doi.org/10.5546/aap.2013.455.

94. Lee J-Y, Han J, Seo JG, Park K-A, Oh SY. Diagnostic value of ganglion cell-inner plexiform layer for early detection of ethambutol-induced optic neuropathy. Br J Ophthalmol. 2019;103(3):379–84.

95. Birmingham MC, Rayner CR, Meagher AK, Flavin SM, Batts DH, Schentag JJ. Linezolid for the treatment of multidrug-resistant, gram-positive infections: experience from a compassionate-use program. Clin Infect Dis. 2003;36(2):159–68. https://doi.org/10.1086/345744.

96. Dempsey SP, Sickman A, Slagle WS. Case report: linezolid optic neuropathy and proposed evidenced-based screening recommendation. Optom Vis Sci. 2018;95(5):468–74. https://doi.org/10.1097/opx.0000000000001216.

97. Purvin V, Kawasaki A, Borruat FX. Optic neuropathy in patients using amiodarone. Arch Ophthalmol. 2006;124(5):696–701. https://doi.org/10.1001/archopht.124.5.696.

98. Chen D, Hedges TR. Amiodarone optic neuropathy—review. Semin Ophthalmol. 2003;18(4):169–73. https://doi.org/10.1080/08820530390895163.

99. Johnson LN, Krohel GB, Thomas ER. The clinical spectrum of amiodarone-associated optic neuropathy. J Natl Med Assoc. 2004;96(11):1477–91.

100. Neufeld A, Warner J. Case of bilateral sequential nonarteritic ischemic optic neuropathy after rechallenge with sildenafil. J Neuroophthalmol. 2018;38(1):123–4.

101. Campbell UB, Walker AM, Gaffney M, Petronis KR, Creanga D, Quinn S, et al. Acute nonarteritic anterior ischemic optic neuropathy and exposure to phosphodiesterase type 5 inhibitors. J Sex Med. 2015;12(1):139–51.

102. Flahavan EM, Li H, Gupte-Singh K, Rizk RT, Ruff DD, Francis JL, et al. Prospective case-crossover study investigating the possible association between nonarteritic anterior ischemic optic neuropathy and phosphodiesterase type 5 inhibitor exposure. Urology. 2017;105:76–84.

103. Margo CE, French DD. Ischemic optic neuropathy in male veterans prescribed phosphodiesterase-5 inhibitors. Am J Ophthalmol. 2007;143(3):538–9.

104. Nathoo NA, Etminan M, Mikelberg FS. Association between phosphodiesterase-5 inhibitors and nonarteritic anterior ischemic optic neuropathy. J Neuroophthalmol. 2015;35(1):12–5.

105. Gaffuri M, Cristofaletti A, Mansoldo C, Biban P. Acute onset of bilateral visual loss during sildenafil therapy in a young infant with congenital heart disease. BMJ Case Rep. 2014;2014:bcr2014204262. https://doi.org/10.1136/bcr-2014-204262.
106. Grzybowski A, Zulsdorff M, Wilhelm H, Tonagel F. Toxic optic neuropathies: an updated review. Acta Ophthalmol. 2015;93(5):402–10. https://doi.org/10.1111/aos.12515.
107. Becker DA, Balcer LJ, Galetta SL. The neurological complications of nutritional deficiency following bariatric surgery. J Obes. 2012;2012:608534. https://doi.org/10.1155/2012/608534.
108. Golnik KC, Schaible ER. Folate-responsive optic neuropathy. J Neuroophthalmol. 1994;14(3):163–9.
109. Grzybowski A, Holder GE. Tobacco optic neuropathy (TON)—the historical and present concept of the disease. Acta Ophthalmol. 2011;89(5):495–9. https://doi.org/10.1111/j.1755-3768.2009.01853.x.
110. Wostyn P, Van Dam D, De Deyn PP. Intracranial pressure and glaucoma: is there a new therapeutic perspective on the horizon? Med Hypotheses. 2018;118:98–102. https://doi.org/10.1016/j.mehy.2018.06.026.
111. Berdahl JP, Allingham RR. Intracranial pressure and glaucoma. Curr Opin Ophthalmol. 2010;21(2):106–11.
112. Kim YW, Kim DW, Jeoung JW, Kim DM, Park KH. Peripheral lamina cribrosa depth in primary open-angle glaucoma: a swept-source optical coherence tomography study of lamina cribrosa. Eye. 2015;29:1368. https://doi.org/10.1038/eye.2015.162. https://www.nature.com/articles/eye2015162#supplementary-information.
113. Downs JC, Roberts MD, Burgoyne CF. The mechanical environment of the optic nerve head in glaucoma. Optom Vis Sci. 2008;85(6):425.
114. Wostyn P, De Groot V, Van Dam D, Audenaert K, De Deyn PP. Senescent changes in cerebrospinal fluid circulatory physiology and their role in the pathogenesis of normal-tension glaucoma. Am J Ophthalmol. 2013;156(1):5–14.e2. https://doi.org/10.1016/j.ajo.2013.03.003.
115. Silverberg GD, Mayo M, Saul T, Rubenstein E, McGuire D. Alzheimer's disease, normal-pressure hydrocephalus, and senescent changes in CSF circulatory physiology: a hypothesis. Lancet Neurol. 2003;2(8):506–11. https://doi.org/10.1016/S1474-4422(03)00487-3.
116. Wostyn P, Killer HE, De Deyn PP. Glymphatic stasis at the site of the lamina cribrosa as a potential mechanism underlying open-angle glaucoma. Clin Exp Ophthalmol. 2017;45(5):539–47. https://doi.org/10.1111/ceo.12915.
117. Mathieu E, Gupta N, Ahari A, Zhou X, Hanna J, Yücel YH. Evidence for cerebrospinal fluid entry into the optic nerve via a glymphatic pathway. Invest Ophthalmol Vis Sci. 2017;58(11):4784–91. https://doi.org/10.1167/iovs.17-22290.
118. Wattjes MP, Rovira À, Miller D, Yousry TA, Sormani MP, de Stefano N, et al. MAGNIMS consensus guidelines on the use of MRI in multiple sclerosis—establishing disease prognosis and monitoring patients. Nat Rev Neurol. 2015;11:597. https://doi.org/10.1038/nrneurol.2015.157.
119. Silver NC, Good CD, Sormani MP, MacManus DG, Thompson AJ, Filippi M, et al. A modified protocol to improve the detection of enhancing brain and spinal cord lesions in multiple sclerosis. J Neurol. 2001;248(3):215–24.
120. Thorpe JW, Kidd D, Moseley IF, Kendall BE, Thompson AJ, MacManus DG, et al. Serial gadolinium-enhanced MRI of the brain and spinal cord in early relapsing-remitting multiple sclerosis. Neurology. 1996;46(2):373–8. https://doi.org/10.1212/wnl.46.2.373.
121. Filippi M, Rocca MA, Ciccarelli O, De Stefano N, Evangelou N, Kappos L, et al. MRI criteria for the diagnosis of multiple sclerosis: magnims consensus guidelines. Lancet Neurol. 2016;15(3):292–303. https://doi.org/10.1016/S1474-4422(15)00393-2.
122. Sati P, Oh J, Constable RT, Evangelou N, Guttmann CR, Henry RG, et al. The central vein sign and its clinical evaluation for the diagnosis of multiple sclerosis: a consensus statement from the North American Imaging in Multiple Sclerosis Cooperative. Nat Rev Neurol. 2016;12(12):714–22. https://doi.org/10.1038/nrneurol.2016.166.

123. Maggi P, Absinta M, Grammatico M, Vuolo L, Emmi G, Carlucci G, et al. Central vein sign differentiates Multiple Sclerosis from central nervous system inflammatory vasculopathies. Ann Neurol. 2018;83(2):283–94. https://doi.org/10.1002/ana.25146.

124. Campion T, Smith RJP, Altmann DR, Brito GC, Turner BP, Evanson J, et al. FLAIR∗ to visualize veins in white matter lesions: a new tool for the diagnosis of multiple sclerosis? Eur Radiol. 2017;27(10):4257–63. https://doi.org/10.1007/s00330-017-4822-z.

125. Dejaco C, Ramiro S, Duftner C, Besson FL, Bley TA, Blockmans D, et al. EULAR recommendations for the use of imaging in large vessel vasculitis in clinical practice. Ann Rheum Dis. 2018;77(5):636–43. https://doi.org/10.1136/annrheumdis-2017-212649.

126. Luqmani R, Lee E, Singh S, Gillett M, Schmidt WA, Bradburn M, et al. The Role of Ultrasound Compared to Biopsy of Temporal Arteries in the Diagnosis and Treatment of Giant Cell Arteritis (TABUL): a diagnostic accuracy and cost-effectiveness study. Health Technol Assess. 2016;20(90):1–238. https://doi.org/10.3310/hta20900.

127. Schmidt WA, Kraft HE, Vorpahl K, Völker L, Gromnica-Ihle EJ. Color duplex ultrasonography in the diagnosis of temporal arteritis. N Engl J Med. 1997;337(19):1336–42. https://doi.org/10.1056/nejm199711063371902.

128. Sammel AM, Fraser CL. Update on giant cell arteritis. Curr Opin Ophthalmol. 2018;29(6):520–7. https://doi.org/10.1097/icu.0000000000000528.

129. Chrysidis S, Duftner C, Dejaco C, Schäfer VS, Ramiro S, Carrara G, et al. Definitions and reliability assessment of elementary ultrasound lesions in giant cell arteritis: a study from the OMERACT Large Vessel Vasculitis Ultrasound Working Group. RMD Open. 2018;4(1):e000598. https://doi.org/10.1136/rmdopen-2017-000598.

130. Duftner C, Dejaco C, Sepriano A, Falzon L, Schmidt WA, Ramiro S. Imaging in diagnosis, outcome prediction and monitoring of large vessel vasculitis: a systematic literature review and meta-analysis informing the EULAR recommendations. RMD Open. 2018;4(1). https://doi.org/10.1136/rmdopen-2017-000612.

131. Halbach C, McClelland CM, Chen J, Li S, Lee MS. Use of noninvasive imaging in giant cell arteritis. Asia Pac J Ophthalmol (Phila). 2018;7(4):260–4. https://doi.org/10.22608/apo.2018133.

132. Rheaume M, Rebello R, Pagnoux C, Carette S, Clements-Baker M, Cohen-Hallaleh V, et al. High-resolution magnetic resonance imaging of scalp arteries for the diagnosis of giant cell arteritis: results of a prospective cohort study. Arthritis Rheumatol. 2017;69(1):161–8. https://doi.org/10.1002/art.39824.

133. Germano G, Muratore F, Cimino L, Lo Gullo A, Possemato N, Macchioni P, et al. Is colour duplex sonography-guided temporal artery biopsy useful in the diagnosis of giant cell arteritis? A randomized study. Rheumatology (Oxford). 2015;54(3):400–4. https://doi.org/10.1093/rheumatology/keu241.

134. Craven A, Robson J, Ponte C, Grayson PC, Suppiah R, Judge A, et al. ACR/EULAR-endorsed study to develop Diagnostic and Classification Criteria for Vasculitis (DCVAS). Clin Exp Nephrol. 2013;17(5):619–21. https://doi.org/10.1007/s10157-013-0854-0.

135. Vincent A, Huda S, Cao M, Cetin H, Koneczny I, Rodriguez-Cruz P, et al. Serological and experimental studies in different forms of myasthenia gravis. Ann N Y Acad Sci. 2018;1413(1):143–53. https://doi.org/10.1111/nyas.13592.

136. Gilhus NE, Skeie GO, Romi F, Lazaridis K, Zisimopoulou P, Tzartos S. Myasthenia gravis—autoantibody characteristics and their implications for therapy. Nat Rev Neurol. 2016;12(5):259–68. https://doi.org/10.1038/nrneurol.2016.44.

137. Fortin E, Cestari DM, Weinberg DH. Ocular myasthenia gravis: an update on diagnosis and treatment. Curr Opin Ophthalmol. 2018;29(6):477–84. https://doi.org/10.1097/icu.0000000000000526.

138. Provenzano C, Marino M, Scuderi F, Evoli A, Bartoccioni E. Anti-acetylcholinesterase antibodies associate with ocular myasthenia gravis. J Neuroimmunol. 2010;218(1–2):102–6. https://doi.org/10.1016/j.jneuroim.2009.11.004.

139. Binks S, Vincent A, Palace J. Myasthenia gravis: a clinical-immunological update. J Neurol. 2016;263(4):826–34. https://doi.org/10.1007/s00415-015-7963-5.
140. Eng H, Lefvert AK. Isolation of an antiidiotypic antibody with acetylcholine-receptor-like binding properties from myasthenia gravis patients. Ann Inst Pasteur Immunol. 1988;139(5):569–80.
141. Rodgaard A, Nielsen FC, Djurup R, Somnier F, Gammeltoft S. Acetylcholine receptor antibody in myasthenia gravis: predominance of IgG subclasses 1 and 3. Clin Exp Immunol. 1987;67(1):82–8.
142. Higuchi O, Hamuro J, Motomura M, Yamanashi Y. Autoantibodies to low-density lipoprotein receptor-related protein 4 in myasthenia gravis. Ann Neurol. 2011;69(2):418–22. https://doi.org/10.1002/ana.22312.
143. Zhang B, Tzartos JS, Belimezi M, Ragheb S, Bealmear B, Lewis RA, et al. Autoantibodies to lipoprotein-related protein 4 in patients with double-seronegative myasthenia gravis. Arch Neurol. 2012;69(4):445–51. https://doi.org/10.1001/archneurol.2011.2393.
144. Achilli A, Iommarini L, Olivieri A, Pala M, Hooshiar Kashani B, Reynier P, et al. Rare primary mitochondrial DNA mutations and probable synergistic variants in Leber's hereditary optic neuropathy. PLoS One. 2012;7(8):e42242. https://doi.org/10.1371/journal.pone.0042242.
145. Gilhus NE, Verschuuren JJ. Myasthenia gravis: subgroup classification and therapeutic strategies. Lancet Neurol. 2015;14(10):1023–36. https://doi.org/10.1016/s1474-4422(15)00145-3.
146. Tsivgoulis G, Dervenoulas G, Kokotis P, Zompola C, Tzartos JS, Tzartos SJ, et al. Double seronegative myasthenia gravis with low density lipoprotein-4 (LRP4) antibodies presenting with isolated ocular symptoms. J Neurol Sci. 2014;346(1–2):328–30. https://doi.org/10.1016/j.jns.2014.09.013.
147. Kerty E, Elsais A, Argov Z, Evoli A, Gilhus NE. EFNS/ENS Guidelines for the treatment of ocular myasthenia. Eur J Neurol. 2014;21(5):687–93. https://doi.org/10.1111/ene.12359.
148. Hoch W, McConville J, Helms S, Newsom-Davis J, Melms A, Vincent A. Auto-antibodies to the receptor tyrosine kinase MuSK in patients with myasthenia gravis without acetylcholine receptor antibodies. Nat Med. 2001;7(3):365–8. https://doi.org/10.1038/85520.
149. Guptill JT, Sanders DB, Evoli A. Anti-MuSK antibody myasthenia gravis: clinical findings and response to treatment in two large cohorts. Muscle Nerve. 2011;44(1):36–40. https://doi.org/10.1002/mus.22006.
150. Stergiou C, Lazaridis K, Zouvelou V, Tzartos J, Mantegazza R, Antozzi C, et al. Titin antibodies in "seronegative" myasthenia gravis—a new role for an old antigen. J Neuroimmunol. 2016;292:108–15. https://doi.org/10.1016/j.jneuroim.2016.01.018.
151. Evoli A, Alboini PE, Damato V, Iorio R, Provenzano C, Bartoccioni E, et al. Myasthenia gravis with antibodies to MuSK: an update. Anne N Y Acad Sci. 2018;1412(1):82–9. https://doi.org/10.1111/nyas.13518.
152. Evoli A, Alboini PE, Iorio R, Damato V, Bartoccioni E. Pattern of ocular involvement in myasthenia gravis with MuSK antibodies. J Neurol Neurosurg Psychiatry. 2017;88(9):761–3. https://doi.org/10.1136/jnnp-2017-315782.
153. Wong SH, Huda S, Vincent A, Plant GT. Ocular myasthenia gravis: controversies and updates. Curr Neurol Neurosci Rep. 2013;14(1):421. https://doi.org/10.1007/s11910-013-0421-9.
154. Huang D, Swanson EA, Lin CP, Schuman JS, Stinson WG, Chang W, et al. Optical coherence tomography. Science (New York, NY). 1991;254(5035):1178–81.
155. Rao HL, Zangwill LM, Weinreb RN, Sample PA, Alencar LM, Medeiros FA. Comparison of different spectral domain optical coherence tomography scanning areas for glaucoma diagnosis. Ophthalmology. 2010;117(9):1692–9, 9.e1. https://doi.org/10.1016/j.ophtha.2010.01.031.
156. Savini G, Bellusci C, Carbonelli M, Zanini M, Carelli V, Sadun AA, et al. Detection and quantification of retinal nerve fiber layer thickness in optic disc edema using stratus OCT. Arch Ophthalmol. 2006;124(8):1111–7. https://doi.org/10.1001/archopht.124.8.1111.

157. Lee MJ, Abraham AG, Swenor BK, Sharrett AR, Ramulu PY. Application of optical coherence tomography in the detection and classification of cognitive decline. J Curr Glaucoma Pract. 2018;12(1):10–8. https://doi.org/10.5005/jp-journals-10028-1238.

158. Kardon RH. Role of the macular optical coherence tomography scan in neuro-ophthalmology. J Neuroophthalmol. 2011;31(4):353–61. https://doi.org/10.1097/WNO.0b013e318238b9cb.

159. Saidha S, Al-Louzi O, Ratchford JN, Bhargava P, Oh J, Newsome SD, et al. Optical coherence tomography reflects brain atrophy in multiple sclerosis: a four-year study. Ann Neurol. 2015;78(5):801–13. https://doi.org/10.1002/ana.24487.

160. Winges KM, Werner JS, Harvey DJ, Cello KE, Durbin MK, Balcer LJ, et al. Baseline retinal nerve fiber layer thickness and macular volume quantified by OCT in the north american phase 3 fingolimod trial for relapsing–remitting multiple sclerosis. J Neuroophthalmol. 2013;33(4):322–9. https://doi.org/10.1097/WNO.0b013e31829c51f7.

161. Werner JS, Keltner JL, Zawadzki RJ, Choi SS. Outer retinal abnormalities associated with inner retinal pathology in nonglaucomatous and glaucomatous optic neuropathies. Eye (Lond). 2011;25(3):279–89. https://doi.org/10.1038/eye.2010.218.

162. La Morgia C, Barboni P, Rizzo G, Carbonelli M, Savini G, Scaglione C, et al. Loss of temporal retinal nerve fibers in Parkinson disease: a mitochondrial pattern? Eur J Neurol. 2013;20(1):198–201. https://doi.org/10.1111/j.1468-1331.2012.03701.x.

163. Roth NM, Saidha S, Zimmermann H, Brandt AU, Isensee J, Benkhellouf-Rutkowska A, et al. Photoreceptor layer thinning in idiopathic Parkinson's disease. Mov Disord. 2014;29(9):1163–70. https://doi.org/10.1002/mds.25896.

164. Archibald NK, Clarke MP, Mosimann UP, Burn DJ. Visual symptoms in Parkinson's disease and Parkinson's disease dementia. Mov Disord. 2011;26(13):2387–95. https://doi.org/10.1002/mds.23891.

165. Garcia-Martin E, Satue M, Otin S, Fuertes I, Alarcia R, Larrosa JM, et al. Retina measurements for diagnosis of Parkinson disease. Retina (Phila). 2014;34(5):971–80. https://doi.org/10.1097/iae.0000000000000028.

166. Satue M, Obis J, Rodrigo MJ, Otin S, Fuertes MI, Vilades E, et al. Optical coherence tomography as a biomarker for diagnosis, progression, and prognosis of neurodegenerative diseases. J Ophthalmol. 2016;2016:8503859. https://doi.org/10.1155/2016/8503859.

167. Garcia-Martin E, Pablo LE, Bambo MP, Alarcia R, Polo V, Larrosa JM, et al. Comparison of peripapillary choroidal thickness between healthy subjects and patients with Parkinson's disease. PLoS One. 2017;12(5):e0177163. https://doi.org/10.1371/journal.pone.0177163.

168. Hagag AM, Gao SS, Jia Y, Huang D. Optical coherence tomography angiography: technical principles and clinical applications in ophthalmology. Taiwan J Ophthalmol. 2017;7(3):115–29. https://doi.org/10.4103/tjo.tjo_31_17.

169. Schmetterer L, Garhofer G. How can blood flow be measured? Surv Ophthalmol. 2007;52(Suppl 2):S134–8. https://doi.org/10.1016/j.survophthal.2007.08.008.

170. Jia Y, Wei E, Wang X, Zhang X, Morrison JC, Parikh M et al. Optical Coherence Tomography Angiography of Optic Disc Perfusion in Glaucoma. Ophthalmol. 2014;121(7):1322–32. https://doi.org/j.ophtha.2014.01.02.

171. Chen JJ, AbouChehade JE, Iezzi R Jr, Leavitt JA, Kardon RH. Optical coherence angiographic demonstration of retinal changes from chronic optic neuropathies. Neuroophthalmology. 2017;41(2):76–83. https://doi.org/10.1080/01658107.2016.1275703.

172. Spain RI, Liu L, Zhang X, Jia Y, Tan O, Bourdette D, et al. Optical coherence tomography angiography enhances the detection of optic nerve damage in multiple sclerosis. Br J Ophthalmol. 2018;102(4):520–4. https://doi.org/10.1136/bjophthalmol-2017-310477.

173. Wang X, Jia Y, Spain R, Potsaid B, Liu JJ, Baumann B, et al. Optical coherence tomography angiography of optic nerve head and parafovea in multiple sclerosis. Br J Ophthalmol. 2014;98(10):1368–73. https://doi.org/10.1136/bjophthalmol-2013-304547.

174. Higashiyama T, Nishida Y, Ohji M. Optical coherence tomography angiography in eyes with good visual acuity recovery after treatment for optic neuritis. PLoS One. 2017;12(2):e0172168. https://doi.org/10.1371/journal.pone.0172168.

175. Takayama K, Ito Y, Kaneko H, Kataoka K, Ra E, Terasaki H. Optical coherence tomography angiography in leber hereditary optic neuropathy. Acta Ophthalmol. 2017;95(4):e344–e5. https://doi.org/10.1111/aos.13244.
176. Kousal B, Kolarova H, Meliska M, Bydzovsky J, Diblik P, Kulhanek J, et al. Peripapillary microcirculation in Leber hereditary optic neuropathy. Acta Ophthalmol. 2019;97(1):e71–6. https://doi.org/10.1111/aos.13817.
177. Borrelli E, Balasubramanian S, Triolo G, Barboni P, Sadda SR, Sadun AA. Topographic macular microvascular changes and correlation with visual loss in chronic leber hereditary optic neuropathy. Am J Ophthalmol. 2018;192:217–28. https://doi.org/10.1016/j.ajo.2018.05.029.
178. Hall S, Persellin S, Lie JT, O'Brien PC, Kurland LT, Hunder GG. The therapeutic impact of temporal artery biopsy. Lancet. 1983;2(8361):1217–20.
179. Stone JH, Tuckwell K, Dimonaco S, Klearman M, Aringer M, Blockmans D, et al. Trial of tocilizumab in giant-cell arteritis. N Engl J Med. 2017;377(4):317–28. https://doi.org/10.1056/NEJMoa1613849.
180. Langford CA, Cuthbertson D, Ytterberg SR, Khalidi N, Monach PA, Carette S, et al. A randomized, double-blind trial of abatacept (CTLA-4Ig) for the treatment of giant cell arteritis. Arthritis Rheumatol. 2017;69(4):837–45. https://doi.org/10.1002/art.40044.
181. Mulero P, Midaglia L, Montalban X. Ocrelizumab: a new milestone in multiple sclerosis therapy. Ther Adv Neurol Disord. 2018;11:1756286418773025. https://doi.org/10.1177/1756286418773025.
182. Falsini B, Chiaretti A, Rizzo D, Piccardi M, Ruggiero A, Manni L, et al. Nerve growth factor improves visual loss in childhood optic gliomas: a randomized, double-blind, phase II clinical trial. Brain. 2016;139(Pt 2):404–14. https://doi.org/10.1093/brain/awv366.
183. Pandit R, Paris L, Rudich DS, Lesser RL, Kupersmith MJ, Miller NR. Long-term efficacy of fractionated conformal radiotherapy for the management of primary optic nerve sheath meningioma. Br J Ophthalmol. 2018. https://doi.org/10.1136/bjophthalmol-2018-313135.
184. Carelli V, Carbonelli M, de Coo IF, Kawasaki A, Klopstock T, Lagreze WA, et al. International consensus statement on the clinical and therapeutic management of leber hereditary optic neuropathy. J Neuroophthalmol. 2017;37(4):371–81. https://doi.org/10.1097/WNO.0000000000000570.
185. Mashima Y, Hiida Y, Oguchi Y. Remission of Leber's hereditary optic neuropathy with idebenone. Lancet (London). 1992;340(8815):368–9.
186. Carelli V, La Morgia C, Valentino ML, Rizzo G, Carbonelli M, De Negri AM, et al. Idebenone treatment in Leber's hereditary optic neuropathy. Brain. 2011;134(Pt 9):e188. https://doi.org/10.1093/brain/awr180.
187. Klopstock T, Yu-Wai-Man P, Dimitriadis K, Rouleau J, Heck S, Bailie M, et al. A randomized placebo-controlled trial of idebenone in Leber's hereditary optic neuropathy. Brain. 2011;134(Pt 9):2677–86. https://doi.org/10.1093/brain/awr170.
188. Manickam AH, Michael MJ, Ramasamy S. Mitochondrial genetics and therapeutic overview of Leber's hereditary optic neuropathy. Indian J Ophthalmol. 2017;65(11):1087–92. https://doi.org/10.4103/ijo.IJO_358_17.
189. Yu-Wai-Man P. Genetic manipulation for inherited neurodegenerative diseases: myth or reality? Br J Ophthalmol. 2016;100(10):1322–31. https://doi.org/10.1136/bjophthalmol-2015-308329.
190. Manfredi G, Fu J, Ojaimi J, Sadlock JE, Kwong JQ, Guy J, et al. Rescue of a deficiency in ATP synthesis by transfer of MTATP6, a mitochondrial DNA-encoded gene, to the nucleus. Nat Genet. 2002;30(4):394–9. https://doi.org/10.1038/ng851.
191. Guy J, Qi X, Pallotti F, Schon EA, Manfredi G, Carelli V, et al. Rescue of a mitochondrial deficiency causing Leber Hereditary Optic Neuropathy. Ann Neurol. 2002;52(5):534–42. https://doi.org/10.1002/ana.10354.
192. Perales-Clemente E, Fernandez-Silva P, Acin-Perez R, Perez-Martos A, Enriquez JA. Allotopic expression of mitochondrial-encoded genes in mammals: achieved goal, unde-

monstrated mechanism or impossible task? Nucleic Acids Res. 2011;39(1):225–34. https://doi.org/10.1093/nar/gkq769.

193. Feuer WJ, Schiffman JC, Davis JL, Porciatti V, Gonzalez P, Koilkonda RD, et al. Gene therapy for leber hereditary optic neuropathy: initial results. Ophthalmology. 2016;123(3):558–70. https://doi.org/10.1016/j.ophtha.2015.10.025.

194. Wan X, Pei H, Zhao MJ, Yang S, Hu WK, He H, et al. Efficacy and safety of rAAV2-ND4 treatment for Leber's hereditary optic neuropathy. Sci Rep. 2016;6:21587. https://doi.org/10.1038/srep21587.

195. Yang S, Ma SQ, Wan X, He H, Pei H, Zhao MJ, et al. Long-term outcomes of gene therapy for the treatment of Leber's hereditary optic neuropathy. EBioMedicine. 2016;10:258–68. https://doi.org/10.1016/j.ebiom.2016.07.002.

196. Hyslop LA, Blakeley P, Craven L, Richardson J, Fogarty NME, Fragouli E, et al. Towards clinical application of pronuclear transfer to prevent mitochondrial DNA disease. Nature. 2016;534(7607):383–6. https://doi.org/10.1038/nature18303.

197. Jurkute N, Yu-Wai-Man P. Leber hereditary optic neuropathy: bridging the translational gap. Curr Opin Ophthalmol. 2017;28(5):403–9. https://doi.org/10.1097/icu.0000000000000410.

198. Kang E, Wu J, Gutierrez NM, Koski A, Tippner-Hedges R, Agaronyan K, et al. Mitochondrial replacement in human oocytes carrying pathogenic mitochondrial DNA mutations. Nature. 2016;540(7632):270–5. https://doi.org/10.1038/nature20592.

199. Rowe F, Brand D, Jackson CA, Price A, Walker L, Harrison S, et al. Visual impairment following stroke: do stroke patients require vision assessment? Age Ageing. 2009;38(2):188–93. https://doi.org/10.1093/ageing/afn230.

200. Ghannam ASB, Subramanian PS. Neuro-ophthalmic manifestations of cerebrovascular accidents. Curr Opin Ophthalmol. 2017;28(6):564–72. https://doi.org/10.1097/icu.0000000000000414.

201. Zhang X, Kedar S, Lynn MJ, Newman NJ, Biousse V. Natural history of homonymous hemianopia. Neurology. 2006;66(6):901–5. https://doi.org/10.1212/01.wnl.0000203338.54323.22.

202. Mansouri B, Roznik M, Rizzo JF 3rd, Prasad S. Rehabilitation of visual loss: where we are and where we need to be. J Neuroophthalmol. 2018;38(2):223–9. https://doi.org/10.1097/wno.0000000000000594.

203. Mueller I, Mast H, Sabel BA. Recovery of visual field defects: a large clinical observational study using vision restoration therapy. Restor Neurol Neurosci. 2007;25(5–6):563–72.

204. Paggiaro A, Birbaumer N, Cavinato M, Turco C, Formaggio E, Del Felice A, et al. Magnetoencephalography in stroke recovery and rehabilitation. Front Neurol. 2016;7:35. https://doi.org/10.3389/fneur.2016.00035.

205. Henriksson L, Raninen A, Nasanen R, Hyvarinen L, Vanni S. Training-induced cortical representation of a hemianopic hemifield. J Neurol Neurosurg Psychiatry. 2007;78(1):74–81. https://doi.org/10.1136/jnnp.2006.099374.

206. Eysel UT. Perilesional cortical dysfunction and reorganization. Adv Neurol. 1997;73:195–206.

207. Sincich LC, Park KF, Wohlgemuth MJ, Horton JC. Bypassing V1: a direct geniculate input to area MT. Nat Neurosci. 2004;7(10):1123–8. https://doi.org/10.1038/nn1318.

208. Darian-Smith C, Gilbert CD. Axonal sprouting accompanies functional reorganization in adult cat striate cortex. Nature. 1994;368(6473):737–40. https://doi.org/10.1038/368737a0.

209. Davies JM, Hopkins LN. Neuroendovascular intervention: evolving at the intersection of neurosurgery and neuro-ophthalmology. J Neuroophthalmol. 2017;37(2):111–2. https://doi.org/10.1097/wno.0000000000000517.

210. Micieli JA, Newman NJ, Barrow DL, Biousse V. Intracranial aneurysms of neuro-ophthalmologic relevance. J Neuroophthalmol. 2017;37(4):421–39. https://doi.org/10.1097/wno.0000000000000515.

211. La Pira B, Brinjikji W, Hunt C, Chen JJ, Lanzino G. Reversible edema-like changes along the optic tract following pipeline-assisted coiling of a large anterior communicating artery aneurysm. J Neuroophthalmol. 2017;37(2):154–8. https://doi.org/10.1097/wno.0000000000000412.

212. Griessenauer CJ, Piske RL, Baccin CE, Pereira BJ, Reddy AS, Thomas AJ, et al. Flow diverters for treatment of 160 ophthalmic segment aneurysms: evaluation of safety and efficacy in a multicenter cohort. Neurosurgery. 2017;80(5):726–32.

213. Adeeb N, Griessenauer CJ, Foreman PM, Moore JM, Motiei-Langroudi R, Chua MH, et al. Comparison of stent-assisted coil embolization and the pipeline embolization device for endovascular treatment of ophthalmic segment aneurysms: a multicenter cohort study. World Neurosurg. 2017;105:206–12.

214. Zu QQ, Liu XL, Wang B, Zhou CG, Xia JG, Zhao LB et al. Recovery of oculomotor nerve palsy after endovascular treatment of ruptured posterior communicating artery aneurysm. Neuroradiol. 2017;59(11):1165–70. https://doi.org/10.1007/s00234-017-1909-9.

215. Hall S, Sadek A-R, Dando A, Grose A, Dimitrov BD, Millar J, et al. The resolution of oculomotor nerve palsy caused by unruptured posterior communicating artery aneurysms: a cohort study and narrative review. World Neurosurg. 2017;107:581–7.

216. Liu KC, Starke RM, Durst CR, Wang TR, Ding D, Crowley RW, et al. Venous sinus stenting for reduction of intracranial pressure in IIH: a prospective pilot study. J Neurosurg. 2017;127(5):1126–33.

217. Matloob SA, Toma AK, Thompson SD, Gan CL, Robertson F, Thorne L, et al. Effect of venous stenting on intracranial pressure in idiopathic intracranial hypertension. Acta Neurochir. 2017;159(8):1429–37.

218. Dinkin MJ, Patsalides A. Venous sinus stenting in idiopathic intracranial hypertension: results of a prospective trial. J Neuroophthalmol. 2017;37(2):113–21. https://doi.org/10.1097/wno.0000000000000426.

219. Miyachi S, Hiramatsu R, Ohnishi H, Takahashi K, Kuroiwa T. Endovascular treatment of idiopathic intracranial hypertension with stenting of the transverse sinus stenosis. Neurointervention. 2018;13(2):138–43. https://doi.org/10.5469/neuroint.2018.00990.

220. Nicholson P, Brinjikji W, Radovanovic I, Hilditch CA, Tsang ACO, Krings T, et al. Venous sinus stenting for idiopathic intracranial hypertension: a systematic review and meta-analysis. J Neurointerv Surg. 2019;11(4):380–5. https://doi.org/10.1136/neurintsurg-2018-014172.

221. Leishangthem L, Sir Deshpande P, Dua D, Satti SR. Dural venous sinus stenting for idiopathic intracranial hypertension: an updated review. J Neuroradiol. 2019;46(2):148–54. https://doi.org/10.1016/j.neurad.2018.09.001.

222. Fargen KM, Liu K, Garner RM, Greeneway GP, Wolfe SQ, Crowley RW. Recommendations for the selection and treatment of patients with idiopathic intracranial hypertension for venous sinus stenting. J Neurointerv Surg. 2018. https://doi.org/10.1136/neurintsurg-2018-014042.

223. Asif H, Craven CL, Siddiqui AH, Shah SN, Matloob SA, Thorne L, et al. Idiopathic intracranial hypertension: 120-day clinical, radiological, and manometric outcomes after stent insertion into the dural venous sinus. J Neurosurg. 2018;129(3):723–31. https://doi.org/10.3171/2017.4.Jns162871.

# Chapter 9
# Recent Advances in Pediatric Ophthalmology

Ken K. Nischal

## The Cornea

Corneal anesthesia can lead to neuropathic keratopathy, corneal scarring and blindness [1]. In children it is a particular problem not only because of the effect on amblyopia but also because children are more likely to cause microtrauma to the cornea [2]. Causes of corneal anesthesia in children include congenital and acquired. The congenital causes are rare and include trigeminal nerve agenesis, Riley-Day syndrome, Goldenhar and Mobius syndrome. Acquired causes are often iatrogenic e.g. after intracranial tumor resection and due to neoplasm damaging the trigeminal nerve [3]. Some of these are unilateral and recent descriptions of the neurotization of the cornea have changed the natural history and course of this condition [4]. Prior to this, all therapies were aimed at keeping the cornea lubricated or protected (with a tarsorrhaphy). Corneal neurotization entails using a sensory nerve such as the sural nerve, as a conduit from the unaffected supratrochlear nerve to the affected cornea. The nerve has to be divided into its fascicular bundles and each fascicle passed under the conjunctiva so as to be equally distributed around the affected cornea at the limbus (see Fig. 9.1). Re-innervation takes several months [4] but results are reproducible, and the technique has been taken up world-wide. Its use in children dramatically changes the prognosis (see Fig. 9.1). Cases where there is bilateral corneal anesthesia have recently been reported and here coaptation of the sural nerve to branches arising from the maxillary division or even the mandibular division of the trigeminal nerves are possible as long as their function is normal or by using the ipsilateral supratrochlear nerves [4].

Congenital corneal opacification has undergone a re-evaluation with respect to nomenclature. The condition is better described as conditions that are due to primary

K. K. Nischal (✉)
UPMC Children's Hospital of Pittsburgh, Pittsburgh, PA, USA
e-mail: nischalkk@upmc.edu

© Springer Nature Switzerland AG 2020
A. Grzybowski (ed.), *Current Concepts in Ophthalmology*,
https://doi.org/10.1007/978-3-030-25389-9_9

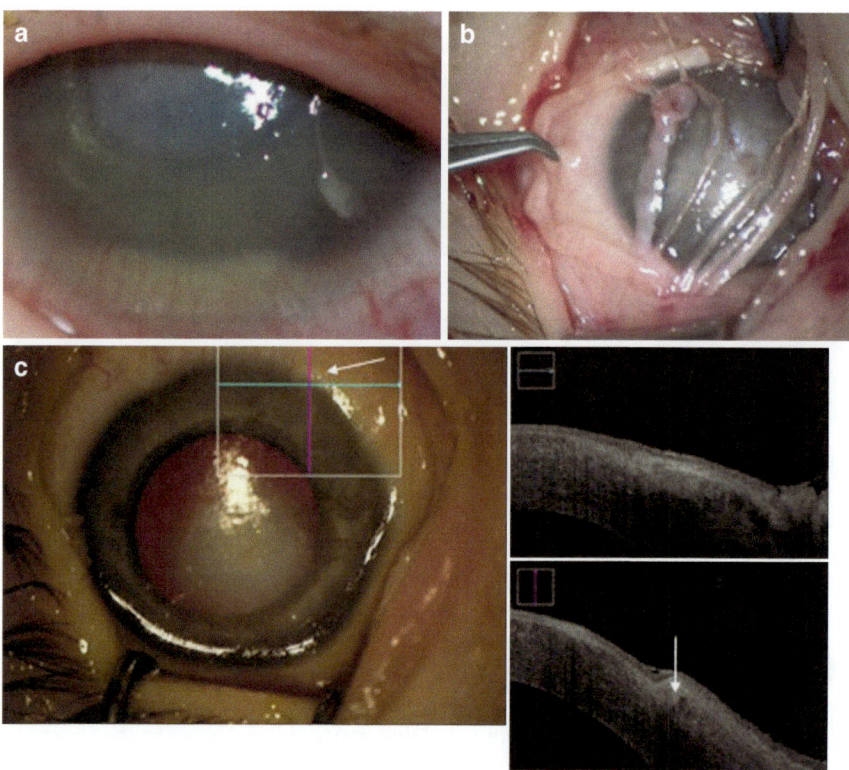

**Fig. 9.1** Shows a child with congenital corneal anesthesia due to aplasia of the trigeminal nerve. (**a**) shows the child at presentation with a neurotrophic ulcer and hypopyon. (**b**) shows the corneal neurotization procedure at the point where the sural nerve is divided into its component fascicles which are then passed under the conjunctiva to the limbus.(**c**) shows an integrated intraoperative OCT of one of the fascicles under the conjunctiva about 3 months after the surgery (white arrow)

corneal disease or secondary corneal disease (see Fig. 9.2) [5–9]. The only primary corneal causes of CCO are corneal dystrophies, such as CHED, PPMD, X-L ECD, corneal dermoids, cornea plana and CYP1B1 cytopathy. Secondary causes of CCO, are due to kerato-irido-lenticular dysgenesis (KILD—see Fig. 9.3) and congenital glaucoma. KILD encompasses iridocorneal adhesions (Peters anomaly I), kerato-lenticular adhesions (Peters II) and other forms of partial or complete lenticular dysgenesis leading to secondary corneal opacity. The importance of this classification is that not only does it allow a more logical approach to these cases but also allows for prognostications which are so important for parents and also the doctors dealing with them.

Perhaps deep phenotyping of CCO allowed identification of those cases where there were only iridocorneal adhesions or only a posterior central defect in endothelium (von Hippel ulcer). It is in such cases that the use of selective endothelial cell removal has resulted in rapid clearing of these congenital corneal opacities

**PRIMARY CORNEAL DISEASE**

A   DEVELOPMENTAL ANOMALIES OF CORNEA

- i. **Corneal dystrophies**
  - CHED,PPMD,CHSD,X-L ECD
- ii. Cornea Plana (sclerocornea)
- iii **Corneal structural defects due to dermoids**
  - Isolated
  - Part of systemic disease eg. Goldenhar, Linear sebaceous nevus
- iv **CYP1B1 Cytopathy**

**SECONDARY CORNEAL DISEASE**

A   DEVELOPMENTAL ANOMALIES OF ANRERIOR SEGMENT

- i **Kerato-Irido-Lenticular Dysgenesis KILD**
  - a. **Iridocorneal adhesions only**
  - b. **Lens fails to separate from cornea**
  - c. Mechanical e.g. due to PHPV
  - d. **Lens separates but fails to form thereafter**
  - e. **Lens fails to from**
- ii **Irido-trabecular Dysgenesis**
  - a. Infantile glaucoma
  - b. Axenfeld-Rieger anomaly
  - c. Aniridia

**SECONDARY CORNEAL DISEASE CONT'D**

B   ACQUIRED CORNEAL DISEASE

- i Metabolic
  - Mucolipidoses
  - Mucopolysaccharidoses
  - Cystinosis
- ii Trauma
- iii Infectious Keratitis
  - Bacterial
  - Viral
  - Protozoal
  - Fungal
- iv Non-infectious Keratitis
  - Exposure
  - Neurotrophic
  - Interstitial e.g. Cogan's disease
  - Steven-Johnson syndrome
  - Epidermolysis hullosa
- v Miscellaneous
  - Keratoconus
  - Keratoglobus
  - Xeroderma pigmentosa

**Fig. 9.2** Classification for congenital corneal opacities. All conditions in red have a poor prognosis for corneal transplant

[10]. IN these subset of CCO, this procedure appears to allow a faster clearing of the cornea than previously seen or expected (see Fig. 9.4). This report is potentially a disruptive moment in this field of pediatric cornea. The fact that corneal opacities in children 'clear with time' is well known but it has always been an issue that the time taken to clear causes so much amblyopia that other therapies (PKP or optical iridectomy) have been sought. IF by selective endothelial removal one is accelerating the corneal opacity clearing, then this may have tremendous benefits. However this technique is unlikely to work if there is a keratolenticular adhesion or a marked loss of posterior corneal stroma. Hence the need for deep phenotyping before applying this technique to a case of CCO.

The advent of intraoperative integrated OCT (i²OCT) has played an enormous role in allowing better accuracy in delivering care for children with corneal disease especially in difficult cases where the view may not be so easy (see Fig. 9.5).

Collagen cross linking (CXL) has been developed to increase the biomechanical rigidity of an ectatic cornea (keratoconus). Initially the application of this technique was in progressive keratoconus in adults but as our understanding of the technique and its applications has improved, its use in children has spread. In children the presence of keratoconus alone is enough to offer CXL. While arguments about epithelium on or

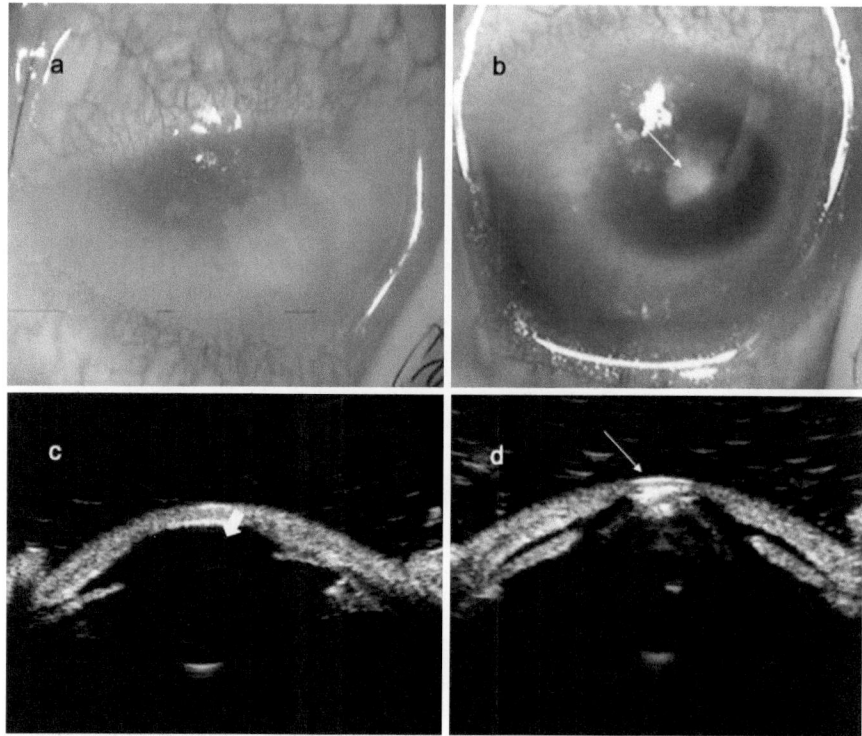

**Fig. 9.3** Shows a child with congenital corneal opacities. The right eye (**a** and **c**) shows no kera-tolenticular adhesions but does show iridocorneal adhesions. The thick white arrow is showing a formed anterior chamber. The left eye shows a clearing centrally but this is due to thinning of the cornea and a keratolenticular adhesion (thin white arrows **b** and **d**)

epithelium off rage in the literature, evidence to date suggests that long-term stability is better achieved with epithelium off using the Dresden protocol in children.

The original Dresden protocol, consists of manual epithelial debridement followed by application of Riboflavin 0.146% with dextran instillation every 2 min for 30 min followed by UV-A irradiation, 3 mW/cm$^2$ for 30 min with continuing riboflavin instillation [11] (see Fig. 9.6).

CXL induces and enhances cross-linking between collagen fibrils. Riboflavin causes photo-sensitisation and UV-A creates cross-linking by generating oxidative products in the presence of oxygen [12]. This process increases the corneal biomechanical strength arresting the progression of biomechanical weakening (ectasia).

Paediatric keratoconus is more aggressive even at presentation with an aggravated progression compared to adults % [13] with a seven-fold increased risk of requiring a penetrating keratoplasty compared to adults [14, 15]. Studies that include no children with allergic eye disease show stabilization of progression with no requirement of any further intervention [14, 16]. In those studies where patients had allergic eye disease [17] 20% of eyes that were followed beyond 4 years showed reversal of keratometric flattening with minimal drop in visual acuity; This regression of cross

**Fig. 9.4** The image shows pre-selective endothelial removal (**a**), then a few weeks later (**b**) and then a few months later (**c**). There is remarkable clearing of the opacity and emphasizes the need for deep phenotyping in these cases so that the correct treatment can be used; e.g. selective endothelial removal could not be used in the eye shown in (**b**). Courtesy of Professor J Mehta

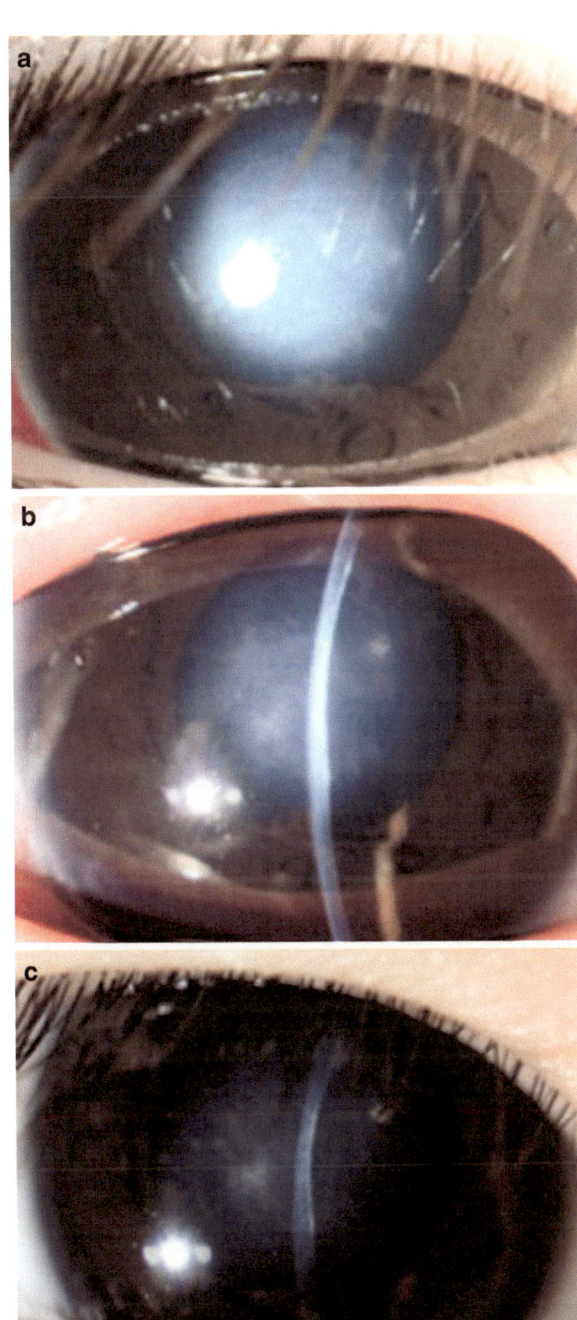

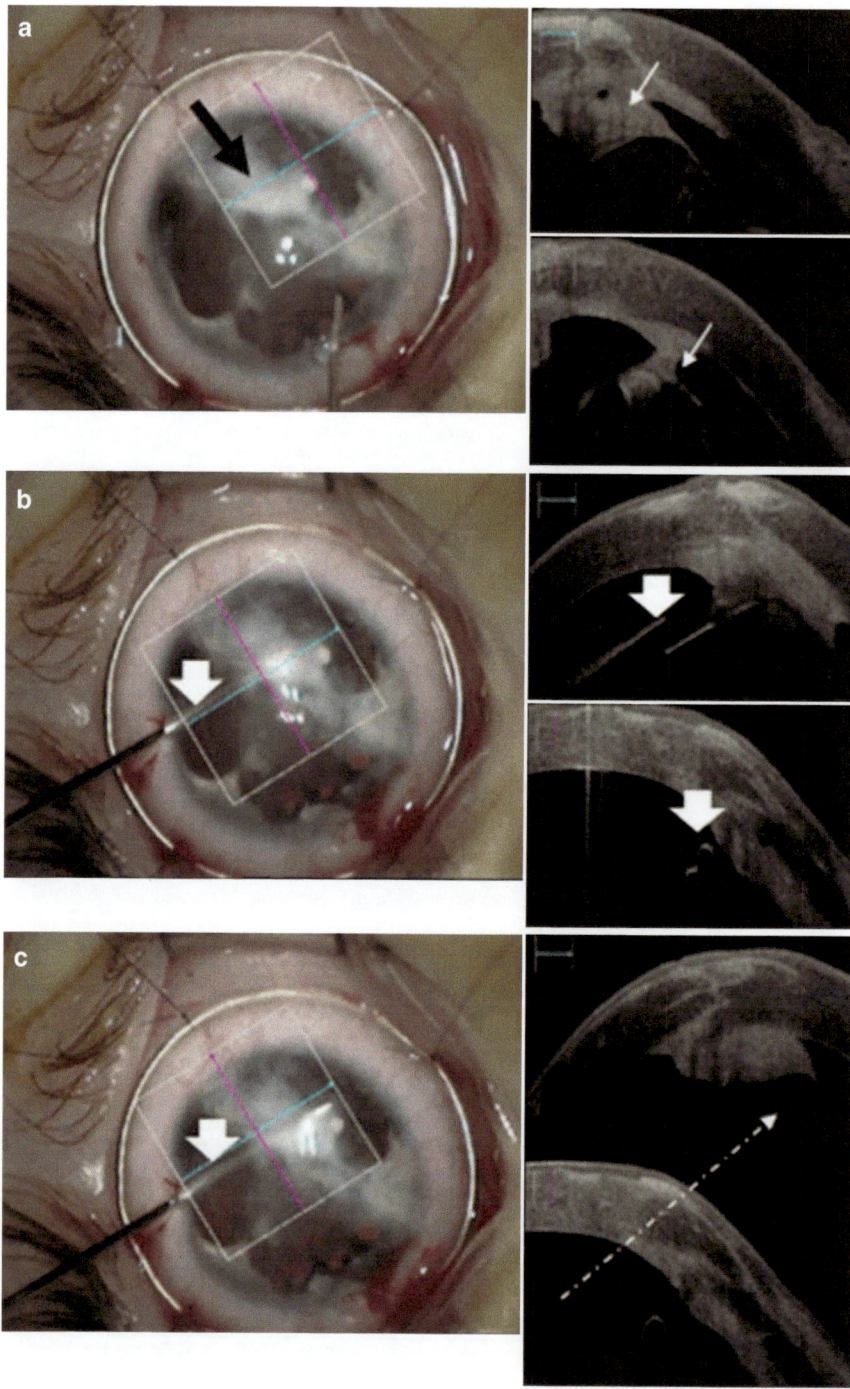

**Fig. 9.5** Shows a child with Bardet Biedl syndrome with retinal dystrophy. The fundus autofluorescence shows hyper fluorescence around the macula (black arrow) while the fundus picture shows marked attenuation of the arterioles (white arrow) without any bony spicule pigmentation

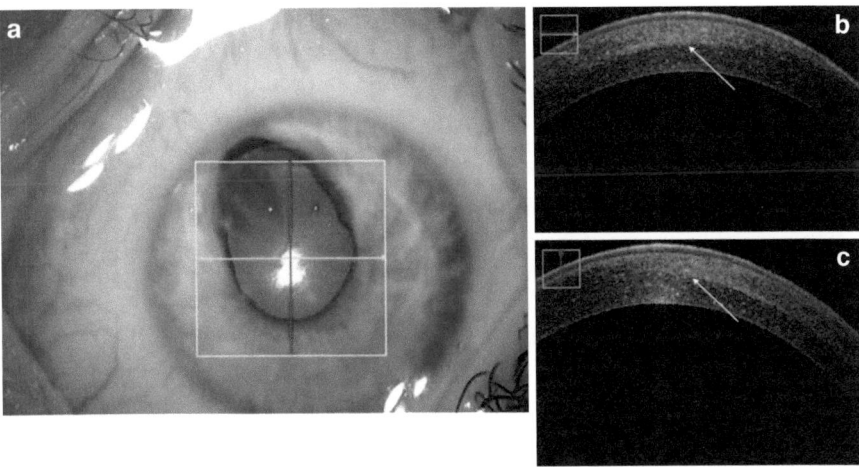

**Fig. 9.6** Shows a child with traumatic corneal scar (**a** black arrow) and traumatic cataract . In order to perform a corneal transplant, cataract removal and primary lens implantation, the integrated intraoperative OCT (i²OCT) was used to cut the keratolenticular adhesion (**a, b**—thin white arrow) using the simultaneous OCT view in the binoculars of the operative microscope (**b, c**—thick white arrow shows the microscissors and the dashed white arrow in (**b**) shows the keratolenticular adhesion cut

linking effect in a small subset of patients was thought to be due to persistent eye rubbing due to allergic eye disease.

In patients of keratoconus older than 15 years, an objective study of quality of life using NEI-VFQ 25 questionnaire by Cingu et al. has shown better quality of life and decreased anxiety related traits 1 year following cross linking [18].

Studies have demonstrated both statistically and clinically that CXL with the Dresden protocol arrests the progression of keratoconus, while causing corneal flattening, variable visual improvement and significantly decreases the requirement of keratoplasty for keratoconus and improves quality of life [16–23].

CXL is associated with minimal sight threatening complications which include infectious keratitis (0.0017%), sterile infiltrates, limbal stem cell damage and an anterior stromal haze not affecting vision with long-term studies showing a regression of CXL effect or failure of up to 8–10% [23–25].

Studies have shown significant progression of the disease in non-cross-linked eyes. Progression is especially higher and rapid in paediatric keratoconus eyes affecting vision significantly and leading to contact lens intolerance and eventually acute hydrops [18, 26, 27].

Other options in moderate to severe keratoconus management include Intra corneal ring segments (Intacs®) and keratoplasty. Intacs, though can partially rehabilitate vision and delay keratoplasty, is associated with poor outcomes with higher grades of keratoconus and has reported risk of extrusion or need for removal [28, 29], which increases the number of procedures, especially in paediatric patients. Pediatric keratoplasty has a higher risk of infections, graft rejection and difficult visual rehabilitation compared to adult keratoplasties [19].

Accelerated CXL (KXL) significantly reduces irradiation time and use of pulsed UV delivery has circumvented the problem of $O_2$ delivery. Long term comparative studies with 48 months follow up in paediatric and adult populations have proven safety and efficacy in halting progression compared to Dresden protocol. Further better outcomes are reported with KXL when Riboflavin with HPMC is used instead of Photrexa viscous [30].

Customised KXL with graded energy delivery to different zones of the cornea with maximum energy at the cone has proven safety and better flattening of cone and visual gain with lesser keratocyte damage in corneal periphery compared to conventional technique [30].

For thinner corneas (less than 400 µm), epi-on trans epithelial CXL, though was initially reported to be inferior to conventional epi-off method, is now showing promise on safety and efficacy with use of modified Riboflavin with other agents as EDTA and use of Iontophoresis for Riboflavin delivery [30].

## Pediatric Cataract

No field in pediatric ophthalmology has advanced at as fast a rate than the area of pediatric cataract surgery surgically. Key studies globally have contributed to a better understanding of surgical outcomes, techniques and decision making for intervention. In the past 5 years.

There have been outcomes of randomized controlled trials (RCT), an individual metanalysis and a Delphi consensus statement, reflecting the integration of real-world evidence, real world data with basic scientific rigor [31–34].

The infant Aphakia Treatment study was the first RCT to be published in the area of pediatric cataract surgery, and specifically looked at unilateral cataract in infants. The conclusion drawn from this study, which has had some criticisms in methodology, were that at 5 year follow up IOL implantation resulted in greater number of re-operations with no difference in vision between the two groups (aphakic corrected with Contact lenses or IOL implantation group corrected with glasses). These conclusions hold true for **unilateral** cataract [31].

Bilateral cataracts are a different type of disease and extrapolations from IATS to applications in bilateral congenital cataract are misleading and misguided. Recently a group in India performed a randomized controlled trial for bilateral congenital cataracts and have shown that the reoperation rates between aphakic and IOL groups were the same and the visual outcomes in the bilateral group with IOL rending to be better than those in the control group [32].

Sixty children (120 eyes) up to 2 years of age undergoing bilateral congenital cataract surgery were randomized to aphakia (n = 30), or primary IOL implantation (pseudophakia) (n = 30). A single surgeon performed all the surgeries with identical surgical technique. All patients were followed up regularly for 5 years. The median age of the patients at time of surgery was 5.11 months (aphakia group) and 6.01 months (pseudophakia group). At 5 year follow up the incidence of glaucoma was about the same (16% aphakic and 13.8% pseudophakic). The incidence of posterior synechiae was significantly higher in the pseudophakia group and visual axis opacification requiring surgery was seen in 8% of the aphakes and 10.3% of the pseudophakes. Mean logMAR visual acuity at 5 years follow-up was 0.59 ± 0.33 and 0.5 ± 0.23. However, more eyes in the pseudophakic group started giving documentable vision earlier in their postoperative follow-ups than the aphakic group [32].

This is understandable for two reasons: firstly almost ALL unilateral cataracts (truly unilateral) are due to some form of persistent fetal vasculature (PFV) and secondly, the IATS included several surgeons (some of whom had small volumes of surgery for pediatric cataract) while the RCT for bilateral disease was performed by a single center high volume pediatric cataract surgeon.

In the only individual metanalysis performed on infant cataract surgery [33], having analyzed 486 eyes the authors concluded that surgery before 4 weeks of age and multiple reoperations increased the risk of glaucoma development while placement of an IOL protected against glaucoma. This last is still controversial; reasons why this should be so, are likely hidden by the fact that each of the surgeons who participated in this metanalysis were experienced high volume cataract surgeons, who had specific indications to abort placement of IOL in even those eyes where parents had been counseled that an IOL would be placed. This of course is real-world evidence. Conducting RCTs for surgical techniques may not be appropriate when the factors that influence a surgeon's decision to place one are not taken into account. In fact some authors suggest that RCTs in such circumstances are in fact dangerous for the participants.

A Delphi process led consensus was reported for management of pediatric cataract [34]. The process consisted of three rounds of anonymous electronic questionnaires followed by a face-to-face meeting, followed by a fourth anonymous electronic questionnaire. The executive committee created questions to be used for the electronic questionnaires. Questions were designed to have unit-based, multiple choice or true–false answers. The questionnaire included issues related to the preoperative, intraoperative and postoperative management of pediatric cataract. Consensus based on 85% of panelists being in agreement for electronic questionnaires or 80% for the face-to-face meeting, and near consensus based on 70%. Sixteen international pediatric cataract participated. Consensus or near consensus was reached for 85/108 (78.7%) questions and non-consensus for the remaining 23 (21.3%) questions.

The first Delphi consensus statement was more valuable in determining where consensus could not be reached rather than where it could. To this end the following remain areas of controversy. There was no consensus on certain topics such as the use of hydrodissection in cases where a pre-existing posterior capsule defect is not suspected, the best formula to use while calculating IOL power and the minimum age for primary IOL implantation.

Surgical techniques for pediatric capsule management continue to improve. While femtosecond laser has been used to describe excellent centration and precision of both anterior and posterior rhexis in children [35, 36], the expense of the procedure has prohibited its widespread use. The zeptosecond capsulotomy device [37] has gained some interest but its use in small eyes is questionable. The Two incision push pull technique continues to gain favor and allows sizing of the anterior and posterior capsulorhexis in pediatric cataract surgery [38]. Continuing this need for precisely sizing the anterior and posterior rhexis, a foldable capsulorhexis ring has been developed specifically for use with the bag-in the lens (BIL). This IOL is designed with a groove around the optic, into which the anterior capsule and posterior capsule fit after capsulorhexes are performed. The beauty of this lens is that the lens epithelial cells are captured and cannot proliferate, resulting in clear visual axes [39].

The use of multifocal implants in children continues to be reported but studies fail to measure contrast sensitivity in children who have had diffractive mutifocal IOLs placed. Without this outcome measure the use of diffractive multifocal IOLs is controversial [40].

The most important and perhaps controversial development has been the report of using a new surgical technique which results in regeneration of the lens itself. This group [41] showed in donor eyes that the younger the patient the greater the ability for LEC's to reproliferate; this is a clinical fact well known to pediatric cataract surgeons. They then showed that the mere act of injury to the capsule would result in a seven-fold increase in LEC proliferation regardless of age. Based on a series of in vitro experiments, followed by surgeries on rabbit and then macaque monkey eyes they described a surgical technique whereby a small peripheral capsule opening was made and the lens fibers removed with as little damage to the proliferating anterior lens epithelial cells. This technique resulted in a regrowth of the lens fibers over a period of several weeks in the animal eyes. This technique was repeated in 24 eyes (12 cases) with congenital cataract in human children and compared to standard cataract surgery in 25 cases (50 eyes) with congenital cataract. The results published show regeneration of the lens using the newer technique over 3–5 months. There are of course many unanswered questions such as, how did an opaque lens regenerate into a clear one and during the period of regeneration how was amblyopia prevented? That said this concept is potentially disruptive if it can be replicated once the unanswered questions are clarified.

## *Refractive Error*

Myopia, commonly called near-sightedness, is the most common human eye disorder in the world, affecting 85–90% of young adults in some Asian countries such as Singapore and Taiwan, and between 25 and 50% of older adults in the United States and Europe. Unlike Western populations where the prevalence of myopia is low (<5%) in children aged 8 years or younger, in Asian children there is a significantly higher prevalence of myopia, affecting 9–15% of preschool children, 24.7% of 7-year-olds, 31.3% of 8-year-olds, and 49.7% of 9-year-old primary school children in Singapore [42]. In 12 year-old children, the prevalence of myopia is 62.0% in Singapore and 49.7% in Guangzhou, China compared with 20.0% in the United States, 11.9% in Australia, 9.7% in urban India and 16.5% in Nepal [43].

The economic cost of myopia is estimated at an annual US$268 billion world-wide. Not only is there a socio-economic burden, there is a significant increased odds ratios for myopic maculopathy, retinal detachment, cataracts, and glaucoma, even for low and moderate levels of myopia and these odds ratios increase further with higher levels of myopia [44].

Evidence supports heritability of the nonsyndromic forms of myopia, especially for high-grade myopia ($-5$ D or higher) and Genome-wide association studies (GWAS) have identified >20 associated loci for myopia. However, the majority of recent studies show that the boom in myopia prevalence reported in different populations is related mostly to environmental factors, including excess in near work especially in young age and low light exposure, especially as outdoor activity.

There has been much interest recently to try and retard myopic progression of childhood. Some interventions that have been used in the past appear not to work. For example under-correction of myopia either increases or has no effect on myopia progression. Under correction does not slow myopia progression and should no longer be advocated [45].

While there is some evidence that bifocal lenses may reduce myopia progression there is some that suggests that they do not [45, 46]. Older studies (PALS, COMET, CLAMP) have shown minimal myopia retardation effect on myopia using traditional contact lenses [45–48].

In overnight orthokeratology the patient wears reverse geometry contact lenses overnight to temporarily flatten the cornea and provide clear vision during the day without any glasses or contact lenses. Reduction in myopia (up to $-6$ D) is achieved by central corneal epithelial thinning, midperipheral epithelial, and stromal thickening. Unfortunately, more than one hundred cases of severe microbial keratitis related to orthokeratology have been reported since 2001. Randomized clinical trials of orthokeratology myopia control demonstrated significantly slower axial elongation in children wearing orthokeratology lenses than children wearing single vision spectacles. Orthokeratology contact lenses can be used to correct central refractive error while leaving peripheral myopic blur, which may act as a putative cue to slow the progression of myopia. Overall, ortho-k results in an approximately 40% reduction in the progression of myopia. There is no good controlled long term study demonstrating sustained myopia control effect and there is no washout data [49, 50].

While there is accumulating evidence for the role of the peripheral retina in the development of refractive errors [51] with initial human studies involving mainly Caucasians suggesting an association between relative peripheral hyperopia and axial myopia, the Peripheral Refraction in Preschool Children (PREP) Study of Singaporean Chinese children and Collaborative Longitudinal Evaluation of Ethnicity and Refractive Error (CLEERE) study showed that relative peripheral hyperopia had little consistent influence on the risk of myopia onset, myopia progression, or axial elongation [52]. Even human clinical trials with treatment strategies aimed at reducing the peripheral retinal hyperopic defocus, there were no statistically significant differences in the rates of myopia progression between children who wore one of three novel spectacle lenses that decreased relative peripheral hyperopia and those who wore the conventional single-vision spectacle lenses.

However, for children aged 6–12 years whose parents are myopic, one of the three spectacle lenses was found to reduce the progression of myopia significantly when higher rates of progression were evident [53, 54].

There has been a tremendous amount of interest in the use of topical atropine. Atropine blocks muscarinic receptors non-selectively. Muscarinic receptors are found in human ciliary muscle, retina and sclera. Although the exact mechanism of atropine in myopia control is not known, it is believed that atropine acts directly or indirectly on the retina or scleral, inhibiting thinning or stretching of the scleral, and thereby eye growth. This was also shown that atropine acts via non-accomodative way. Studies have shown some clinical effect on slowing the progression of myopia in children. The Atropine for the Treatment of Myopia studies (ATOM 1 and 2) were randomized, double-masked, placebo-controlled trials each involving 400 Singapore children. The ATOM1 study suggested 1% atropine eyedrops nightly in one eye over a 2-year period slowed myopic progression by 77% and reduced the axial length elongation (mean axial length increase of 0.39 mm in controls versus no growth in atropine group). The ATOM2 study demonstrated a dose-related response with 0.5%, 0.1% and 0.01% atropine slowing myopia progression by an estimated 75%, 70% and 60% with SE changes of 0.30D,0.38D and 0.48D, respectively over 2-years. However, when atropine was stopped, there was an inverse increase in myopia, with rebound being greater in the children previously on higher doses. This resulted in myopia progression being significantly lower in children previously assigned to the 0.01% group at 36 months compared with that in the 0.1 and 0.5% groups. Younger children and those with greater myopic progression in year 1 were more likely to require re-treatment. By the end of 5 years, myopia progression remained lowest in the 0.01% group. It was estimated that, overall, atropine 0.01% slowed myopia progression by at least 50%. The efficacy of lower dose atropine is corroborated by Taiwanese cohort studies. However, there may be children who are poor responders to atropine. In ATOM1, 12.1% of children (younger, with higher myopia, and greater tendency of myopic progression) had myopia progression of more than 0.5D after 1 year of treatment with atropine 1%. Atropine 0.01% caused minimal pupil dilation (0.8 mm), minimal loss of accommodation (2–3 D), and no near visual loss compared with higher doses. Children on atropine 0.01% did not need progressive additional lenses, and they did not need photochromatic lenses because of photophobia [55–58].

Finally, there have been many studies showing that outdoor activity, what was shown to be exposition to natural light, decreased the onset of myopia and neutralized the effect of parental myopia and near-distance work. The role of outdoor activity to myopia progression is not as clear since different studies shown conflicting results. The recent interventional studies showed effectiveness in reducing the myopia onset after increasing outdoor activity time in school. The notion that at least 2 h daylight exposure can be preventive against myopic progression of childhood has gained favour and in some countries is influencing the design of classrooms to increase daylight exposure while indoors [59–62].

## Molecular Genetics

There is of course always something new in the field of molecular genetics but in terms of overarching concepts the two that are the most important and relatively new are nonsense suppression therapy and ciliopathies.

Nonsense mutations are single base pair substitutions in the DNA that create one of three stop codon sequences, UAA, UAG, or UGA, called premature termination codons (PTC). These types of mutations often result in truncated protein products which may be subject to nonsense-mediated mRNA decay (NMD). NMD is an evolutionarily-conserved surveillance pathway designed to eliminate abnormal mRNA transcripts before abnormally truncated proteins can be synthesized [63, 64]. Interference in the NMD pathway may stabilize abnormal transcripts, promote "read-through" of PTCs, and increase the amount of functioning protein [65].

"Read-through" is the misreading of stop codon during translation, allowing an amino acid to be incorporated into the growing polypeptide [66, 67] and occurs at a frequency of less than 0.1% at normally positioned stop codons and less than 1% at PTCs [66–70]. Nonsense suppression therapy (NST) is promotion of read-through and is potentially very impactful since nonsense mutations account for about 30% of ocular genetic disease [71].

Ataluren is classified as an orphan drug by the European Medicines Agency and U.S. Food and Drug Administration for treatment of Duchenne Muscular Dystrophy and cystic fibrosis as a form of NST [72–76]. Despite its successes, the in vivo and in vitro effectiveness of ataluren has been questioned and the potential complication of action on non-targeted genes and stop codons has been raised [71, 77, 78].

In ophthalmology ataluren has been used to treat aniridia [79]. Aniridia is a congenital, progressive, panocular condition characterized by partial or complete absence of iris, nystagmus, corneal opacification, glaucoma, cataract, and foveal hypoplasia. The condition is due to mutations in the *PAX6* gene, which plays a central role in early ocular development of the cornea, iris, lens, and retina [80, 81].

Using a mouse model of aniridia with a naturally occurring nonsense mutation, notated Gly194Term, in *PAX6*, Gregory-Evans et al. administered daily subcutaneous injections of ataluren (30 μg/g) from postnatal days 4 to 14 [79]. In untreated mice, the baseline ocular phenotype included a thickened cornea connected to a lenticular stalk and a thickened retina with abnormal infolding. By day 14, the phenotype progressed to globe distortion, further retinal infolding, and an abnormally small lens. In ataluren-treated mice, the retinal infolding was corrected and the lens was 70% larger compared to controls. Functional improvements were also apparent by postnatal day 60 when measured by electroretinography (ERG), where untreated mice had non-recordable ERG tracings at and treated mice had relatively substantial ERG responses. Of note, the ERG responses in treated mice were improved but not normalized. Anterior segment examinations revealed an abnormally thick corneal stroma with epithelial thinning, which was not statistically different from untreated mice. Extending injections to postnatal day 60 did not significantly improve the corneal phenotype. The authors concluded that systemic injection may limit delivery to the cornea and that improvement in the corneal phenotype may be also be limited as other *PAX6*-independent factors contribute to anterior segment development and would not be responsive to ataluren. Modification of the study for topical delivery rescued the corneal abnormalities, demonstrated a greater reversal of lens and retina defects compared to systemic injection, and improved retinal function by ERG and behavioral optokinetic tracking. This study was the first to demonstrate that an abnormal ocular phenotype could be subject to remodeling and rescue of a near-normal or normal phenotype after birth in an animal model. These remarkable research outcomes have led to the design and implementation of an ongoing clinical trial of ataluren in children and adults with aniridia (NCT02647359).

To date, research of the read-through efficacy of aminoglycosides or ataluren in cell and animal models has included aniridia, ocular coloboma, Usher Syndrome Type 1C, choroideremia, and various forms of retinitis pigmentosa [82–84]. Given the frequency of nonsense mutations in certain ocular disorders and the optimized delivery system of ataluren that can penetrate both anterior and posterior segment tissues, the success of nonsense suppression therapy with ataluren has the potential to be extended and positively impact the phenotype of patients.

For optimal patient management and consideration for the ongoing clinical trial, patients with aniridia should have a comprehensive testing including *PAX6* sequencing and *PAX6/WT1* deletion/duplication studies. *PAX6* sequencing will allow detection of intragenic mutations, including nonsense mutations that would establish the patient's eligibility for the clinical trial of ataluren, and *PAX6/WT1* deletion/duplication studies are essential to rule out involvement of the nearby *WT1* gene that increases the risk for Wilms Tumor to 45–57% [85, 86]. In the case of *WT1* involvement or in the absence of any *PAX6* analyses, children with aniridia should undergo renal ultrasound every 3 months until age 8 years when the development of Wilms Tumor is rare. Late-onset Wilms Tumor, delayed involvement of the contralateral kidney, and high incidence of renal failure with or without a history of Wilms Tumor justifies a low threshold for ultrasonography, kidney function tests, and nephrology referral [86–89].

Cilia are highly conserved organelles that exist and function as either motile or non-motile structures. Motile cilia are primarily found in the ventricles, middle ear, respiratory tract, and fallopian tubes, where they protrude from the cellular surface and move in a coordinated, wave-like motion [90–93]. A dysfunction of motile cilia result in certain diseases in these tissues, such as hydrocephalus, airway disease, and infertility, or cause a broader effect such as situs inversus totalis [90–92]. Non-motile, or primary, cilia are expressed in nearly every cell type and therefore have the potential to result in multisystem dysfunction [91, 93].

The motile and non-motile cilia are structurally similar in that they are both anchored by a basal body and have a projection, referred to as the axoneme. The axonemes contain nine paired microtubule structures, where the motile cilia have an additional, central pair of microtubules. These microtubule configurations are referred to as 9 + 0 for non-motile cilia and 9 + 2 for motile cilia [94]. Within the cilia, there are hundreds of proteins responsible for its functions. The synthesis of these proteins does not occur within the cilium; rather, they are transported through a process referred to as intraflagellar transport (IFT). IFT is achieved through complexes within the base and along the cilium, which are essential for the protein trafficking to form and maintain cilia [95, 96].

Cilia have essential mechanical, developmental, and sensory roles that, if dysfunctional, result in a spectrum of symptoms and disorders referred to as ciliopathies. The following is a summary of these overlapping roles as they occur in normal cilia and an example of their effect on a disease process.

1. *Mechanosensation.* External stimuli including fluid flow, osmotic pressure, heat shock, touch, and extracellular movement can impact primary cilia [97–100]. In response, signaling inside the cilium result in changes in length and stiffness which alter how the cilia interact with their immediate environment. The mechanical properties and relation to disease are most understood in the setting of cystic kidney diseases including polycystic kidney disease and nephronophthisis. The relevant proteins (referred to as cystoproteins), have been localized to the cilia and centrioles and are mislocalized or absent in models in animal models of cystic kidney diseases [101–104]. Studies have demonstrated the mechanical role of cilia in these diseases, where bending of kidney epithelial cilia initiates a calcium-mediated response that subsequently affects several signaling pathways related to cell proliferation and cystogenesis [104]. As an example, mutations in *NPHP1* account for approximately 20% of cases nephronophthisis, resulting in cyst formation and subsequent renal failure [105, 106].

2. *Development.* The role of primary cilia in various signaling pathways is still emerging, but previous work demonstrates that primary cilia modulate Sonic hedgehog, canonical and non-canonical Wnt, platelet-derived growth factor (PDGFR), and mTOR pathways [91, 93]. A relevant disease model is Joubert Syndrome. Mutations in *AHI1* account for up to 10% of cases of Joubert Syndrome and, in humans, primarily causes a neurologic and ocular phenotype [107]. *AHI1* mutations result in cerebellar vermis hypoplasia and the characteristic "molar tooth sign" on MRI, rod-cone dystrophy, and progressive renal disease, among other symptoms [107].

3. *Sensory.* The sensory role of cilium is most prominent in the form of retinal photoreceptors, which are modified primary cilia composed of an outer segment (OS) and inner segment (IS) bridged by the connecting cilium (CC) and a synaptic ending [108]. Phototransduction occurs in the outer segment and cascades to the CC and inner segment, which relies on the integrity of IFT [108]. Mutations in ciliary genes may disrupt the structure or sensory function of the photoreceptor, resulting in nonsyndromic or syndromic retinal dystrophy [109]. As an example, mutations in *BBS2* result in Bardet-Biedl Syndrome or, rarely, nonsyndromic retinitis pigmentosa [110]. The BBS2 protein is localized to the basal body of the cilium and mutations in this protein may explain *BBS2*-related retinitis pigmentosa as well as offer insight to the underlying defect of other retinal ciliopathies, in humans.

Although the individual syndromes are rare, ciliopathies may affect up to 1 in 2000 individuals [111]. Syndromes now recognized as ciliopathies include Alstrom syndrome, Bardet-Biedl syndrome (BBS) (see Fig. 9.7), Ellis van Creveld syndrome (EVC), Jeune asphyxiating thoracic syndrome (JATD), Joubert syndrome and

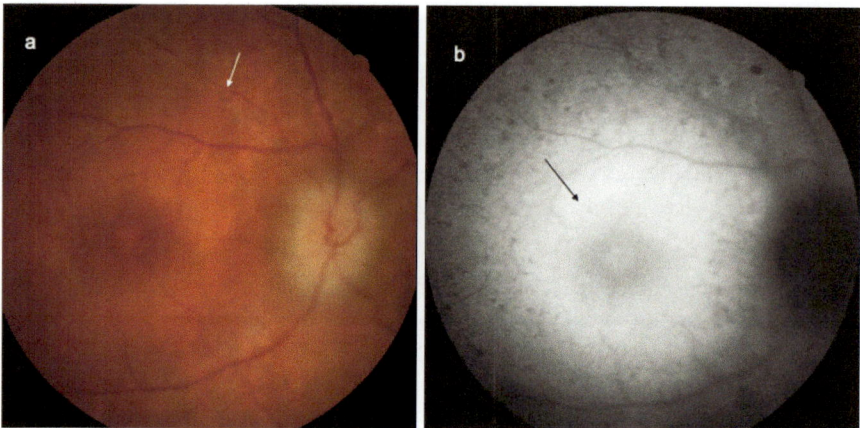

**Fig. 9.7** Shows a child post collagen cross linking 3 months; the integrated intraoperative OCT shows the interface where the UV light penetrated to (white arrows) This shows the cross-linking

related disorders (JSRD), Leber Congenital Amaurosis (LCA), McKusick-Kaufman syndrome (MKKS), Meckel Syndrome (MKS), nephronophthisis (NPHP), orofaciodigital syndromes (OFD), Senior-Loken Syndrome (SNLS), Sensenbrenner syndrome, Short-rib polydactyly syndromes (SRPS), and Usher syndrome [112, 113].

Traditionally, the syndromes now recognized as ciliopathies were diagnosed based on the involved tissues and overall phenotype. With time, it has become obvious that the overlap between these syndromes is striking and that mutations in genes associated with these syndromes can even result in a nonsyndromic phenotype. This variability has the potential to have a profound impact on medical management and genetic testing and counseling. Therefore, a low threshold for pursuing relevant systemic investigations such as renal ultrasound, audiometric testing, echocardiogram, intracranial imaging, and skeletal survey, in addition to genetic testing should be considered in all early onset retinal dystrophies.

## Retina

Recently, there have been revolutions in the development of both gene medicine therapy and genome surgical treatments for inherited disorders. Much of this progress has been centered on hereditary retinal dystrophies, because the eye is an immune-privileged and anatomically ideal target. Gene therapy treatments, already demonstrated to be safe and efficacious in numerous clinical trials, are benefitting from the development of new viral vectors, such as dual and triple adeno-associated virus (AAV) vectors. CRISPR/Cas9, which revolutionized the field of gene editing, is being adapted into more precise "high fidelity" and catalytically dead variants. Newer CRISPR endonucleases, such as CjCas9 and Cas12a, are generating excitement in the field as well. Stem cell therapy has emerged as a promising alternative, allowing human embryo-derived stem cells and induced pluripotent stem cells to be edited precisely in vitro and then reintroduced into the body [114–117].

## Nystagmus

The field of nystagmus evaluation and management has enjoyed a period of increased understanding and an expansion of the armamentarium of possible treatments. The value of using drugs including topical dorzolamide, systemic gabapentin and memantine has gained favor but again not all types of nystagmus benefit from these treatments [118].The use of molecular investigation has revealed that most cases of X-linked infantile nystagmus are due to mutations in the FRMD7 gene [118]. While surgical regimens for abnormal head posture due to eccentric null position have been around for many years the advent of the Dell'Osso-Hertle procedure (horizontal tenotomy and reattachment) has been shown to be as effective as retroequatorial recessions of the horizontal muscles for infantile nystagmus without a definite null position [119]. The utility of this new horizontal four-muscle tenotomy and reattachment his that it is an effective procedure for reducing nystagmus, broadening the null position, and improving visual acuity in primary position for patients with nystagmus [120–122].

## Neurophysiology

Previous visual neuroscience research with non-human animal subjects suggests that visual deprivation early in life results in permanent visual function deficit (amblyopia) leading to the idea of a 'critical period' for acquiring visual function. The implication of this idea is that children who have been blind since early in life due to cataracts or other conditions, will not be able to gain functional vision if treated late in childhood. Hence, there is the belief that such treatments will not result in improvements in their quality of life. A group from Boston examined the development of contrast sensitivity in a group of children who had been visually deprived due to cataracts before the age of 1 year and had had prolonged visual deprivation until their cataracts were operated upon. Contrast sensitivity is a fundamental metric of visual performance that describes the sensitivity of neurons and observers and its neural substrate is found in early visual cortex. It is the primary visual limitation in a variety of tasks, including mobility, reading, and face and object recognition. In both brain and behavior, contrast sensitivity functions exhibit a characteristic shape and there is a direct relationship between behavioral and neural contrast sensitivity. Contrast sensitivity therefore provides a valuable barometer for visual development and examination of its change following deprivation may provide fundamental insights into the critical periods of neural plasticity. The group reported marked improvements in contrats sensitivity functions of a sample of sight restoration patients who experienced early-onset visual deprivation that remained untreated for an extended duration (the minimum age at treatment was 8 years). These patients exhibited extremely poor presurgical acuity of, at most, finger counting at a distance of 1 m. Their findings corroborate studies in animals, demonstrating that visual development is experience dependent and that critical periods can be extended through delayed exposure to light [123–127].

In a follow up questionnaire study the participants of the original study reported improved or newly acquired abilities to travel on their own. Positive improvements were also seen in other domains, including social interactions and societal attitudes towards the children and their families. This again showed that treatment for blindness, even at a late age, can result in significant improvements in a child's quality of life [124–126].

The take home message therefore is that in bilateral visual deprivation affecting the anterior segment, it is never too late tom operate and improve visual function.

# References

1. Dua HS, Said DG, Messmer EM, Rolando M, Benitez-Del-Castillo JM, Hossain PN, Shortt AJ, Geerling G, Nubile M, Figueiredo FC, Rauz S, Mastropasqua L, Rama P, Baudouin C. Neurotrophic keratopathy. Prog Retin Eye Res. 2018;66:107–31.
2. Ramappa M, Chaurasia S, Chakrabarti S, Kaur I. Congenital corneal anesthesia. J AAPOS. 2014;18(5):427–32. https://doi.org/10.1016/j.jaapos.2014.05.011. Epub 2014 Oct 21. PubMed PMID: 25439301.
3. Mantelli F, Nardella C, Tiberi E, Sacchetti M, Bruscolini A, Lambiase A. Congenital corneal anesthesia and neurotrophic keratitis: diagnosis and management. Biomed Res Int. 2015;2015:805876. https://doi.org/10.1155/2015/805876. Epub 2015 Sep 16. Review.
4. Elbaz U, Bains R, Zuker RM, Borschel GH, Ali A. Restoration of corneal sensation with regional nerve transfers and nerve grafts: a new approach to a difficult problem. JAMA Ophthalmol. 2014;132(11):1289–95.
5. Nischal KK. Genetics of congenital corneal opacification--impact on diagnosis and treatment. Cornea. 2015;34(Suppl 10):S24–34.
6. Mataftsi A, Islam L, Kelberman D, Sowden JC, Nischal KK. Chromosome abnormalities and the genetics of congenital corneal opacification. Mol Vis. 2011;17:1624–40. Epub 2011 Jun 17.
7. Kelberman D, Islam L, Jacques TS, Russell-Eggitt I, Bitner-Glindicz M, Khaw PT, Nischal KK, Sowden JC. CYP1B1-related anterior segment developmental anomalies novel mutations for infantile glaucoma and von Hippel's ulcer revisited. Ophthalmology. 2011;118(9):1865–73.
8. Nischal KK. Congenital corneal opacities—a surgical approach to nomenclature and classification. Eye (Lond). 2007;21(10):1326–37.
9. Nischal KK. A new approach to the classification of neonatal corneal opacities. Curr Opin Ophthalmol. 2012;23(5):344–54.
10. Soh YQ, Mehta JS. Selective endothelial removal for peters anomaly. Cornea. 2018;37(3):382–5.
11. Wollensak G, Spoerl E, Seiler T. Riboflavin/ultraviolet-a-induced collagen crosslinking for the treatment of keratoconus. Am J Ophthalmol. 2003;135(5):620–7.
12. Meek KM, Hayes S. Corneal cross-linking—a review. Ophthal Physiol Opt. 2013;33(2):78–93.
13. Zotta PG, Diakonis VF, Kymionis GD, Grentzelos M, Moschou KA. Long-term outcomes of corneal cross-linking for keratoconus in pediatric patients. J AAPOS. 2017;21(5):397–401.
14. Mazzotta C, Traversi C, Baiocchi S, Bagaglia S, Caporossi O, Villano A, et al. Corneal collagen cross-linking with riboflavin and ultraviolet a light for pediatric keratoconus: ten-year results. Cornea. 2018;37(5):560–6.

15. Padmanabhan P, Rachapalle Reddi S, Rajagopal R, Natarajan R, Iyer G, Srinivasan B, et al. Corneal collagen cross-linking for keratoconus in pediatric patients-long-term results. Cornea. 2017;36(2):138–43.
16. Nicula C, Nicula D, Pop RN. Results at 7 years after cross-linking procedure in keratoconic patients. J Fr Ophtalmol. 2017;40(7):535–41.
17. Raiskup F, Theuring A, Pillunat LE, Spoerl E. Corneal collagen crosslinking with riboflavin and ultraviolet-a light in progressive keratoconus: ten-year results. J Cataract Refract Surg. 2015;41(1):41–6.
18. Leoni-Mesplie S, Mortemousque B, Touboul D, Malet F, Praud D, Mesplie N, et al. Scalability and severity of keratoconus in children. Am J Ophthalmol. 2012;154(1):56–62.e1.
19. Vanathi M, Panda A, Vengayil S, Chaudhuri Z, Dada T. Pediatric keratoplasty. Surv Ophthalmol. 2009;54(2):245–71.
20. Cingu AK, Bez Y, Cinar Y, Turkcu FM, Yildirim A, Sahin A, et al. Impact of collagen cross-linking on psychological distress and vision and health-related quality of life in patients with keratoconus. Eye Contact Lens. 2015;41(6):349–53.
21. Beshtawi IM, Akhtar R, Hillarby MC, O'Donnell C, Zhao X, Brahma A, et al. Biomechanical properties of human corneas following low- and high-intensity collagen cross-linking determined with scanning acoustic microscopy. Invest Ophthalmol Vis Sci. 2013;54(8):5273–80.
22. Vinciguerra R, Romano V, Arbabi EM, Brunner M, Willoughby CE, Batterbury M, et al. In vivo early corneal biomechanical changes after corneal cross-linking in patients with progressive keratoconus. J Refract Surg. 2017;33(12):840–6.
23. Shetty R, Kaweri L, Nuijts RM, Nagaraja H, Arora V, Kumar RS. Profile of microbial keratitis after corneal collagen cross-linking. Biomed Res Int. 2014;2014:340509.
24. Evangelista CB, Hatch KM. Corneal collagen cross-linking complications. Semin Ophthalmol. 2018;33(1):29–35.
25. Sharma A, Nottage JM, Mirchia K, Sharma R, Mohan K, Nirankari VS. Persistent corneal edema after collagen cross-linking for keratoconus. Am J Ophthalmol. 2012;154(6):922–6 e1.
26. Tuft SJ, Gregory WM, Buckley RJ. Acute corneal hydrops in keratoconus. Ophthalmology. 1994;101(10):1738–44.
27. Romano V, Vinciguerra R, Arbabi EM, Hicks N, Rosetta P, Vinciguerra P, et al. Progression of keratoconus in patients while awaiting corneal cross-linking: a prospective clinical study. J Refract Surg. 2018;34(3):177–80.
28. Alio JL, Shabayek MH, Artola A. Intracorneal ring segments for keratoconus correction: long-term follow-up. J Cataract Refract Surg. 2006;32(6):978–85.
29. Colin J, Malet FJ. Intacs for the correction of keratoconus: two-year follow-up. J Cataract Refract Surg. 2007;33(1):69–74.
30. Shetty R, Kaweri L, Pahuja N, Nagaraja H, Wadia K, Jayadev C, et al. Current review and a simplified "five-point management algorithm" for keratoconus. Indian J Ophthalmol. 2015;63(1):46–53.
31. Plager DA, Lynn MJ, Buckley EG, Wilson ME, Lambert SR, Infant Aphakia Treatment Study Group. Complications in the first 5 years following cataract surgery in infants with and without intraocular lens implantation in the Infant Aphakia Treatment Study. Am J Ophthalmol. 2014;158(5):892–8.
32. Vasavada AR, Vasavada V, Shah SK, Praveen MR, Vasavada VA, Trivedi RH, Rawat F, Koul A. Five-year postoperative outcomes of bilateral aphakia and pseudophakia in children up to 2 years of age: a randomized clinical trial. Am J Ophthalmol. 2018;193:33–44.
33. Mataftsi A, Haidich AB, Kokkali S, Rabiah PK, Birch E, Stager DR Jr, Cheong-Leen R, Singh V, Egbert JE, Astle WF, Lambert SR, Amitabh P, Khan AO, Grigg J, Arvanitidou M, Dimitrakos SA, Nischal KK. Postoperative glaucoma following infantile cataract surgery: an individual patient data meta-analysis. JAMA Ophthalmol. 2014;132(9):1059–67.
34. Serafino M, Trivedi RH, Levin AV, Wilson ME, Nucci P, Lambert SR, Nischal KK, Plager DA, Bremond-Gignac D, Kekunnaya R, Nishina S, Tehrani NN, Ventura MC. Use of the Delphi process in paediatric cataract management. Br J Ophthalmol. 2016;100(5):611–5.
35. Dick HB, Schultz T. Femtosecond laser-assisted cataract surgery in infants. J Cataract Refract Surg. 2013;39(5):665–8.

36. Dick HB, Schelenz D, Schultz T. Femtosecond laser-assisted pediatric cataract surgery: Bochum formula. J Cataract Refract Surg. 2015;41(4):821–6.
37. Khokhar SK, Pillay G, Agarwal E, Mahabir M. Innovations in pediatric cataract surgery. Indian J Ophthalmol. 2017;65(3):210–6.
38. Hamada S, Low S, Walters BC, Nischal KK. Five-year experience of the 2-incision push-pull technique for anterior and posterior capsulorrhexis in pediatric cataract surgery. Ophthalmology. 2006;113(8):1309–14.
39. Van Looveren J, Ní Dhubhghaill S, Godts D, Bakker E, De Veuster I, Mathysen DG, Tassignon MJ. Pediatric bag-in-the-lens intraocular lens implantation: long-term follow-up. J Cataract Refract Surg. 2015;41(8):1685–92.
40. Lapid-Gortzak R, van der Meulen IJ, Jellema HM, Mourits MP, Nieuwendaal CP. Seven-year follow-up of unilateral multifocal pseudophakia in a child. Int Ophthalmol. 2017;37(1):267–70.
41. Lin H, Ouyang H, Zhu J, Huang S, Liu Z, Chen S, Cao G, Li G, Signer RA, Xu Y, Chung C, Zhang Y, Lin D, Patel S, Wu F, Cai H, Hou J, Wen C, Jafari M, Liu X, Luo L, Zhu J, Qiu A, Hou R, Chen B, Chen J, Granet D, Heichel C, Shang F, Li X, Krawczyk M, Skowronska-Krawczyk D, Wang Y, Shi W, Chen D, Zhong Z, Zhong S, Zhang L, Chen S, Morrison SJ, Maas RL, Zhang K, Liu Y. Lens regeneration using endogenous stem cells with gain of visual function. Nature. 2016;531(7594):323–8.
42. Saw SM, Katz J, Schein OD, et al. Epidemiology of myopia. Epidemiol Rev. 1996;18:175–87.
43. Saw SM, Carkeet A, Chia KS, Stone RA, Tan DT. Component dependent risk factors for ocular parameters in Singapore Chinese children. Ophthalmology. 2002;109:2065–71.
44. Saw SM, Tong L, Chua WH, Chia KS, Koh D, Tan DT, et al. Incidence and progression of myopia in Singaporean school children. Invest Ophthalmol Vis Sci. 2005;46:51–7.
45. Mak CY, Yam JC, Chen LJ, Lee SM, Young AL. Epidemiology of myopia and prevention of myopia progression in children in East Asia: a review. Hong Kong Med J. 2018;24(6):602–9.
46. Cheng D, Woo GC, Drobe B, Schmid KL. Effect of bifocal and prismatic bifocal spectacles on myopia progression in children: three-year results of a randomized clinical trial. JAMA Ophthalmol. 2014;132(3):258–64.
47. Gwiazda JE, Hyman L, Everett D, Norton T, Kurtz D, Manny R. Five-year results from the correction of myopia evaluation trial (COMET). Invest Ophthalmol Vis Sci. 2006;47:E–abstract 1166.
48. Katz J, Schein OD, Levy B, et al. A randomized trial of rigid gas permeable contact lenses to reduce progression of children's myopia. Am J Ophthalmol. 2003;136:82–90.
49. Charm J, Cho P. High myopia-partial reduction ortho-k: a 2-year randomized study. Optom Vis Sci. 2013;90(6):530–9.
50. Cho P, Cheung SW. Retardation of myopia in Orthokeratology (ROMIO) study: a 2-year randomized clinical trial. Invest Ophthalmol Vis Sci. 2012;53(11):7077–85.
51. Mutti D, Sinnott L, Mitchell G, et al. Relative peripheral refractive error and the risk of onset and progression of myopia in children. Invest Ophthalmol Vis Sci. 2011;52:199–205.
52. Mutti DO, Sinnott LT, Mitchell GL, Jones-Jordan LA, Moeschberger ML, Cotter SA, Kleinstein RN, Manny RE, Twelker JD, Zadnik K, CLEERE Study Group. Relative peripheral refractive error and the risk of onset and progression of myopia in children. Invest Ophthalmol Vis Sci. 2011;52(1):199–205.
53. Kanda H, Oshika T, Hiraoka T, Hasebe S, Ohno-Matsui K, Ishiko S, Hieda O, Torii H, Varnas SR, Fujikado T. Effect of spectacle lenses designed to reduce relative peripheral hyperopia on myopia progression in Japanese children: a 2-year multicenter randomized controlled trial. Jpn J Ophthalmol. 2018;62(5):537–43.
54. Benavente-Pérez A, Nour A, Troilo D. Axial eye growth and refractive error development can be modified by exposing the peripheral retina to relative myopic or hyperopic defocus. Invest Ophthalmol Vis Sci. 2014;55(10):6765–73.
55. Chua WH, Balakrishnan V, Chan YH, et al. Atropine for the treatment of childhood myopia. Ophthalmology. 2006;113:2285–91.

56. Chia A, Chua WH, Cheung YB, et al. Atropine for the treatment of childhood myopia: safety and efficacy of 0.5%, 0.1%, and 0.01% doses (ATOM2). Ophthalmology. 2012;119:347–54.
57. Chia A, Chua WH, Li W, et al. Atropine for the treatment of childhood myopia: changes after stopping atropine 0.01%, 0.1% and 0.5% (ATOM2). Am J Ophthalmol. 2014;157:451–7.
58. Chia A, Lu QS, Tan D. Five-year clinical trial on atropine for the treatment of myopia 2: myopia control with atropine 0.01% eyedrops. Ophthalmology. 2016;123(2):391–9.
59. Wu PC, Chen CT, Lin KK, Sun CC, Kuo CN, Huang HM, Poon YC, Yang ML, Chen CY, Huang JC, Wu PC, Yang IH, Yu HJ, Fang PC, Tsai CL, Chiou ST, Yang YH. Myopia prevention and outdoor light intensity in a school-based cluster randomized trial. Ophthalmology. 2018;125(8):1239–50.
60. Zhou Z, Chen T, Wang M, Jin L, Zhao Y, Chen S, Wang C, Zhang G, Wang Q, Deng Q, Liu Y, Morgan IG, He M, Liu Y, Congdon N. Pilot study of a novel classroom designed to prevent myopia by increasing children's exposure to outdoor light. PLoS One. 2017;12(7):e0181772.
61. Galvis V, Tello A, Camacho PA, Parra MM, Merayo-Lloves J. Bio-environmental factors associated with myopia: an updated review. Arch Soc Esp Oftalmol. 2017;92(7):307–25.
62. Torii H, Kurihara T, Seko Y, Negishi K, Ohnuma K, Inaba T, Kawashima M, Jiang X, Kondo S, Miyauchi M, Miwa Y, Katada Y, Mori K, Kato K, Tsubota K, Goto H, Oda M, Hatori M, Tsubota K. Violet light exposure can be a preventive strategy against myopia progression. EBioMedicine. 2017;15:210–9.
63. Conte E, Izaurralde E. Nonsense-mediated mRNA decay: molecular insights and mechanistic variations across species. Curr Opin Cell Biol. 2005;17:316–25.
64. Lejeune F. Nonsense-mediated mRNA decay at the crossroads of many cellular pathways. BMB Rep. 2017;50:175–85.
65. Welch EM, Barton ER, Zhuo J, Tomizawa Y, Friesen WJ, Trifillis P, et al. PTC124 targets genetic disorders caused by nonsense mutations. Nature. 2007;447:87–91.
66. Cassan M, Rousset JP. UAG readthrough in mammalian cells: effect of upstream and downstream stop codon contexts reveal different signals. BMC Mol Biol. 2001;2:3.
67. McCaughan KK, Brown CM, Kalphin ME, Berry MJ, Tate WP. Translational termination efficiency in mammals is influenced by the base following the stop codon. Proc Natl Acad Sci U S A. 1992;92:5431–5.
68. Tate WP, Poole ES, Horsfield JA, Mannering SA, Brown CM, Moffat JG, et al. Translational termination efficiency in both bacteria and mammals is regulated by the base following the stop codon. Biochem Cell Biol. 1995;73:1095–03.
69. Manuvakhova M, Keeling K, Bedwell DM. Aminogylcoside antibiotics mediate context-dependent suppression of termination codons in a mammalian translation system. RNA. 2000;6:1044–55.
70. Mendell JT, Dietz HC. When the message goes awry: disease-producing mutations that influence mRNA content and performance. Cell. 2001;107:411–4.
71. Richardson R, Smart M, Tracey-white D, Webster AR, Moosajee M. Mechanism and evidence of nonsense suppression therapy for genetic eye disorders. Exp Eye Res. 2017;155:24–37.
72. Kerem E, Hirawat S, Armoni S, Yaakov Y, Shoseyov D, Cohen M, et al. Effectiveness of PTC124 treatment of cystic fibrosis caused by nonsense mutations: a prospective phase II trial. Lancet. 2008;372:719–27.
73. Kerem E, Konstan MW, De Boeck K, Accurso FJ, Sermet-Gaudelus I, Wilschanski M, et al. Ataluren for the treatment of nonsense-mutation cystic fibrosis, a randomized double-blind, placebo-controlled phase 3 trial. Lancet Respir Med. 2014;2:539–47.
74. Sermet-Gaudelus I, Boeck KD, Casimir GJ, Vermeulen F, Leal T, Mogenet A, et al. Ataluren (PTC124) induces cystic fibrosis transmemebrane conductance regulator protein expression and activity in children with nonsense mutation cystic fibrosis. Am J Respir Crit Care Med. 2010;182:1262–72.
75. Wilschanski M, Miller LL, Shoseyov D, BLau H, Rivlin J, Aviram M, et al. Chronic ataluren (PTC124) treatment of nonsense mutation cystic fibrosis. Eur Respir J. 2011;38:59–69.

76. Bushby K, Finkel R, Wong B, Barohn R, Campbell C, Comi GP, et al. Ataluren treatment of patients with nonsense mutation dystrophinopathy. Muscle Nerve. 2014;50:477–87.
77. McElroy K, Auld DS. Mechanism of PTC124 activity in cell-based luciferase assays of nonsense codon suppression. Proc Natl Acad Sci U S A. 2009;11:e1001593.
78. Sahel JA, Marazova K. Toward postnatal reversal of ocular congenital malformations. J Clin Invest. 2014;124:81–4.
79. Gregory-Evans CY, Wang X, Wasan KM, Zhao J, Metcalfe AL, Gregory-Evans K. Postnatal manipulation of Pax6 dosage reverses congenital tissue malformation defects. J Clin Invest. 2014;124:111–6.
80. Van Heyningen V, Williamson KA. PAX6 in sensory development. Hum Mol Genet. 2002;11:1161–7.
81. Simpson TI, Price DJ. PAX6: a pleitropic player in development. Bioessays. 2002;24:1041–51.
82. Goldmann T, Overlack N, Wolfrum U, Nagel-Wolfrum K. PTC124-mediated translational readthrough of a nonsense mutation causing Usher syndrome type 1C. Hum Gen Ther. 2011;22:537–47.
83. Goldmann T, Overlack N, Noller F, Belakhov V, van Wyk M, Baasov T, et al. A comparative evaluation of NB30, NB54, and PTC124 in translational read-through efficacy for treatment of an USH1C nonsense mutation. EMBO Mol Med. 2012;4:1196–9.
84. Moosajee M, Gregory-Evans K, Ellis CD, Seabra MC, Gregory-Evans CY. Translational bypass of nonsense mutations in zebrafish rep1, pax2.1, and lamb1 highlights a viable therapeutic option for untreatable genetic eye disease. Hum Mol Genet. 2008;17:3987–4000.
85. Muto R, Yamamori S, Ohashi H, Osawa M. Prediction by FISH analysis of the occurrence of Wilms tumor in aniridia patients. Am J Med Genet. 2009;108:285–9.
86. Fischbach BV, Trout KL, Lewis J, Luis CA, Sika M. WAGR syndrome: a clinical review of 54 cases. Pediatrics. 2005;116:984–8.
87. Breslow NE, Olshan A, Beckwith JB, Green DM. Epidemiology of Wilms' tumor. Med Pediatr Oncol. 1993;21:172–81.
88. Breslow NE, Takashima JR, Ritchey ML, Strong LC, Green DM. Renal failure in the Denys-Drash and Wilms' Tumor Aniridia-syndromes. Cancer Res. 2000;60:4030–2.
89. Breslow NE, Norris R, Norkool P, et al. Characteristics and outcomes of children with the Wilms' Tumor-Aniridia syndrome: a report from the National Wilms' Tumor Study Group. J Clin Oncol. 2003;24:4579–85.
90. Toriello HV, Parisi MA. Cilia and the ciliopathies: an introduction. Am J Med Genet C Semin Med Genet. 2009;15:261–2.
91. Baker K, Beales PL. Making sense of cilia in disease: the human ciliopathies. Am J Med Genet C Semin Med Genet. 2009;151C:281–9515.
92. Mitchison HM, Valente EM. Motile and non-motile cilia in human pathology: from function to phenotypes. J Pathol. 2017;241:294–309.
93. Mitchison TJ, Mitchison HM. Cell biology: how cilia beat. Nature. 2010;463:308–9.
94. Rosenbaum JL, Witman GB. Intraflagellar transport. Nat Rev Mol Cell Biol. 2002;3:813–25.
95. Goetz SC, Anderson KV. The primary cilium: a signaling centre during vertebrate development. Nat Rev Genet. 2010;11:331–44.
96. Gerdes JM, Davis EE, Katsanis N. The vertebrate primary cilium in development, homeostasis, and disease. Cell. 2009;137:32–45.
97. Hildebrant F, Benzing T, Natsanis N. Ciliopathies. N Engl J Med. 2011;364:1533–43.
98. Satir P, Pedersen LB, Christensen ST. The primary cilium at a glance. J Cell Sci. 2010;123:499–503.
99. Hoey DA, Downs ME, Jacobs CR. The mechanics of the primary cilium: an intricate structure with complex function. J Biomech. 2012;45:17–26.
100. Basten SG, Giles RH. Functional aspects of primary cilia in signaling, cell cycle, and tumorigenesis. Cilia. 2013;2:6.

101. Pazour GJ, San Agustin JT, Follit JA, Rosenbaum JL, Witman GB. Polycystin-2 localizes to kidney cilia and the ciliary level is elevated in orpk mice with polycystic kidney disease. Curr Biol. 2002;12:R378–80.
102. Yoder BK, Hou X, Guay-Woodford LM. The polycystic kidney disease proteins, polycystin-1, polycystin-2, polaris, and cystin, are co-localized in the renal cilia. J Am Soc Nephrol. 2002;13:2508–16.
103. Lin F, Hiesberger T, Cordes K, Sinclair AM, Goldstein LS, Somlo S, et al. Kidney-specific inactivation of the KIF3A subunit of kinesin-II inhibits renal ciliogenesis and produces polycystic kidney disease. Proc Natl Acad Sci U S A. 2003;100:5286–91.
104. Yokoyama T. Ciliary subcompartments and cysto-proteins. Anat Sci Int. 2017;92:207–14.
105. Hildebrant F, Attanasio M, Otto E. Nephronophthisis: disease mechanisms of a ciliopathy. J Am Soc Nephrol. 2009;20:23–35.
106. Srivastava S, Sayer JA. Nephronophthisis. J Pediatr Genet. 2014;3:103–14.
107. Parisi MA, Doherty D, Eckert ML, Shaw DW, Ozyurek H, Aysun S, et al. AHI1 mutations cause both retinal dystrophy and renal cystic disease in Joubert syndrome. J Med Genet. 2006;43:334–9.
108. Mockel A, Perdomo Y, Stutzmann F, Letsch J, Marion V, Dollfus H. Retinal dystrophy in Bardet-Biedl syndrome and related syndromic ciliopathies. Prog Retin Eye Res. 2011;30:258–74.
109. Bujakowska KM, Liu Q, Pierce EA. Photoreceptor cilia and retinal ciliopathies. Cold Spring Harb Perspect Biol. 2017;13:a028274.
110. Nishimura DY, Searby CC, Carmi R, Elbedour K, Van Maldergem L, Fulton AB, et al. Positional cloning of a novel gene on chromosome 16q causing Bardet-Biedl syndrome (BBS). Hum Mol Genet. 2001;10:865–74.
111. Quinlan RJ, Tobin JL, Beales PL. Modeling ciliopathies: primary cilia in development and disease. Curr Top Dev Biol. 2008;84:249–310.
112. Tobin JL, Beales PL. The nonmotile ciliopathies. Genet Med. 2009;11:386–402.
113. Waters AM, Beales PL. Ciliopathies: an expanding disease spectrum. Pediatr Nephrol. 2011;26:1039–56.
114. Campa C, Gallenga CE, Bolletta E, Perri P. The role of gene therapy in the treatment of retinal diseases: a review. Curr Gene Ther. 2017;17(3):194–213.
115. Xue K, Groppe M, Salvetti AP, MacLaren RE. Technique of retinal gene therapy: delivery of viral vector into the subretinal space. Eye (Lond). 2017;31(9):1308–16.
116. MacLaren RE, Bennett J, Schwartz SD. Gene therapy and stem cell transplantation in retinal disease: the new frontier. Ophthalmology. 2016;123(10S):S98–S106.
117. Pierce EA, Bennett J. The status of RPE65 gene therapy trials: safety and efficacy. Cold Spring Harb Perspect Med. 2015;5(9):a017285.
118. Papageorgiou E, McLean RJ, Gottlob I. Nystagmus in childhood. Pediatr Neonatol. 2014;55(5):341–51.
119. Singh A, Ashar J, Sharma P, Saxena R, Menon V. A prospective evaluation of retro-equatorial recession of horizontal rectus muscles and Hertle-Dell'Ossotenotomy procedure in patients with infantile nystagmus with no definite null position. J AAPOS. 2016;20(2):96–9.
120. Greven MA, Nelson LB. Four-muscle tenotomy surgery for nystagmus. Curr Opin Ophthalmol. 2014;25(5):400–5.
121. Hertle RW, Dell'Osso LF, FitzGibbon EJ, Yang D, Mellow SD. Horizontal rectus muscle tenotomy in children with infantile nystagmus syndrome: a pilot study. J AAPOS. 2004;8(6):539–48.
122. Hertle RW, Dell'Osso LF, FitzGibbon EJ, Thompson D, Yang D, Mellow SD. Horizontal rectus tenotomy in patients with congenital nystagmus: results in 10 adults. Ophthalmology. 2003;110(11):2097–105.

123. Kalia A, Gandhi T, Chatterjee G, Swami P, Dhillon H, Bi S, Chauhan N, Gupta SD, Sharma P, Sood S, Ganesh S, Mathur U, Sinha P. Assessing the impact of a program for late surgical intervention in early-blind children. Public Health. 2017;146:15–23.
124. Ganesh S, Arora P, Sethi S, Gandhi TK, Kalia A, Chatterjee G, Sinha P. Results of late surgical intervention in children with early-onset bilateral cataracts. Br J Ophthalmol. 2014;98(10):1424–8.
125. Kalia A, Lesmes LA, Dorr M, Gandhi T, Chatterjee G, Ganesh S, Bex PJ, Sinha P. Development of pattern vision following early and extended blindness. Proc Natl Acad Sci U S A. 2014;111(5):2035–9.
126. Sinha P, Chatterjee G, Gandhi T, Kalia A. Restoring vision through "Project Prakash": the opportunities for merging science and service. PLoS Biol. 2013;11(12):e1001741.
127. Mower GD, Christen WG, Caplan CJ. Very brief visual experience eliminates plasticity in the cat visual cortex. Science. 1983;221(4606):178–80.

# Chapter 10
# Recent Developments in Ocular Oncology

Bertil Damato

Ocular oncology is advancing rapidly thanks to accelerating progress in genetics, pathology, ocular and systemic therapies, ocular imaging, and other fields. Because of the exponential growth of knowledge, it is increasingly difficult for general ophthalmologists and other non-oncologists to keep abreast of developments in ocular oncology especially with more common diseases prioritizing their attention. The aim of this article is to describe recent trends and achievements in ocular oncology. This review is not meant to be encyclopedic, as it assumes that the reader is already reasonably knowledgeable about ocular oncology.

## Uveal Melanoma

### Prognostication

The most important development, in the author's opinion, is the discovery that metastatic disease from uveal melanoma occurs almost exclusively in patients whose tumor shows chromosome 3 loss, this genetic abnormality being strongly associated with high mortality [1]. Extensive research has since revealed a variety of other genetic aberrations that are associated with metastasis. The most important of these are chromosome 8q gain, 'class 2' gene expression profile, epigenetic alteration, aberrant expression of preferentially expressed antigen in melanoma (PRAME), and BRCA1-associated protein 1 (*BAP1*) mutation [2, 3]. These abnormalities merely indicate that the tumor has metastatic potential; however, prognostication

B. Damato, MD, PhD (✉)
Nuffield Department of Clinical Neurosciences, University of Oxford, John Radcliffe Hospital, Oxford, UK
https://www.ndcn.ox.ac.uk/team/bertil-damato
e-mail: Bertil.Damato@NHS.net

© Springer Nature Switzerland AG 2020                                        275
A. Grzybowski (ed.), *Current Concepts in Ophthalmology*,
https://doi.org/10.1007/978-3-030-25389-9_10

also requires an estimate of life expectancy. The American Joint Commission on Cancer (AJCC) has recently updated the TNM (Tumor, Node, Metastasis) staging system for choroidal melanomas, which categorizes these tumors according to tumor basal diameter, tumor thickness, ciliary body involvement and extraocular spread [4]. Survival predictions based only on anatomic findings are only approximate, however, so that they are relevant only to large groups of patients, as in clinical trials. As long ago as 2007, the author improved the accuracy of survival prediction by performing multivariable analysis combining genetic, histologic and anatomic data, also taking the patient's age and sex into account [5]. He and associates have developed predictive tools that are available on the Internet (www.ocularmelanomaonline.org) [6]. The genetic tumor typing has become more successful thanks to improved methods of tumor analysis, such as multiplex ligation-dependent probe amplification (MLPA), next generation sequencing (NGS), and immunohistochemical analysis of nuclear BAP1 expression [2, 7, 8]. Highly reliable prognostication has made it possible to confidently reassure patients with a good prognosis while targeting more intensive systemic surveillance and counseling at high-risk individuals. These benefits have led to prognostic tumor biopsy of uveal melanoma becoming routine in a growing number of centers. This, in turn, has resulted in better biopsy techniques so that experienced surgeons can reliably sample choroidal tumors with a thickness of less than 1 mm [9–12]. Some have expressed concerns that biopsy and other surgical manipulations may disseminate tumor cells around the body to cause metastatic disease. Although the author considers this unlikely, he and associates have shown that genetic tumor analysis is successful even when biopsy is performed soon after radiotherapy, at least with MLPA and NGS [13].

## Surveillance for Metastatic Disease

Systemic surveillance for early detection of metastatic disease has changed dramatically over the past few years, with liver function tests and chest x-ray being largely superseded by liver imaging. Many centers favor magnetic resonance imaging, which unlike ultrasonography does not depend on the skill of the examiner for its success and which does not expose the patient to ionizing radiation, unlike computerized tomography [14]. Magnetic resonance imaging is expensive, however, and also detects abnormalities that are not metastases [15]. These problems are less troublesome if this investigation is targeted at patients whose genetic tumor typing indicates a high risk of metastasis [16].

## Treatment for Metastasis

Metastases from uveal melanoma are less responsive than cutaneous melanomas to dacarbazine and other forms of chemotherapy. Interest in agents targeting the MAPK and PI3K pathways was stimulated by the finding that in uveal melanomas these pathways are usually activated by GNAQ and GNA11 mutations; however, clinical trials investigating agents such as selumetinib and trametinib have proved disappointing [17]. With cutaneous melanomas, dramatic remissions have been achieved with immune checkpoint inhibitors, such ipilimumab and nivolumab, which inhibit CTLA-4 and PD-1 respectively, thereby enabling cytotoxic T cells to kill melanoma cells; however, these agents are less effective with uveal melanomas, which are less immunogenic than cutaneous melanomas because they have fewer mutations [17]. Encouraging results have recently been reported with Tebentafusp (IMCgp100) (Immunocore, Abingdon, UK), a synthetic molecule that binds T-lymphocytes to melanoma cells, causing tumor cell death [18]. Promising results have also been reported with percutaneous isolated hepatic perfusion with melphalan (Delcath Systems Inc., New York, US) [19]. Prolonged survival occurs in some patients following partial hepatectomy for isolated liver metastases, but whether this is the result of treatment or merely selection bias is not known [20]. Other forms of therapy for hepatic metastases include radiofrequency ablation, radioembolization with yttrium-90 microspheres, and adoptive transfer of tumor infiltrating lymphcytes (TILs) [17]. Patients receiving systemic adjuvant sunitinib have apparently lived longer than historical controls, but randomized clinical trials are needed to determine whether this treatment is actually beneficial [21].

## *Ocular Treatment*

It is still not known whether ocular treatment for uveal melanoma influences survival and, if so, in whom [22]. The Collaborative Ocular Melanoma Study concluded that plaque radiotherapy is as 'safe' as enucleation [23]. This is obviously true in patients whose tumor has already metastasized by the time of diagnosis, and in those who are fortunate enough never to develop lethal mutations in their tumor, even if this is left untreated. However, failure of ocular radiotherapy to sterilize uveal melanoma is well known to be associated with increased mortality and it is not known whether this is because recurrent tumor actually results in metastasis or whether tumor recurrence is merely an indicator of increased malignancy. It is also not known whether it is safe for treatment of small uveal melanomas to be deferred for months or years until tumor growth is documented [22]. The author had a patient whose tumor rapidly grew after years of indolent behavior, with the older, basal part of the tumor showing disomy 3, spindle cells and the newer, apical region showing monosomy 3, epithelioid cells; the patient developed metastases, which might have been prevented if she had been treated without delay [24]. The author also reported a higher prevalence of monosomy 3 melanoma in older patients, hypothesizing that this is the result of delayed presentation and treatment [25].

Most choroidal melanomas are treated with brachytherapy [26, 27]. Iodine-125 continues to be the preferred isotope for plaque radiotherapy in the US, whereas ruthenium-106 plaques are more widely used in Europe. With iodine-125 brachytherapy, collateral damage to healthy ocular tissues has diminished with the development of highly collimated plaques, which are tailored to each individual tumor using 3-D printing [28]. With ruthenium applicators, irradiation of optic nerve and fovea is reduced by positioning the plaque eccentrically in relation to the tumor, with its posterior edge aligned with the posterior tumor margin (Fig. 10.1) [29]. This requires a high degree of accuracy, which is achieved with the use of a template having perforations in which the tip of a right-angled 20-gauge transilluminator is placed while performing binocular indirect ophthalmoscopy.

Trans-scleral local resection of choroidal melanomas involves removal of the tumour en bloc through a scleral trapdoor. This operation is not widely performed, because of technical difficulty and because of the need for hypotensive anesthesia (Fig. 10.2). In expert hands, rhegmatogenous retinal detachment has become less common with the development of surgical techniques for preventing retinal tears and preserving the pars plana epithelium [30]. Local tumor recurrence has become rarer with adjunctive brachytherapy if this is administered with a 25 mm ruthenium applicator. The author has found that iris conservation during iridocyclectomy are improved by administering meiotics instead of mydriatics before

**Fig. 10.1** Choroidal melanoma successfully treated with an eccentrically placed ruthenium plaque (**a**) before treatment, and (**b**) months after treatment. The tumoricidal radiation dose extends beyond the visible choroidal atrophy

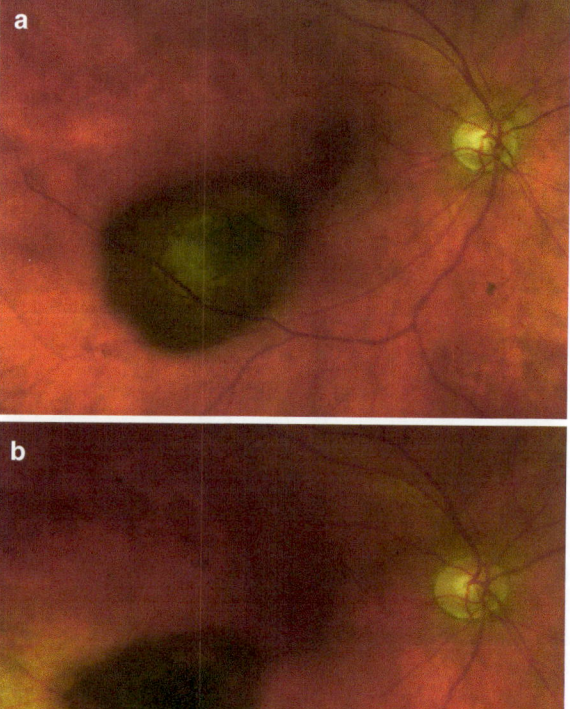

**Fig. 10.2** Choroidal melanoma (**a**) before and (**b**) after trans-scleral local resection (also known as 'exoresection')

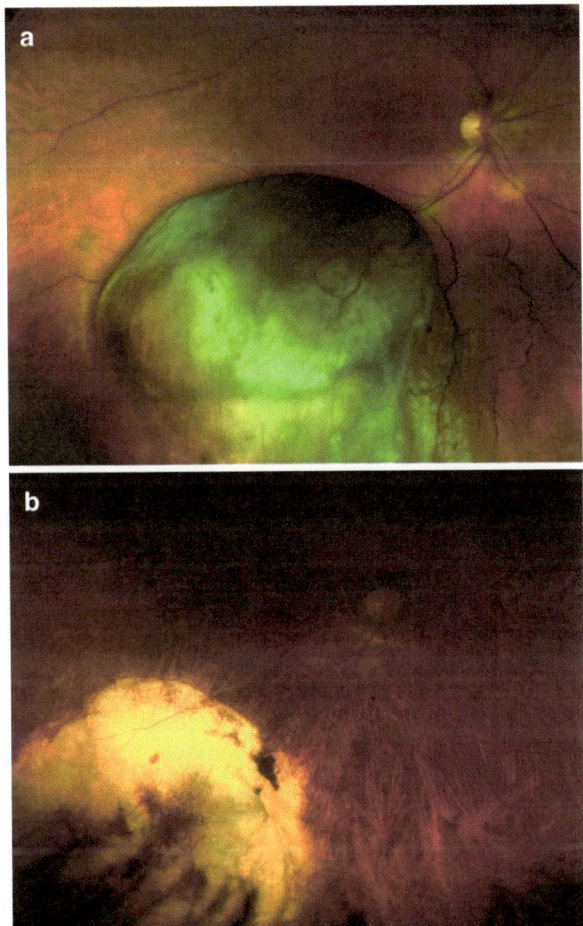

surgery and by excising the tumor postero-anteriorly or circumferentially instead of antero-posteriorly [31]. With endoresection, the tumour is removed piecemeal with a vitreous cutter that is passed through the retina, preventing recurrence with adjunctive laser therapy and, in some cases, radiotherapy. Long-term studies of endoresection of choroidal melanoma have reported good rates of local tumor control [32]; however, some authors continue to advocate neoadjuvant radiotherapy [33]. With trans-retinal endoresection of choroidal melanoma, the most important development is the use of heavy liquid instead of air to flatten the retina, this change being prompted by a fatal case of air embolism, which occurred because of the escape of air through a vortex vein [34].

In some centers, proton beam radiotherapy has replaced resection and plaque radiotherapy for iris melanoma [35, 36]. Proton beam radiotherapy for more posterior uveal melanomas has changed little in recent years, except in patients whose upper eyelid margin cannot be fully retracted out of the radiation field. These cases are now treated by trans-palpebral proton beam radiotherapy, administered through the closed eyelid to avoid irradiating the lid margin, hence preventing keratinization of the palpebral conjunctiva, which causes painful keratopathy [37]. Proton beam radiotherapy is becoming more widely available as less expensive technology is developed.

There is growing use of stereotactic radiotherapy as an alternative to proton beam radiotherapy and brachytherapy, and several authors have reported good results with this modality [38].

After radiotherapy, many eyes develop macular edema and exudative retinal detachment, with some also developing iris neovascularization and neovascular glaucoma [39]. Several years ago, the author found that these complications can be treated by photoablation or excision of the irradiated tumor, coining the term 'toxic tumor syndrome' for this condition (Fig. 10.3) [39, 40]. Others have reported successful prevention and treatment for less severe disease with intraocular injections of steroids or anti-angiogenic agents, especially in patients who do not have extensive loss of macular vascularity on optical coherence tomography angiography [41–43].

## Detection and Diagnosis

Any opportunities for conserving the eye and vision, and perhaps preventing metastasis are enhanced by early treatment, when the tumor is still small. Ocular oncologists have a wide range of imaging modalities to differentiate choroidal nevi from melanomas [44]; however, these facilities are not widely available in the community. The author has devised the acronym, MOLES (M, mushroom shape; O, orange pigment; L, large size; E, enlargement; and S, subretinal fluid) to distinguish choroidal nevi from melanomas and this is currently under evaluation. He has also

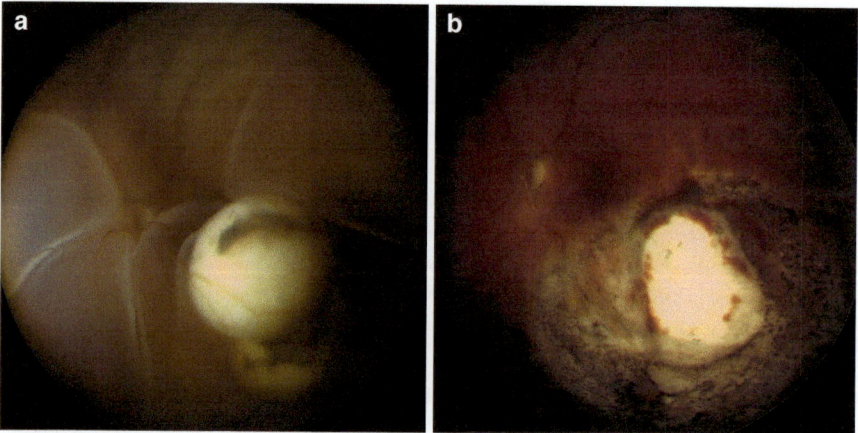

**Fig. 10.3** Successful treatment of toxic tumour syndrome by endoresection. (**a**) choroidal melanoma with extensive retinal detachment and (**b**) post-operative result, with a flat retina

developed an online atlas, which organizes tumors according to their location in the eye and their color in the hope of enabling practitioners to diagnose conditions they never knew existed (www.oculonco.com).

## Quality of Life

A study on more than 1400 patients suggests that irrespective of type of treatment (i.e., enucleation or radiotherapy), quality of life after treatment for choroidal melanoma is not significantly worse than the general population, once factors such as general health, social support and employment are taken into account [45]. There is scope for studies evaluating quality of life in patients who have developed severe radiation-induced ocular morbidity to help predict which patients do better after primary enucleation.

## Further Studies

Clinical trials are under way to evaluate photodynamic therapy for choroidal melanoma using intravitreal injections of AU-011, which consists of a phthalocyanine photosensitizer conjugated with a novel recombinant papillomavirus-like particle [46]. Improved methods for detecting circulating tumor cells and DNA in the blood are raising hopes for 'liquid biopsy', which if successful would avoid the need for invasive sampling of intraocular tumors [47, 48]. As mentioned, various forms of systemic adjuvant therapy for patients with high-risk melanoma are under evaluation. These include Vorinostat, a histone deacetylase (HDAC) inhibitor, as well as immune checkpoint inhibitors, tyrosine kinase inhibitors, and autologous dendritic cell vaccines [17]. Studies on germline *BAP1* mutation in patients with uveal melanoma are in progress following the discovery that some of these tumors develop as part of the *BAP1* tumor predisposition syndrome, which also causes renal cancer, cutaneous melanoma, mesothelioma and other tumors [49, 50].

## Retinoblastoma

### Treatment

A major advance in the treatment of retinoblastoma is intravitreal chemotherapy for eyes with vitreous seeds, which respond poorly to other forms of therapy [51]. This has greatly improved chances of ocular conservation in patients with advanced disease. Tumor seeding into extraocular tissues is prevented by a variety of measures, such as using fine needle to inject the drug into the eye and administering cryotherapy to the injection site on withdrawing the needle from the eye. A system for classifying vitreous seeds has been developed (i.e., dust, spheres, clouds), which helps to predict the efficacy of intra-vitreal chemotherapy [51]. There has also been progress in intra-arterial chemotherapy, with improvements in technique and the use of drugs other than melphalan, such as topotecan [52]. There is ongoing debate as to how intra-arterial and systemic therapy compare with respect to preventing pineoblastoma and metastatic disease.

## Classification

There are several classification systems for retinoblastoma, the Reese-Ellsworth method having become less relevant since external beam radiotherapy was superseded by chemotherapy. The most widely used is the International Retinoblastoma Classification (IRC), which categorizes retinoblastomas according to size, extent, proximity to disc and fovea, seeding and secondary effects; however, different versions of the IRC exist [53]. The TNM staging system has recently undergone several refinements, one of which defines heritability of the disease. A limitation of current staging systems is that they classify whole eyes and not individual tumors in eyes harboring multiple lesions. There is a need for improved documentation so that classification systems can evolve in response to advances in imaging and treatment [54].

## Genetic Analysis

Advances in genetic techniques makes it possible to identify RB1 mutations that were previously undetectable [55]. This improved sensitivity has enhanced the detection of mosicism. A relatively recent discovery is that some retinoblastomas develop with high levels of MYC amplification in the absence of detectable RB1, these tumors occurring unilaterally and tending to be highly aggressive, presenting at a median age of 4 months [56].

## Survival

Pineoblastoma is the most common cause of death in the first decade of life in countries with high-quality care. Survival rates have improved greatly with the development of aggressive treatment protocols if started early so that patients with germline retinoblastoma now undergo screening with 6-monthly brain MRI until the age of around 5 years. In later life, mortality occurs because of osteosarcomas and other second malignant neoplasms, especially in patients who have received external beam radiotherapy, which is why this modality has been abandoned. Early results suggest that proton beam radiotherapy does not cause second malignant neoplasms, but further studies are needed [57].

There is a need for greater efforts to detect second cancers earlier. There is also a need for improved awareness of the late physical and emotional effects of retinoblastoma and its treatment so that these problems can be addressed in a timely manner.

## Uveal Metastases

The epidemiology of uveal metastasis is changing with improvements in therapy and longer survival times [58].

### *Diagnosis*

The diagnosis of choroidal metastases has become easier with optical coherence tomography, which shows the surface of these tumors to have a characteristic 'lumpy-bumpy' appearance (Fig. 10.4) [59]. Diagnosis has also been enhanced by improvements in tumor biopsy and immunohistochemistry. In some centers, biopsy

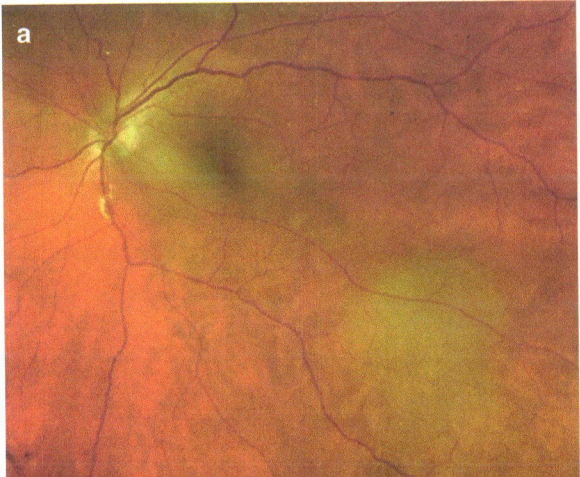

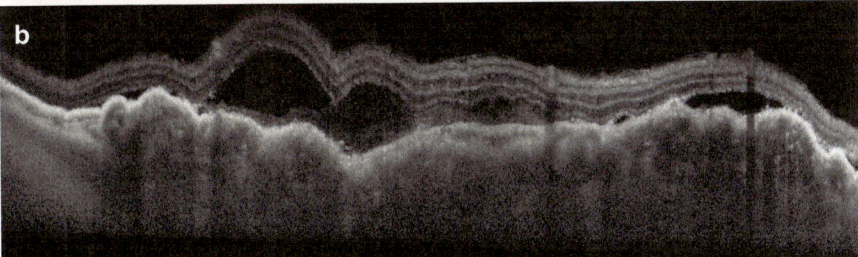

**Fig. 10.4** Inferotemporal choroidal metastasis in the left eye. (**a**) color photograph showing amelanotic tumor. (**b**) Optical coherence tomography (OCT) showing a lumpy appearance

is performed without delay, to confirm the diagnosis and to seek clues to the location of the primary tumor, if this is not already known [60]. In other centers, intraocular tumor biopsy is performed only as a last resort, if systemic investigations are uninformative.

## Treatment

Previously, patients underwent immediate radiotherapy whereas now there is now a growing tendency to administer this form of treatment only if systemic therapy fails to control the ocular tumor [61].

# Drug-Induced Ocular Disease

Novel anti-cancer therapies have resulted in a wide variety of adverse effects. Examples include: blepharitis, poliosis, eyelash trichomegaly, conjunctivitis and keratopathy from cetuximab, a monoclonal antibody that targets epidermal growth factor receptor; uveitis and vein occlusion from vemurafenib, a BRAF inhibitor; conjunctivitis, scleritis and uveitis from ipilimumab, an anti-CLTA-4 monoclonal antibody, which enhances T-cell responses against cancer cells; uveitis from nivolumab and pembrolizumab, which are anti-PD-1/PD-L1 monoclonal antibodies; and serous retinal detachment and retinal vein occlusion from trametinib, a MEK inhibitor [62–64]. The management of patients with these adverse effects is an expanding role in ocular oncology as is indeed the case with paraneoplastic syndromes, such as bilateral diffuse uveal melanocytic proliferation (BDUMP), cancer-associated retinopathy (CAR) and vitrelliform maculopathy, to mention but a few.

# Retinal Lymphoma

## Terminology

This terms 'vitreoretinal lymphoma' and 'retinal lymphoma' have replaced 'primary intraocular lymphoma (PIOL)', because intraocular lymphomas comprise both retinal lymphomas, which are aggressive and highly lethal because of CNS involvement, as well as indolent uveal lymphomas, which are associated with a very good survival probability [65]. Retinal lymphoma is becoming more common.

## *Investigation*

Ocular assessment has improved thanks to optical coherence tomography, which demonstrates lymphoma deposits between the retinal pigment epithelium and Bruch's membrane [66]. Another useful development is fundus autofluorescence imaging, with hyper-autofluorescence indicating active disease and hypo-autofluorescence corresponding to areas of inactive RPE atrophy (Fig. 10.5) [67]. Vitreous biopsy often fails to detect lymphoma cells, because these are so fragile, but diagnosis can still be achieved by detecting immunoglobulin heavy chain rearrangements, measuring interleukin-10 protein levels, detecting myeloid differentiation primary response 88 (MYD88) L265P mutation and measuring levels of particular microRNAs [68, 69]. It can be difficult to differentiate lymphoma from uveitis, but this task has become easier with the development of metagenomic deep sequencing, which detects any non-human DNA, also identifying the species of any infectious organism [70].

## *Treatment*

In many centers, the standard treatment for retinal lymphoma consists of ocular radiotherapy or intra-vitreal methotrexate and/or rituximab injections [71]. Encouraging results have recently been reported with intravitreal melphalan injections, which need to be administered less frequently than methotrexate [72]. Although ocular therapy suppresses the intraocular disease, it does not prevent mortality from central

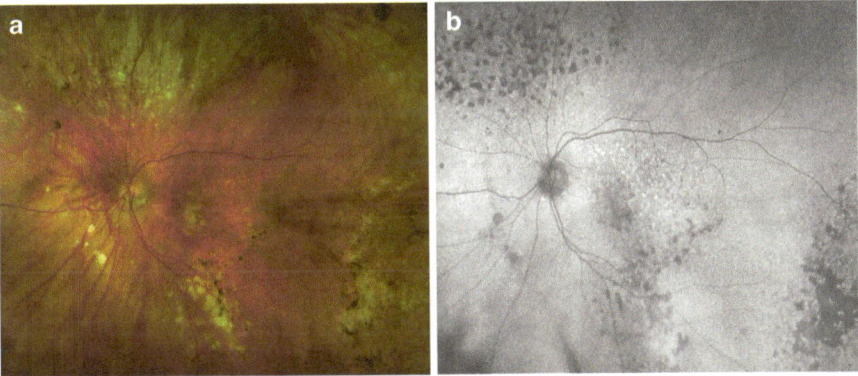

**Fig. 10.5** Fundus autofluorescence imaging in retinal lymphoma showing hyper-fluorescent sub-RPE lymphoma deposits and hypofluorescent, atrophic RPE scars. (**a**) color photograph and (**b**) autofluorescence image

nervous system disease. Some studies have concluded that systemic therapy does not prolong survival [73]; however, the author and associates have achieved encouraging ocular and systemic outcomes with systemic chemotherapy combined with maintenance therapy using immunomodulators. These include lenalidomide, which is effective only in activated B-cell (ABC) lymphoma subtype, and CC-122, which also induces regression of the germinal center B-cell lymphoma subtype [74, 75]. The author and associates have found that systemic therapy is relatively ineffective for vitreous infiltrates unless combined with 'therapeutic vitrectomy' [76].

## Conjunctival Melanoma

There is some evidence that the incidence of conjunctival melanoma is increasing [77].

## *Grading and Staging*

As with other ocular tumors, such as uveal melanoma and retinoblastoma, the Tumor, Node, Metastasis (TNM) staging of conjunctival melanomas has been refined. One significant improvement is the incorporation of *in-situ* melanoma in this classification (Tis). A scoring system has been developed to grade conjunctival melanocytic intra-epithelial neoplasia (otherwise known as primary acquired melanosis [PAM] with atypia) more objectively according to the density of melanoma cells in the epithelium and the degree of cellular atypia [78]. Sentinel lymph node biopsy is reported to improve prognostication but has yet to be accepted widely [79].

## *Treatment*

Many centers continue to treat invasive conjunctival melanoma by excision with wide margins, adjunctive cryotherapy, and amniotic membrane grafting [80]; however, the author prefers excision with narrow safety margins and wound closure by primary intention without grafting, administering adjunctive radiotherapy and, in patients with diffuse intra-epithelial disease, adjunctive mitomycin C drops [81]. The author has found that comfort and compliance are improved by prescribing this topical chemotherapy for only 1 week per month for 4 months, instead of two 14-day courses over 6 weeks, as originally recommended. Successful treatment with interferon alpha-2a has also been reported [82, 83].

BRAF mutation is found in about 40% of conjunctival melanomas, many of which are responsive to systemic treatment with a BRAF inhibitor, such as vemurafenib (Zelboraf) [84, 85]. As with cutaneous melanoma, metastases from conjunctival melanoma can respond to systemic treatment with immune check-point inhibitors [86, 87].

## Conjunctival Carcinoma

Conjunctival squamous intra-epithelial neoplasias and invasive carcinomas are common, especially in hot, sunny climates [88].

### *Investigation*

The development of optical coherence tomography has made it easier to differenti-ate CISN/CCIN from other conditions; however, most surgeons continue to perform biopsy to establish the diagnosis [89].

### *Treatment*

Invasive conjunctival carcinomas are treated by excision, with adjunctive cryo-therapy or radiotherapy. In many centers, the preferred treatment for primary or secondary in-situ disease is topical interferon, administered 4 times per day continuously for 3–6 months [90]. The author has achieved good results with 5-FU drops, administered four times daily for only 4 days a month for 4 months [91]. The 5-FU drops are less expensive than interferon and do not require refrigeration.

## Other Developments

Increasingly, patients with ocular malignancy are being treated at specialist ocu-lar oncology centers. This is because of the need for specialized equipment and expertise, and also because of a greater awareness of the need for holistic care, best provided by experienced multidisciplinary teams, which address psychologi-cal and general health issues in addition to treating the ocular tumor. Patients' expectations are increasing so that they are dissatisfied if they are not adequately informed of all the risks and benefits of every management option, in a caring manner, and if the emotional support they receive is deficient. The Internet has led to the formation of patient advocacy groups so that patients and their families are better informed about their condition and the standards of care being delivered in different centers.

## Conclusion

Patients expect their local, non-specialist ophthalmologist to be knowledgeable about their disease when their tumor is first detected and during long-term follow up after completion of their treatment at an ocular oncology center. It is hoped that the present update will be helpful in this respect.

## References

1. Prescher G, Bornfeld N, Hirche H, Horsthemke B, Jockel KH, Becher R. Prognostic implications of monosomy 3 in uveal melanoma. Lancet. 1996;347:1222–5.
2. Dogrusoz M, Jager MJ. Genetic prognostication in uveal melanoma. Acta Ophthalmol. 2018;96:331–47.
3. Robertson AG, Shih J, Yau C, Gibb EA, Oba J, Mungall KL, Hess JM, Uzunangelov V, Walter V, Danilova L, Lichtenberg TM, Kucherlapati M, Kimes PK, Tang M, Penson A, Babur O, Akbani R, Bristow CA, Hoadley KA, Iype L, Chang MT, Network TR, Cherniack AD, Benz C, Mills GB, Verhaak RGW, Griewank KG, Felau I, Zenklusen JC, Gershenwald JE, Schoenfield L, Lazar AJ, Abdel-Rahman MH, Roman-Roman S, Stern MH, Cebulla CM, Williams MD, Jager MJ, Coupland SE, Esmaeli B, Kandoth C, Woodman SE. Integrative analysis identifies four molecular and clinical subsets in uveal melanoma. Cancer Cell. 2018;33:151.
4. Kivela TT, Piperno-Neumann S, Desjardins L, Schmittel A, Bechrakis N, Midena E, Leyvraz S, Zografos L, Grange JD, Ract-Madoux G, Marshall E, Damato B, Eskelin S. Validation of a prognostic staging for metastatic uveal melanoma: a collaborative study of the European Ophthalmic Oncology Group. Am J Ophthalmol. 2016;168:217–26.
5. Damato B, Duke C, Coupland SE, Hiscott P, Smith PA, Campbell I, Douglas A, Howard P. Cytogenetics of uveal melanoma: a 7-year clinical experience. Ophthalmology. 2007;114:1925–31.
6. Eleuteri A, Taktak AFG, Coupland SE, Heimann H, Kalirai H, Damato B. Prognostication of metastatic death in uveal melanoma patients: a Markov multi-state model. Comput Biol Med. 2018;102:151–6.
7. Kalirai H, Dodson A, Faqir S, Damato BE, Coupland SE. Lack of BAP1 protein expression in uveal melanoma is associated with increased metastatic risk and has utility in routine prognostic testing. Br J Cancer. 2014;111:1373–80.
8. Smit KN, van Poppelen NM, Vaarwater J, Verdijk R, van Marion R, Kalirai H, Coupland SE, Thornton S, Farquhar N, Dubbink HJ, Paridaens D, de Klein A, Kilic E. Combined mutation and copy-number variation detection by targeted next-generation sequencing in uveal melanoma. Mod Pathol. 2018;31(5):763–71.
9. Kim RS, Chevez-Barrios P, Divatia M, Bretana ME, Teh B, Schefler AC. Yield, techniques, and complications of transvitreal and transscleral biopsies in small uveal melanoma. JAMA Ophthalmol. 2018;136(5):482–8.
10. Angi M, Kalirai H, Taktak A, Hussain R, Groenewald C, Damato BE, Heimann H, Coupland SE. Prognostic biopsy of choroidal melanoma: an optimised surgical and laboratory approach. Br J Ophthalmol. 2017;101:1143–6.
11. Finn AP, Materin MA, Mruthyunjaya P. Choroidal tumor biopsy: a review of the current state and a glance into future techniques. Retina. 2018;38(Suppl 1):S79–87.
12. Bagger MM. Intraocular biopsy of uveal melanoma risk assessment and identification of genetic prognostic markers. Acta Ophthalmol. 2018;96(Suppl A112):1–28.

13. Hussain RN, Kalirai H, Groenewald C, Kacperek A, Errington RD, Coupland SE, Heimann H, Damato B. Prognostic biopsy of choroidal melanoma after proton beam radiation therapy. Ophthalmology. 2016;123:2264–5.
14. Wen JC, Sai V, Straatsma BR, McCannel TA. Radiation-related cancer risk associated with surveillance imaging for metastasis from choroidal melanoma. JAMA Ophthalmol. 2013;131:56–61.
15. Francis JH, Catalanotti F, Landa J, Barker CA, Shoushtari AN, Abramson DH. Hepatic abnormalities identified by staging MRI and accuracy of MRI of patients with uveal melanoma. Br J Ophthalmol. 2018. https://doi.org/10.1136/bjophthalmol-2018-312612. pii: bjophthalmol-2018-312612. [Epub ahead of print]
16. Marshall E, Romaniuk C, Ghaneh P, Wong H, McKay M, Chopra M, Coupland SE, Damato BE. MRI in the detection of hepatic metastases from high-risk uveal melanoma: a prospective study in 188 patients. Br J Ophthalmol. 2013;97:159–63.
17. Yang J, Manson DK, Marr BP, Carvajal RD. Treatment of uveal melanoma: where are we now? Ther Adv Med Oncol. 2018;10:1758834018757175.
18. Damato B, Dukes J, Goodall H, Carvajal RD. Tebentafusp: T cell Redirection for the Treatment of Metastatic Uveal Melanoma. Cancers. (In Press).
19. Karydis I, Gangi A, Wheater MJ, Choi J, Wilson I, Thomas K, Pearce N, Takhar A, Gupta S, Hardman D, Sileno S, Stedman B, Zager JS, Ottensmeier C. Percutaneous hepatic perfusion with melphalan in uveal melanoma: a safe and effective treatment modality in an orphan disease. J Surg Oncol. 2018;117:1170–8.
20. Gomez D, Wetherill C, Cheong J, Jones L, Marshall E, Damato B, Coupland SE, Ghaneh P, Poston GJ, Malik HZ, Fenwick SW. The Liverpool uveal melanoma liver metastases pathway: outcome following liver resection. J Surg Oncol. 2014;109:542–7.
21. Valsecchi ME, Orloff M, Sato R, Chervoneva I, Shields CL, Shields JA, Mastrangelo MJ, Sato T. Adjuvant sunitinib in high-risk patients with uveal melanoma: comparison with institutional controls. Ophthalmology. 2018;125:210–7.
22. Damato B. Ocular treatment of choroidal melanoma in relation to the prevention of metastatic death—a personal view. Prog Retin Eye Res. 2018;66:187–99.
23. Collaborative Ocular Melanoma Study G. The COMS randomized trial of iodine 125 brachytherapy for choroidal melanoma: V. Twelve-year mortality rates and prognostic factors: COMS report No. 28. Arch Ophthalmol. 2006;124:1684–93.
24. Callejo SA, Dopierala J, Coupland SE, Damato B. Sudden growth of a choroidal melanoma and multiplex ligation-dependent probe amplification findings suggesting late transformation to monosomy 3 type. Arch Ophthalmol. 2011;129:958–60.
25. Damato BE, Heimann H, Kalirai H, Coupland SE. Age, survival predictors, and metastatic death in patients with choroidal melanoma: tentative evidence of a therapeutic effect on survival. JAMA Ophthalmol. 2014;132:605–13.
26. Reichstein D, Karan K. Plaque brachytherapy for posterior uveal melanoma in 2018: improved techniques and expanded indications. Curr Opin Ophthalmol. 2018;29:191–8.
27. Milam RW Jr, Batson SA, Breazzano MP, Ayala-Peacock DN, Daniels AB. Modern and novel radiotherapy approaches for the treatment of uveal melanoma. Int Ophthalmol Clin. 2017;57:11–27.
28. Le BHA, Kim JW, Deng H, Rayess N, Jennelle RL, Zhou SY, Astrahan MA, Berry JL. Outcomes of choroidal melanomas treated with eye physics plaques: a 25-year review. Brachytherapy. 2018;17:981–9.
29. Russo A, Laguardia M, Damato B. Eccentric ruthenium plaque radiotherapy of posterior choroidal melanoma. Graefes Arch Clin Exp Ophthalmol. 2012;250:1533–40.
30. Damato BE, Stewart JM, Afshar AR, Groenewald C, Foulds WS. Surgical resection of choroidal melanoma. In: Schachat AP, editor. Ryan's retina, vol. 3. Philadelphia: Elsevier; 2018. p. 2591–600.
31. Rospond-Kubiak I, Damato B. The surgical approach to the management of anterior uveal melanomas. Eye. 2014;28:741–7.

32. Konstantinidis L, Groenewald C, Coupland SE, Damato B. Long-term outcome of primary endoresection of choroidal melanoma. Br J Ophthalmol. 2014;98:82–5.
33. Bechrakis NE, Foerster MH. Neoadjuvant proton beam radiotherapy combined with subsequent endoresection of choroidal melanomas. Int Ophthalmol Clin. 2006;46:95–107.
34. Rice JC, Liebenberg L, Scholtz RP, Torr G. Fatal air embolism during endoresection of choroidal melanoma. Retin Cases Brief Rep. 2014;8:127–9.
35. Damato B, Kacperek A, Chopra M, Sheen MA, Campbell IR, Errington RD. Proton beam radiotherapy of iris melanoma. Int J Radiat Oncol Biol Phys. 2005;63:109–15.
36. Konstantinidis L, Roberts D, Errington RD, Kacperek A, Damato B. Whole anterior segment proton beam radiotherapy for diffuse iris melanoma. Br J Ophthalmol. 2013;97(4):471–4.
37. Konstantinidis L, Roberts D, Errington RD, Kacperek A, Heimann H, Damato B. Transpalpebral proton beam radiotherapy of choroidal melanoma. Br J Ophthalmol. 2015;99:232–5.
38. Wackernagel W, Holl E, Tarmann L, Mayer C, Avian A, Schneider M, Kapp KS, Langmann G. Local tumour control and eye preservation after gamma-knife radiosurgery of choroidal melanomas. Br J Ophthalmol. 2014;98:218–23.
39. Damato B. Vasculopathy after treatment of choroidal melanoma. In: Joussen A, Gardner TW, Kirchhof B, Ryan SJ, editors. Retinal vascular disease. Berlin: Springer; 2007. p. 582–91.
40. Konstantinidis L, Groenewald C, Coupland SE, Damato B. Trans-scleral local resection of toxic choroidal melanoma after proton beam radiotherapy. Br J Ophthalmol. 2014;98:775–9.
41. Seibel I, Hager A, Riechardt AI, Davids AM, Boker A, Joussen AM. Antiangiogenic or corticosteroid treatment in patients with radiation maculopathy after proton beam therapy for uveal melanoma. Am J Ophthalmol. 2016;168:31–9.
42. Matet A, Daruich A, Zografos L. Radiation maculopathy after proton beam therapy for uveal melanoma: optical coherence tomography angiography alterations influencing visual acuity. Invest Ophthalmol Vis Sci. 2017;58:3851–61.
43. Mantel I, Schalenbourg A, Bergin C, Petrovic A, Weber DC, Zografos L. Prophylactic use of bevacizumab to avoid anterior segment neovascularization following proton therapy for uveal melanoma. Am J Ophthalmol. 2014;158:693–701 e692.
44. Dalvin LA, Shields CL, Ancona-Lezama DA, Yu MD, Di Nicola M, Williams BK, Jr., Lucio-Alvarez JA, Ang SM, Maloney SM, Welch RJ, Shields JA. Combination of multimodal imaging features predictive of choroidal nevus transformation into melanoma. Br J Ophthalmol. 2018. https://doi.org/10.1136/bjophthalmol-2018-312967. pii: bjophthalmol-2018-312967. [Epub ahead of print]
45. Damato B, Hope-Stone L, Cooper B, Brown S, Salmon P, Heimann H, Dunn L. Patient-reported outcomes and quality of life after treatment of choroidal melanoma: a comparison of enucleation vs radiotherapy in 1596 patients. Am J Ophthalmol. 2018;193:230–51.
46. Kines RC, Varsavsky I, Choudhary S, Bhattacharya D, Spring S, McLaughlin R, Kang SJ, Grossniklaus HE, Vavvas D, Monks S, MacDougall JR, de Los Pinos E, Schiller JT. An infrared dye-conjugated virus-like particle for the treatment of primary uveal melanoma. Mol Cancer Ther. 2018;17:565–74.
47. Bidard FC, Madic J, Mariani P, Piperno-Neumann S, Rampanou A, Servois V, Cassoux N, Desjardins L, Milder M, Vaucher I, Pierga JY, Lebofsky R, Stern MH, Lantz O. Detection rate and prognostic value of circulating tumor cells and circulating tumor DNA in metastatic uveal melanoma. Int J Cancer. 2014;134:1207–13.
48. Tura A, Lueke J, Grisanti S. Liquid biopsy for uveal melanoma. In: Scott JF, Gerstenblith MR, editors. Noncutaneous melanoma. Brisbane: Codon Publications; 2018.
49. Abdel-Rahman MH, Pilarski R, Cebulla CM, Massengill JB, Christopher BN, Boru G, Hovland P, Davidorf FH. Germline BAP1 mutation predisposes to uveal melanoma, lung adenocarcinoma, meningioma, and other cancers. J Med Genet. 2011;48:856–9.
50. Masoomian B, Shields JA, Shields CL. Overview of BAP1 cancer predisposition syndrome and the relationship to uveal melanoma. J Curr Ophthalmol. 2018;30:102–9.

51. Munier FL. Classification and management of seeds in retinoblastoma. Ellsworth Lecture Ghent August 24th 2013. Ophthalmic Genet. 2014;35:193–207.
52. Francis JH, Levin AM, Zabor EC, Gobin YP, Abramson DH. Ten-year experience with ophthalmic artery chemosurgery: ocular and recurrence-free survival. PLoS One. 2018;13: e0197081.
53. Dimaras H, Corson TW, Cobrinik D, White A, Zhao J, Munier FL, Abramson DH, Shields CL, Chantada GL, Njuguna F, Gallie BL. Retinoblastoma. Nat Rev Dis Primers. 2015;1:15021.
54. Damato B, Afshar AR, Everett L, Banerjee A, Hetts SW. The University of California, San Francisco documentation system for retinoblastoma: preparing to improve staging methods for this disease. Ocul Oncol Pathol. 2019;5:36–45.
55. Soliman SE, Racher H, Zhang C, MacDonald H, Gallie BL. Genetics and molecular diagnostics in retinoblastoma—an update. Asia Pac J Ophthalmol (Phila). 2017;6:197–207.
56. Ewens KG, Bhatti TR, Moran KA, Richards-Yutz J, Shields CL, Eagle RC, Ganguly A. Phosphorylation of pRb: mechanism for RB pathway inactivation in MYCN-amplified retinoblastoma. Cancer Med. 2017;6:619–30.
57. Sethi RV, Shih HA, Yeap BY, Mouw KW, Petersen R, Kim DY, Munzenrider JE, Grabowski E, Rodriguez-Galindo C, Yock TI, Tarbell NJ, Marcus KJ, Mukai S, MacDonald SM. Second nonocular tumors among survivors of retinoblastoma treated with contemporary photon and proton radiotherapy. Cancer. 2014;120:126–33.
58. Shields CL, Welch RJ, Malik K, Acaba-Berrocal LA, Selzer EB, Newman JH, Mayro EL, Constantinescu AB, Spencer MA, McGarrey MP, Knapp AN, Graf AE, Altman AJ, Considine SP, Shields JA. Uveal metastasis: clinical features and survival outcome of 2214 tumors in 1111 patients based on primary tumor origin. Middle East Afr J Ophthalmol. 2018;25: 81–90.
59. Al-Dahmash SA, Shields CL, Kaliki S, Johnson T, Shields JA. Enhanced depth imaging optical coherence tomography of choroidal metastasis in 14 eyes. Retina. 2014;34:1588–93.
60. Konstantinidis L, Rospond-Kubiak I, Zeolite I, Heimann H, Groenewald C, Coupland SE, Damato B. Management of patients with uveal metastases at the Liverpool Ocular Oncology Centre. Br J Ophthalmol. 2014;98:92–8.
61. Konstantinidis L, Damato B. Intraocular metastases—a review. Asia Pac J Ophthalmol (Phila). 2017;6:208–14.
62. Stjepanovic N, Velazquez-Martin JP, Bedard PL. Ocular toxicities of MEK inhibitors and other targeted therapies. Ann Oncol. 2016;27:998–1005.
63. Abdel-Rahman O, Oweira H, Petrausch U, Helbling D, Schmidt J, Mannhart M, Mehrabi A, Schob O, Giryes A. Immune-related ocular toxicities in solid tumor patients treated with immune checkpoint inhibitors: a systematic review. Expert Rev Anticancer Ther. 2017;17:387–94.
64. Dalvin LA, Shields CL, Orloff M, Sato T, Shields JA. Checkpoint inhibitor immune therapy: systemic indications and ophthalmic side effects. Retina. 2018;38:1063–78.
65. Coupland SE, Damato B. Understanding intraocular lymphomas. Clin Exp Ophthalmol. 2008;36:564–78.
66. Barry RJ, Tasiopoulou A, Murray PI, Patel PJ, Sagoo MS, Denniston AK, Keane PA. Characteristic optical coherence tomography findings in patients with primary vitreoretinal lymphoma: a novel aid to early diagnosis. Br J Ophthalmol. 2018;102:1362–6.
67. Mapelli C, Invernizzi A, Barteselli G, Pellegrini M, Tabacchi E, Staurenghi G, Viola F. Multimodal imaging of vitreoretinal lymphoma. Ophthalmologica. 2016;236:166–74.
68. Dawson AC, Williams KA, Appukuttan B, Smith JR. Emerging diagnostic tests for vitreoretinal lymphoma: a review. Clin Exp Ophthalmol. 2018;46:945–54.
69. Araujo I, Coupland SE. Primary vitreoretinal lymphoma—a review. Asia Pac J Ophthalmol (Phila). 2017;6:283–9.
70. Gonzales J, Doan T, Shantha JG, Bloomer M, Wilson MR, DeRisi JL, Acharya N. Metagenomic deep sequencing of aqueous fluid detects intraocular lymphomas. Br J Ophthalmol. 2018;102:6–8.

71. Pulido JS, Johnston PB, Nowakowski GS, Castellino A, Raja H. The diagnosis and treatment of primary vitreoretinal lymphoma: a review. Int J Retina Vitreous. 2018;4:18.

72. Shields CL, Sioufi K, Mashayekhi A, Shields JA. Intravitreal melphalan for treatment of primary vitreoretinal lymphoma: a new indication for an old drug. JAMA Ophthalmol. 2017;135:815–8.

73. Riemens A, Bromberg J, Touitou V, Sobolewska B, Missotten T, Baarsma S, Hoyng C, Cordero-Coma M, Tomkins-Netzer O, Rozalski A, Tugal-Tutkun I, Guex-Crosier Y, Los LI, Bollemeijer JG, Nolan A, Pawade J, Willermain F, Bodaghi B, ten Dam-van Loon N, Dick A, Zierhut M, Lightman S, Mackensen F, Moulin A, Erckens R, Wensing B, le Hoang P, Lokhorst H, Rothova A. Treatment strategies in primary vitreoretinal lymphoma: a 17-center European collaborative study. JAMA Ophthalmol. 2015;133:191–7.

74. Rubenstein JL, Treseler PA, Stewart PJ. Regression of refractory intraocular large B-cell lymphoma with lenalidomide monotherapy. J Clin Oncol Off J Am Soc Clin Oncol. 2011;29:e595–7.

75. Hagner PR, Man HW, Fontanillo C, Wang M, Couto S, Breider M, Bjorklund C, Havens CG, Lu G, Rychak E, Raymon H, Narla RK, Barnes L, Khambatta G, Chiu H, Kosek J, Kang J, Amantangelo MD, Waldman M, Lopez-Girona A, Cai T, Pourdehnad M, Trotter M, Daniel TO, Schafer PH, Klippel A, Thakurta A, Chopra R, Gandhi AK. CC-122, a pleiotropic pathway modifier, mimics an interferon response and has antitumor activity in DLBCL. Blood. 2015;126:779–89.

76. Bever GJ, Kim DJ, Afshar AR, Rubenstein JL, Damato BE. Therapeutic vitrectomy as an adjunct treatment to systemic chemotherapy for intraocular lymphoma. Retin Cases Brief Rep. 2017. https://doi.org/10.1097/ICB.0000000000000668. [Epub ahead of print]

77. Larsen AC. Conjunctival malignant melanoma in Denmark: epidemiology, treatment and prognosis with special emphasis on tumorigenesis and genetic profile. Acta Ophthalmol. 2016;94 Thesis 1:1–27.

78. Damato B, Coupland SE. Conjunctival melanoma and melanosis: a reappraisal of terminology, classification and staging. Clin Exp Ophthalmol. 2008;36:786–95.

79. Pfeiffer ML, Ozgur OK, Myers JN, Peng A, Ning J, Zafereo ME, Thakar S, Thuro B, Prieto VG, Ross MI, Esmaeli B. Sentinel lymph node biopsy for ocular adnexal melanoma. Acta Ophthalmol. 2017;95:e323–8.

80. Shields CL, Chien JL, Surakiatchanukul T, Sioufi K, Lally SE, Shields JA. Conjunctival tumors: review of clinical features, risks, biomarkers, and outcomes—the 2017 J. Donald M. Gass lecture. Asia Pac J Ophthalmol (Phila). 2017;6:109–20.

81. Damato B, Coupland SE. An audit of conjunctival melanoma treatment in Liverpool. Eye. 2009;23:801–9.

82. Wong JR, Nanji AA, Galor A, Karp CL. Management of conjunctival malignant melanoma: a review and update. Expert Rev Ophthalmol. 2014;9:185–204.

83. Kim SE, Salvi SM. Immunoreduction of ocular surface tumours with intralesional interferon alpha-2a. Eye. 2018;32:460–2.

84. Lake SL, Jmor F, Dopierala J, Taktak AF, Coupland SE, Damato BE. Multiplex ligation-dependent probe amplification of conjunctival melanoma reveals common BRAF V600E gene mutation and gene copy number changes. Invest Ophthalmol Vis Sci. 2011;52:5598–604.

85. Larsen AC. Conjunctival malignant melanoma in Denmark. Epidemiology, treatment and prognosis with special emphasis on tumorigenesis and genetic profile. Acta Ophthalmol. 2016;94:842.

86. Sagiv O, Thakar SD, Kandl TJ, Ford J, Sniegowski MC, Hwu WJ, Esmaeli B. Immunotherapy with programmed cell death 1 inhibitors for 5 patients with conjunctival melanoma. JAMA Ophthalmol. 2018;136:1236–41.

87. Kini A, Fu R, Compton C, Miller DM, Ramasubramanian A. Pembrolizumab for recurrent conjunctival melanoma. JAMA Ophthalmol. 2017;135:891–2.

88. Cicinelli MV, Marchese A, Bandello F, Modorati G. Clinical management of ocular surface squamous neoplasia: a review of the current evidence. Ophthalmol Ther. 2018;7:247–62.

89. Nanji AA, Mercado C, Galor A, Dubovy S, Karp CL. Updates in ocular surface tumor diagnostics. Int Ophthalmol Clin. 2017;57:47–62.
90. Siedlecki AN, Tapp S, Tosteson AN, Larson RJ, Karp CL, Lietman T, Zegans ME. Surgery versus interferon alpha-2b treatment strategies for ocular surface squamous neoplasia: a literature-based decision analysis. Cornea. 2016;35:613–8.
91. Kenawy N, Garrick A, Heimann H, Coupland SE, Damato BE. Conjunctival squamous cell neoplasia: the Liverpool Ocular Oncology Centre experience. Graefes Arch Clin Exp Ophthalmol. 2015;253:143–50.

# Index

**A**

Abatacept, 229
Abicipar pegol (Allergan), 155
Accommodating IOLs, 63
Accommodative lenses, 5
Acrylic lenses, 62
AcrySof Cachet pIOL, 24
AcrySof® Restor® SN6AD3, 11, 12
Acute disseminated encephalomyelopathy
       (ADEM), 203
Acute retinal necrosis (ARN), 123, 131
Adalimumab, 128
Adaptive optics (AO), 103
Adaptive Optics OCT (AO-OCT) devices, 145
Adaptive optics scanning light
       ophthalmoscopy (AO-SLO), 103
Adeno-associated virus (AAV), 156
Aflibercept, 154, 155
Age related macular degeneration (AMD), 146
Air-viscobubble (AVB) dissection, 42, 43
Alcon Accurus machine, 171
Alcon Constellation machine, 172
Alzheimer disease, 219
Ametropia, 64
Amiodarone, 212
Amiodarone-associated optic
       neuropathy (AAON), 212
Aneurysms, 233
Angiogenesis, 154
Angiotensin converting enzyme (ACE), 125
Angle fixated pIOL, 24
Aniridia, 263
Anterior chamber IOL, 63, 86
Anterior uveitis (AU), 124
Anterior-chamber pIOL, 23
Antiplatelet, 56, 57

Aphakic glasses, 86
Apodized diffractive lenses, 6
Artificial intelligence, 149
Artiflex phakic IOL, 24, 25
Artisan, 24
Artisan/Verisyse toric pIOL, 24, 25
AT LISA® tri 839 MP, 6, 7
Ataluren, 263

**B**

Bardet Biedl syndrome, 256
Barotraumatic phenomenon, 214
Bausch + Lomb hypersonic
       vitrector, 175
Bausch + Lomb Millenium Microsurgical
       System, 170
Bausch + Lomb Stellaris Elite, 175
Bausch + Lomb Stellaris PC., 174
Beaver Dam Eye Study, 64
Behcet's disease (BD), 125, 126
Bevacizumab, 154
Bilateral cataracts, 258
Bimanual phacoemulsification, 72
Bimatoprost ocular ring, 108
Bimatoprost sustained-release (SR)
       intracameral implant, 108, 109
BiocomFold 89A, 14
Biometry
   contact A-mode biometry, 58
   optical biometry, 58, 59
   ultrasound, 58
Boston Kpro type I, 50
Boston Kpro type II, 50
Brolucizumab, 155
Buettner, Helmut, 166

© Springer Nature Switzerland AG 2020
A. Grzybowski (ed.), *Current Concepts in Ophthalmology*,
https://doi.org/10.1007/978-3-030-25389-9

**C**
Calcification, 85
Cannula Big Bubble, 42
Capsular contraction syndrome, 14
Cataract surgery
    AMD, 65
    and anticoagulants, 56, 57
    benchmarking, 62
    biometry
        contact A-mode biometry, 58
        corneal indentation, 58
        optical biometry, 58, 59
        ultrasound, 58
    combined surgeries
        anesthesia, 66, 67
        bilateral operation, 68
        combined phacoemulsification and
            vitrectomy, 65
        combined phacoemulsification with
            intraocular lens implantation and
            keratoplasty, 65, 66
        complications, 67
        lens opacification, 65
        settings, 66
    corneal power assessment, 57, 58
    and glaucoma, 64
    intraoperative considerations
        dropless cataract surgery, 77
        FLACS, 71
        ICCE vs. ECCE, 68–70
        intraoperative complications,
            74–76
        MICS, 71, 72
        phacoemulsification, 70
        posterior capsulotomy, 77
        retained lens fragments and nucleus
            luxation, 76, 77
        wound construction, 72–74
    IOL calculation formula, 60, 61
    IOL types, 62–64
    postoperative complications
        Aphakic management, 86
        IOP spikes, 83, 84
        late postoperative IOL opacifications,
            84–86
        PCME, 79, 80
        PCO, 81
        postoperative day 1 (POD1), 78, 79
        postoperative endophthalmitis (POE),
            81–83
        prevalence, 78
        TASS, 82
    postoperative examinations, 78
    preoperative examinations, 56

Cenegermin, 35, 36
Central serous chorioretinopathy, 152
Chang, Stanley, 187
Charles, Steven, 185
Choroidal melanoma, 278, 279
Choroidal neovascularization (CNV), 122
Chronic relapsing inflammatory optic
    neuropathy (CRION), 206
Ciliopathies, 263, 265
Clear corneal incision (CCI), 57, 72–74
Collagen cross linking (CXL), 37, 253
Color vision deficiencies, 208
Congenital corneal anesthesia, 252
Congenital corneal opacities, 254
Conjunctival carcinoma
    investigation, 287
    treatment, 287
Conjunctival limbal autograft, 48
Conjunctival melanoma
    grading and staging, 286
    treatment, 286
Constellation Vision System, 184
Contact A-mode biometry, 58
Contrast sensitivity function, 7
Conventional fundus photography, 122
Convergence insufficiency, 209
Cornea
    corneal infections
        collagen cross-linking (CXL), 37
        diagnostic investigation, 36
        povidone-iodine (PVI), 37
    dry eye disease, 37, 38
    neurotrophic keratopathy,
        NGF treatment, 35, 36
Corneal endothelial dysfunction, 46
Corneal inlays
    advantages and disadvantages, 2
    corneal curvature, 2
    corneal reshaping inlays, 2
    intracorneal inlays, 4
    multifocality, 4, 5
    refractive inlays, 2
        Flexivue Microlens™, 3
        Icolens™, 3, 4
    small aperture inlays, 2–4
Corneal neurotization procedure, 252
Corneal opacities, 67
Corneal tomography, 57, 58
Corneal topography, 58
Corneal transplantation
    artificial cornea (keratoprosthesis)
        surgery, 39
    DALK (*see* Deep anterior lamellar
        keratoplasty)

endothelial keratoplasty (*see* Endothelial keratoplasty)
limbal stem cell deficiency (LSCD), 47
ocular surface reconstruction, 39
ocular surface transplantation
    conjunctival limbal autograft, 48
    ex-vivo cultured graft, 50
    keratolimbal allograft, 48
    keratoprosthesis, 50
    lr-CLAU, 49
    ocular surface diseases
        classification, 47, 48
    procedure selection, 47
    SLET, 48
penetrating keratoplasty (PK), 38
techniques comparison, 39–41
Corneal tunnel incisions, 72
Corticosteroids, 127
CrystaLens®, 13, 14
Cultivated limbal epithelial transplantation (CLET), 50
Cultivated oral mucosal epithelial transplantation (COMET), 50
C-Well, 15
CyPass Micro-Stent, 111, 112

**D**
de Juan , Eugene, 167
Deep anterior lamellar keratoplasty (DALK), 39
    advantages, 43
    AVB, 42, 43
    cannula Big Bubble, 42
    corneal stromal layer disorders, 39
    dangerous infectious stromal keratitis, 39
    Descemet membrane, 41
    endothelium cells, 43
    epithelial rejection, 43
    graft survival, 43
    indications, 39
    intraoperative and postoperative complications, 43
    Keratoconus, 39
    needle Big Bubble technique, 41
    rejection rate, 43
    stromal rejection, 43
    subepithelial rejection, 43
Dell'Osso-Hertle procedure, 267
Delphi process, 259
Descemet membrane (DM), 41, 45
Descemet Membrane Endothelial Keratoplasty (DMEK), 45, 46
Descemet stripping automated endothelial Keratoplasty (DSAEK), 44

Descemetorhexis, 46
Diagnostic and Classification Criteria in Vasculitis Study (DCVAS), 217
Diagnostic techniques, 124
Diathermy, 187
Dodo, Tsugio, 165
DORC EVA machine, 173
Dropless cataract surgery, 77
Drug-induced ocular disease, 284
Dry eye disease (DED), 37, 38
Dual optic IOL, 15, 16
Dual-optic lenses, 16

**E**
Eckardt, Claus, 167
Electroadaptive accommodating IOL, 19
Endolasers, 186
Endothelial keratoplasty (EK), 39
    advantages and disadvantages, 43, 44
    DMEK, 45, 46
    DSAEK, 44
    endothelium disfunction treatment, 43
    ROCK inhibitor, 46
European Society of Cataract and Refractive Surgeons (ESCRS) study, 83
Extended depth-of-focus (EDOF) lenses, 5
    MiniWell, 9, 10
    strategies, 9
    Wichterle Intraocular Lens-Continuous Focus (WIOL-CF), 10
Extendible Diamond Dusted Sweeper, 185
Extracapsular cataract extraction (ECCE), 69, 70
Extrusion cannulas, 186
Ex-vivo cultured graft, 50

**F**
Femtosecond Laser-Assisted Cataract Surgery (FLACS), 71
FineVision® Micro F, 7
Flexivue Microlens™, 3
FluidVision®, 16
Fluorescein angiography (FA), 122, 141, 143
Forceps, 185
Four-dimensional (4-D) OCT imaging, 191
Fuchs endothelial corneal dystrophy (FECD), 46
Fujii, Gildo, 167
Fundus autofluorescence (FAF) imaging, 147, 149

**G**
Ganglion cell layer (GCL), 100
Ganglion cell-inner plexiform layer (GC-IPL),
        100
Gene therapy, 156, 158, 231
Genome-wide association studies (GWAS), 261
Giant cell arteritis (GCA), 216, 228, 229
Glaucoma
    bilateral blindness, 99
    imaging
        adaptive optics, 103
        OCT (*see* Optical coherence
            tomography)
    irreversible blindness, 99
    laser and surgery
        laser iridotomy, 109
        lens extraction, angle-closure
            glaucoma, 110
        minimally invasive glaucoma surgery,
            110–113
        primary trabeculectomy/tube surgery, 110
    medical therapy
        bimatoprost ocular ring, 108
        bimatoprost sustained-release implant,
            108, 109
        iDose, 109
        latanoprostene bunod, 107
        ROCK inhibitors, 106, 107
        travoprost punctum plug, 108
    visual field testing
        free tablet-based perimetry
            application, 106
        fundus-tracked
            perimetry/microperimetry, 105
        home-based perimetry, 106
        Humphrey Field Analyzer, 106
        portable perimetry, 106
        tablet-based perimetry, 106
        testing strategies and novel
            thresholding algorithms, 104, 105
Glaucomatous optic neuropathy, 219
Glial fibrillary acidic protein (GFAP),
        205, 206
Glistening, 84, 85
Gradient-Oriented Automated Natural
        Neighbor Approach (GOANNA),
        104


**H**
Hagen-Poiseuille equation, 112
Heintz, Ralph, 166
Hickingbotham, Dyson, 166
Horizontal scissors, 186

Hybrid lenses
    AcrySof® Restor® SN6AD3, 11, 12
    Lentis® Mplus LS-313, 12, 13
    Panoptix®, 12
    Tecnis® Symfony, 13
Hydrodelineation, 74
Hydrophobic acrylic IOL
    gross photograph, 85
    light photomicrograph, 84
Hydrus Microstent, 111


**I**
IC-8 small-aperture IOL, 10, 11
Icolens™, 3, 4
Idebenone, 230
iDose, 109
Iluvien implant, 155
Immediate sequential bilateral cataract surgery
        (ISBCS), 68
*In vivo* confocal microscopy, 36
Indocyanine green angiography (ICGA), 143
Infant Aphakia Treatment study, 258
Infliximab, 128
InnFocus MicroShunt, 112, 113
Internal limiting membrane (ILM) forceps, 185
Intracapsular cataract extraction
        (ICCE), 68–70
Intraflagellar transport (IFT), 265
Intranasal neurostimolator, 38
Intraocular lens (IOL)
    banking, 56
    calculation formula, 60, 61
    hydrophobic acrylic IOL
        gross photograph, 84, 85
        light photomicrograph, 84
    late postoperative IOL opacifications,
        84–86
    MemoryLens IOL,
        light photomicrograph, 85
    optical properties, 63
    types, 62–64
Intraocular pressure (IOP), 214
    reduction, 102
    spikes, 83, 84
Intraoperative floppy iris syndrome (IFIS), 75
Intravitreal anti-vascular endothelial growth
        factor, 80
Iris-fixated or "iris claw" lens, 24, 25
iStent, 111


**J**
Juvene accommodating IOL, 17, 18

**K**

Kamra Inlay™, 3, 4
Kasner, David, 165
Kelman Duet Implant Phakic IOL, 24
Keratolimbal allograft (KLAL), 48
Keratoprosthesis, 50

**L**

Laser-assisted in situ keratomileusis
 (LASIK), 20, 21
Laser iridotomy, 109
Latanoprost, 107
Latanoprostene bunod, 107
Leber hereditary optic neuropathy (LHON),
 211, 230
Leber's Congenital Amaurosis (LCA), 157
Lensectomy, 184
Lentis® Mplus LS-313, 12, 13
Lentiviral vectors, 156
Lidocaine, 75
Light Adjustable Lens (LAL), 64
Limbal stem cell deficiency (LSCD), 47
Linezolide, 212
LiquiLens, 19
Living related conjunctival limbal allograft
 (lr- CLAL), 49
Long-term corticosteroid implants, 129
Lumina®, 18, 19

**M**

Machemer, Robert, 166
Macular Edema Ranibizumab *vs.* Intravitreal
 Anti-inflammatory Therapy
 (MERIT) trial, 130
Maculopathies
 intravitreal treatments, 153, 155, 156
 non-surgical treatments, 156, 158, 159
 retinal imaging techniques
  fluorescein angiography (FA), 141
  fundus autofluorescence (FAF)
   imaging, 147
  indocyanine green angiography
   (ICGA), 143
  optical coherence tomography (OCT),
   144, 145
  optical coherence tomography
   angiography (OCTA), 146
Magnet-driven active shift IOL, 19
Magnetic Resonance Imaging in MS
 (MAGNIMS) committee, 215
Manual small incision cataract surgery
 (MSICS), 69, 70

McDonald Criteria, 202
Mechanosensation, 265
Membrane scrapers, 185
MemoryLens IOL, 85
Methanol toxicity, 211
M-Flex 630F, 9
Micro-incisional cataract surgery
 (MICS), 71, 72
Minimally invasive glaucoma surgery
 (MIGS), 110–113
Minimum distance band (MDB), 100
MiniWell, 9, 10
Mitochondrial replacement therapy
 (MRT), 231
Monofocal IOLs, 63
Multicenter Uveitis Steroid Treatment
 (MUST) trial, 129
Multifocal IOLs, 63
Multiple sclerosis (MS), 202, 215, 222, 225
Myasthenia gravis (MG) antibodies, 217, 218
Myelin oligodendrocyte glycoprotein (MOG),
 203–205
Myopia control, 261, 262

**N**

Nanoparticles (NPs), 157
Near-infrared autofluorescence imaging
 (NIR-AF), 147
Needle Big Bubble technique, 41
Netarsudil, 107
Neuroadaptation, 5
Neuro-degenerative diseases, 208
Neuro endovascular intervention
 aneurysms, 233
 venous sinus stenting in PTC, 235
Neuro-immunology, 201
Neuromyelitis Optica (NMO), 202
Neurophysiology, 267, 268
Neurostimulation, 38
Neurotrophic keratopathy (NK), 35, 36
Ngenuity 3-D viewing system, 181
NMO spectrum disorder (NMOSD), 203
Non-infectious uveitis, 124, 125
Nonsense suppression therapy
 (NST), 263, 264
"Normal-tension glaucoma" (NTG), 214
NuLens®, 17
Nutritional optic neuropathies, 213

**O**

O'Malley, Conor, 166
Ocular glymphatic system, 215

Ocular myasthenia gravis (OMG), 217
Ocular surface transplantation
    conjunctival limbal autograft, 48
    ex-vivo cultured graft, 50
    keratolimbal allograft, 48
    keratoprosthesis, 50
    lr-CLAU, 49
    ocular surface diseases classification, 47
    procedure selection, 47
    SLET, 48
1CU®, 14, 15
OPAL, 15
Open sky technique, 165
Optical biometry, 58, 59
Optical coherence tomography (OCT), 80,
        144, 145
    diagnosis and monitoring, 219
    neurodegenerative disease, 219
    OCT-A, 101–103
    optic disc elevation, 219
    three-dimensional optical coherence
        tomography, 100, 101
    wide-field swept-source optical coherence
        tomography, 101
Optical coherence tomography angiography
        (OCTA), 101–103, 122, 146
    in LHON, 226, 227
    in multiple sclerosis, 225
    in optic neuropathies, 225
Optic disc elevation, 219
Optic disc margin, 100
Optic nerve sheath meningioma
        (ONSM), 229, 230
Optic pathway gliomas, 229
Oral corticosteroids, 127
Orthokeratology contact lenses, 261
Osteo-odonto-keratoprosthesis (OOKP), 50


P
Paediatric keratoconus, 254
Panoptix®, 12
Parel, Jean-Marie, 166, 167
Parkinson disease (PD), 222
    color vision, 208
    convergence insufficiency, 209
    progressive supranuclear palsy, 209
    saccades, 208
    smooth pursuit eye movements, 208
    stereopsis, 209
    visual contrast sensitivity, 208
Pars plana vitrectomy (PPV), 76, 77, 166, 168
Pediatric capsule management, 259
Pediatric keratoplasty, 257

Pediatric ophthalmology
    cornea, 251, 254, 258
    molecular genetics, 263–265
    neurophysiology, 267, 268
    nystagmus evaluation and
        management, 267
    pediatric cataract, 258, 260
    refractive error, 260–262
    retina, 266
Penetrating keratoplasty (PK), 38
Perfluorocarbon, 187
Perfluorocarbon liquid, 187
Peribulbar anesthesia, 169
Periocular and Intravitreal Corticosteroids for
        Uveitis Macular Edema (POINT)
        trial, 130
Peripheral iridotomies, 24
Peyman, Gholam, 166, 167
Phacoemulsification, 70, 184
Phacoemulsification cataract surgery
        (PCS), 56
Phakic Intraocular Lenses (pIOL), 23–25
Phosphodiesterase-5 (PDE-5) inhibitors, 213
Photorefractive keratectomy (PRK), 20
Pirenoxine eyedrops, 2
Polarization-sensitive OCT (PS-OCT), 146
Polymerase chain reaction (PCR), 36, 131
Polymethyl methacrylate (PMMA), 50
Position-changing IOL, 13, 14
Posterior capsule opacification (PCO), 81
Posterior capsule rupture (PCR), 74
Posterior capsulotomy, 77
Posterior chamber lenses, 62
Posterior-chamber pIOL, 25
Postoperative endophthalmitis (POE), 81–83
Povidone-iodine (PVI), 37
Power-changing IOL, 18, 19
Premature termination codons (PTC), 263
Primary angle closure (PAC), 110
Primary open-angle glaucoma (POAG), 214
Primary tube versus trabeculectomy
        (PTVT), 110
Progressive supranuclear palsy, 209
Pseudoexfoliation syndrome (XFS), 76
Pseudophakic ametropias, 64
Pseudophakic cystoid macular edema
        (PCME), 64, 79, 80
Pseudophakic presbyopic IOL
    accommodative lenses, 5
    bifocal IOL's, 5
    EDOF, 5
    multifocal IOL's, 5
    neuroadaptation, 5
    optical profiles

accommodating IOLs, 13–19
   diffractive multifocal IOL's, 6, 7
   EDOF lenses, 9, 10
   hybrid lenses, 11–13
   refractive multifocal IOL's, 8, 9
  preoperative evaluation and planning, 5
  rotationally asymmetric or varifocal
    IOLs, 5
  rotationally symmetrical IOL's, 5
  trifocal IOL's, 5
Pseudotumor cerebri (PTC), 236


**R**
Raindrop™, 2
Randomized controlled trials (RCT), 258
Ranibizumab, 154, 155
Ray-tracing, 61
Recurrent optic neuritis, 206
Refractive laser procedures
  excimer laser, 19
  femtosecond laser, 20
  LASIK, 20, 21
  photorefractive keratectomy (PRK), 20
  SMILE, 22
Refractive surgery
  ablative, 19
  ammetropia, 1
  Corneal inlays (*see* Corneal inlays)
  laser procedure (*see* Refractive laser
    procedure)
  phakic intraocular lenses (pIOL), 23–25
  presbyopia, pharmacologic treatment, 1, 2
  pseudophakic presbyopic IOL's
    (*see* Pseudophakic presbyopic
    IOL's)
Retinal detachments, 187
Retinal ischemia, 123
Retinal nerve fiber layer (RNFL), 100
Retinal pigment epithelium (RPE), 100
Retinitis pigmentosa, 157
Retinoblastoma
  classification, 282
  genetic analysis, 282
  survival, 282
  treatment, 281, 282
Retrobulbar anesthesia, 168–169
Rezoom, 8, 9
Rho kinase (ROCK) inhibitor, 46
  corneal endothelial dysfunction, 46
  glaucoma, 106, 107
Ripasudil, 107
Routine preoperative non-ophthalmic medical
   testing, 56

**S**
Saccades, 208
Sarcoidosis, 124, 125
Sarfarazi®, 16, 17
Sarilumab, 128
Scleral buckling (SB), 189
Scleral incisions, 72–74
Scleral tunnel incisions, 72
Secondary piggyback IOLs, 64
Secukinumab, 128
SeeLens, 7
Sensory, 265
Shape-changing IOL, 16, 18
Silicone lenses, 62
Simple limbal epithelial transplant (SLET), 48
Single-piece IOLs, 62
Small Incision Lenticule Extraction
   (SMILE), 22
SN6AD3 model, 11, 12
Soft-tip extrusion cannulas, 186
Space flight-associated neuro-ocular syndrome
   (SANS), 210
Spatially Weighted Likelihoods in Zippy
   Estimation by Sequential Testing
   (SWeLZ), 104
Spondyloarthritis, 124
Squalamine, 155
Standardization of Uveitis Nomenclature
   (SUN), 121, 122
Stellaris Elite Vision Enhancement System, 171
Stereopsis, 209
Storz Daisy machine, 170
Structure Estimation of Minimum Uncertainty
   (SEMU), 104, 105
Subretinal injections, 188
Subretinal microphotodiode-array, 158
Subsurface nanoglistenings (SSNGs), 84
Sub-Tenon's space, 169
Swept-source optical coherence tomography
   (SS-OCT), 101, 123
Synchrony®, 15, 16


**T**
Tecnis® Symfony, 13
Tek-Clear, 15
Telemedicine, 149
Tetraflex®, 14, 15
Three-piece IOLs, 62
Time-domain technology (TD-OCT), 145
Timolol, 107
Tocilizumab, 228
Topical anesthesia, 169
Toxic anterior segment syndrome (TASS), 82

Toxic-nutritional optic neuropathies (TNON)
  alcohol and tobacco, role of, 214
  medication-induced optic neuropathies, 212, 213
  nutritional optic neuropathies, 213
  toxins, 211
Toxic tumour syndrome, 280
Toxoplasmosis, 132
Traumatic cataract, 257
Traumatic corneal scar, 257
Travoprost punctum plug (OTX-TP), 108
TriMoxi, 77
TriMoxiVanc, 77
Tuberculosis (TB), 132

**U**
Ultra-wide-field (UWF) imaging, 122
Uncorrected distance visual acuity (UDVA), 2
Uncorrected near visual acuity (UNVA), 2
Uveal melanoma
  detection and diagnosis, 280
  metastatic disease, systemic surveillance for, 276
  ocular treatment, 277, 280
  prognostication, 275
  quality of life, 281
  treatment for metastasis, 276
Uveal metastasis
  diagnosis, 283
  treatment, 284
Uveitis
  acute retinal necrosis (ARN), 131
  anterior uveitis (AU), 124
  Behcet's disease (BD), 126
  imaging modalities, 122, 124
  non-infectious uveitis treatment, 127, 129, 130
  sarcoidosis, 124, 125
  spondyloarthritis, 124
  standardization of nomenclature, 121
  Standardization of Uveitis Nomenclature (SUN), 122
  toxoplasmosis, 132
  tuberculosis (TB), 132

**V**
Valved cannulas, 176
Venous sinus stenosis, 236
Vertical scissors, 186

Visian ICL, 25, 26
Visual rehabilitation, 65
Visual restoration therapy, 231, 232
Vitrectomized eyes, 45
Vitreo-retinal lymphoma
  investigation, 285
  terminology, 284
  treatment, 285
Vitreo-retinal surgery
  cannula-trocar systems, 172
  four-dimensional (4-D) OCT imaging, 191
  history of, 165, 167
  instrumentation, 184, 187
  lensectomy and phacoemulsification, 184
  perfluorocarbon liquid, 187
  postoperative considerations and complications, 168, 191
  robotics in, 191
  scleral buckling (SB), 189
  subretinal injections, 188
  tamponade agents, 190
  viewing systems
    chromovitrectomy, 183
    illumination and filters, 181
    lens, 178
    microscopes, 176
    three-dimensional (3-D) viewing techniques, 179
  vitrectomy systems, 169
Vitreous infusion suction cutter (VISC), 167
Vitrophage, 167
Vogt-Koyanagi-Harada syndrome (VKH), 123
Voretigene neparvovec-rzyl, 157
Voretigene therapy, 157

**W**
Wichterle Intraocular Lens-Continuous Focus (WIOL-CF), 10
Wide-field swept-source optical coherence tomography, 101

**X**
X-linked infantile nystagmus, 267
Xtrafocus Pinhole Implant, 10, 11

**Z**
ZB5M lens, 24
ZSAL4, 24